Mental Health and PSYCHIATRIC NURSING for GNM Students

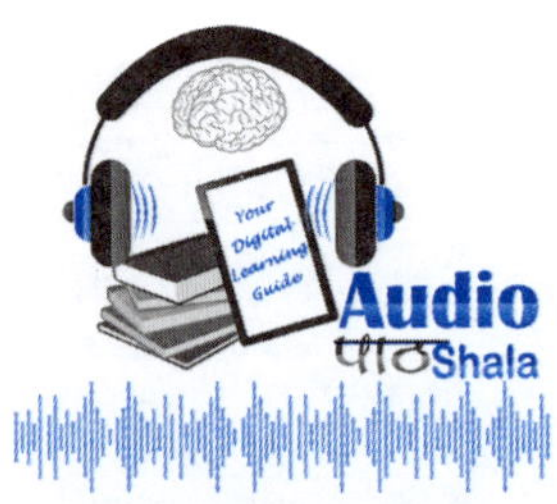

Your Digital Learning Guide

Audio पाठShala *seamlessly integrates audio lessons, offering a comprehensive learning experience. Audio पाठShala not only fosters a deeper understanding of subjects but also caters to diverse learning styles, making education more inclusive and enjoyable.*

Topics for **Audio** पाठShala

1.	Mental Health and Mental Health Nursing	15.	Disorders of Insight and Judgement
2.	Defense Mechanisms	16.	Electroconvulsive Therapy (ECT)
3.	Disorders of Consciousness	17.	Schizophrenia
4.	Disorders of Attention and Concentration	18.	Mood Disorders
5.	Disorders of Orientation	19.	Phobic Anxiety Disorder
6.	Volitional Disturbances	20.	Panic Disorder
7.	Disorders of Motor Activity	21.	Generalized Anxiety Disorder
8.	Disturbances of Posture and Expression	22.	Obsessive Compulsive Disorder
9.	Disturbances of Motor Speech	23.	Conversion Disorder
10.	Disorders of Perception	24.	Dissociative Disorder
11.	Disorders of Mood	25.	Somatoform Disorders
12.	Disorders of Memory	26.	Substance Abuse
13.	Disorders of Thought	27.	Personality Disorder
14.	Disorders of Intelligence	28.	Sexual Disorder
		29.	Eating Disorder
		30.	Mental Retardation

Mental Health and PSYCHIATRIC NURSING for GNM Students

As per the INC Syllabus

R Sreevani PhD (Psychiatric Nursing)
Professor and Head
Department of Psychiatric Nursing
Dharwad Institute of Mental Health and Neurosciences (DIMHANS)
Dharwad, Karnataka, India

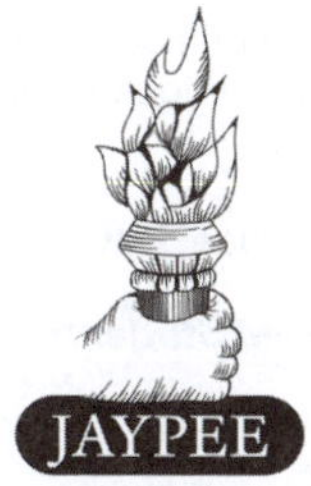

JAYPEE BROTHERS MEDICAL PUBLISHERS
The Health Sciences Publisher
New Delhi | London

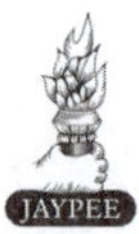 **Jaypee Brothers Medical Publishers (P) Ltd**

Headquarters

EMCA House, 23/23-B
Ansari Road, Daryaganj
New Delhi 110 002, India
Landline: +91-11-23272143, +91-11-23272703
+91-11-23282021, +91-11-23245672
e-mail: jaypee@jaypeebrothers.com

Corporate Office

4838/24, Ansari Road, Daryaganj
New Delhi 110 002, India
Phone: +91-11-43574357
Fax: +91-11-43574314
e-mail: jaypee@jaypeebrothers.com

Overseas Office

JP Medical Ltd.
83, Victoria Street, London
SW1H 0HW (UK)
Phone: +44-20 3170 8910
e-mail: info@jpmedpub.com

EU GPSR Authorised Representative

Logos Europe, 9 rue Nicolas Poussin
17000, La Rochelle, France
Phone: +33 (0) 6 67 93 73 78
e-mail: contact@logoseurope.eu

Website: www.jaypeebrothers.com
Website: www.jaypeedigital.com

© 2024, Jaypee Brothers Medical Publishers

Inquiries for bulk sales may be solicited at: jaypee@jaypeebrothers.com

Mental Health and Psychiatric Nursing for GNM Students

First Edition: **2024**

Reprint : 2025, **2026**

ISBN: 978-93-5696-655-0

Printed in India at Sterling Graphics Pvt. Ltd.

Dedicated to

My Husband

Preface

The well-being of a human being has two facets, namely physical and mental health. Physical health is a state of the body, while mental health is a state of the mind, feelings, and emotions. Physical health includes getting enough sleep at night, eating balanced meals, and staying active while mental health refers to the ability to process information. However, the physical health of an individual has gained greater importance over the mental health aspect. Although mental health and mental illness impact nearly every family, stigma causes much shame, fear, doubt, isolation, and misunderstanding, keeping the people from seeking treatment so richly needed and deserved. Ignorance of mental health concepts and related ailments is also a major cause for lower awareness levels among the masses. It is only in the recent years that due emphasis has been laid on mental health needs, and practices. Accordingly, syllabi have been revised and upgraded at various levels and qualified people identified and appointed in appropriate places for better monitoring of mental healthcare needs and providing inputs to healthcare teams by conducting seminars and workshops. The time has now come to move past the existing stigma and see physical and mental health equally.

This textbook is an earnest effort to include all such information required for a nurse student at the GNM level. It covers various psychiatric disorders in an exhaustive manner. Topics such as evolution of mental health services and treatment, development of modern psychiatric nursing, prevalence and incidence of mental disorders, and psychiatric emergencies have also been included to provide a comprehensive idea on the subject. Theoretical aspects have been well complemented by practical aspects where necessary, enabling the students to equip themselves better for their future endeavors. The book also includes a drug guide apart from an exhaustive glossary of various terms used in describing common psychiatric disorders, which is a must for gaining a broad understanding of the subject. Each chapter is followed by important questions pulled out from the previous examinations for self-evaluation purposes.

The matter has been presented using simple and lucid language, which comprehensively caters to the needs of an average student at the GNM level. After going through the book, the students should be able to not only manage their exams on Psychiatric Nursing but also meet the mental healthcare needs of patients more effectively.

All constructive suggestions from the readers in making this guide more valuable and helpful will be earnestly solicited.

R Sreevani

Acknowledgments

I would like to begin by thanking the Almighty God, who bestowed upon me the spiritual strength and perseverance to make it all happen.

I would like to thank the publishers M/s Jaypee Brothers Medical Publishers (P) Ltd, New Delhi, for being supportive all through. I extend my special thanks to Shri Jitendar P Vij (Group Chairman), Mr Ankit Vij (Managing Director), and Mr MS Mani (Group President) for continuing to repose strong faith in me.

Nobody has been more important to me in the pursuit of this title than the members of my family. I would like to thank my grandparents, parents, and in-laws, whose love and guidance are with me in whatever I pursue. They are the ultimate role models. While I wish to thank my loving and supportive husband Mr Giridhar who has been a source of constant support. I would also like to specially acknowledge the contribution made by my elder son Pranith Ambati in organizing and conceptualizing the visual material and reading through the complete text during the manuscript preparation and proofing stage. A word of appreciation is due to my younger son Daivik Ambati for exhibiting keen interest in the complete process from beginning to the end.

I extend my sincere thanks to Dr Madhu Choudhary (Director–Educational Publishing), Ms Pooja Bhandari [Director–Production (Books and Journals)], Mr Ajay Sharma [Deputy General Manager–Production (Books and Journals)], Ms Sunita Katla (Executive Assistant to Group Chairman and Publishing Manager), Ms Samina Khan (Executive Assistant to Director–Educational Publishing), Ms Alisha Talwar (Team Lead–Nursing), Mr Rajesh Sharma (Production Coordinator), Ms Seema Dogra (Cover Visualizer), Ms Neha Verma (Graphic Designer), Ms Uma Adhikari (Typesetter), Ms Geeta Barik (Proofreader), Mr Manoj Pahuja (Sr Graphic Designer), and their team members for the wonderful back office support.

Contents

Syllabus

MENTAL HEALTH NURSING

Placement: Second Year **Time:** 70 hours

Course description: This course is designed to help students develop the concept of mental health and mental illness, its causes, symptoms, prevention, treatment modalities and nursing management of mentally ill for individual, family and community.

General objectives:

Upon completion of this course, the students shall be able to:

1. Describe the concept of mental health and mental illness and the emerging trends in psychiatric nursing.
2. Explain the causes and factors of mental illness, its prevention and control.
3. Identify the symptoms and dynamics of abnormal human behavior in comparison with normal human behavior.
4. Demonstrate a desirable attitude and skills in rendering comprehensive nursing care to the mentally ill.

Unit	Learning objectives	Content	Hours	Teaching learning activities	Methods of assessment
I	Describe the concept of mental health and mental illness in relation to providing comprehensive care to the patients.	**Introduction** a. Concept of mental health and mental illness b. Misconceptions related to mental illness c. Principles of mental health nursing d. Definition of terms used in psychiatry e. Review of defense mechanisms f. Mental health team	5	Lecture-cum-discussion Structured discussion Group interaction	Short answers Objective type
II	Narrate the historical development of psychiatry and psychiatric nursing.	**History of psychiatry** a. History of psychiatric nursing—India and at international level b. Trends in psychiatric nursing c. National mental health program	4	Lecture-cum-discussion	Short answer Objective type
III	Describe mental health assessment.	**Mental health assessment** a. Psychiatry history taking b. Mental status examination c. Interview technique	4	Lecture-cum-discussion Demonstration	Short answer Objective type Return demonstration

Unit	Learning objectives	Content	Hours	Teaching learning activities	Methods of assessment
IV	Describe therapeutic relationship. Demonstrate skills in process recording.	**Therapeutic nurse—patient relationship:** a. Therapeutic nurse–patient relationship: Definition, components and phases, importance b. Communication skills: Definition elements, types, factors influencing communication, barriers (therapeutic impasses)	5	Lecture-cum-discussions Role play Videos Demonstration of process recording	Short answers Return demonstration

V	List various mental disorders and describe their mental and psychiatric and nursing management.	**Mental disorders and nursing interventions**
		a. Psycho-pathophysiology of human behavior
		b. Etiological theories (genetics, biochemical, psychological, etc.)
		c. Classification of mental disorders
		d. Disorders of thought, motor activity, perception, mood, speech, memory, concentration, judgment
		e. Prevalence, etiology, signs and symptoms, prognosis, medical and nursing management
		f. Personality and types of personality related to psychiatric disorder
		g. Organic mental disorders: Delirium, dementia
		h. Psychotic disorders:
		  – Schizophrenic disorders
		  – Mood (affective) disorders: Mania depression, bipolar affective disorders (BPAD)
		i. Neurotic disorders: Phobia, anxiety disorders, obsessive compulsive disorders, depressive neurosis, conversion disorders, dissociative reaction, psychosomatic disorders, post-traumatic stress disorder
			25	Lecture-cum-discussions
				
				Case study
				
				Case presentation
				
				Process recording
				
				Videos
				
				Role plays
				
				Field visits—De-addiction centers, Alcohol Anonyms group, Adolescent clinics, Child guidance centers, etc.
					Short answers
					
					Essay types
					
					Case study
					
					Case presentation

Unit	Learning objectives	Content	Hours	Teaching learning activities	Methods of assessment
		j. Substance use and de-addiction: Alcohol, tobacco and other psychoactive substance k. Child and adolescent psychiatric disorder: – Sleep disorder – Eating disorders – Sexual disorders l. Nursing management: Nursing process and process recording in caring for patients with various psychiatric disorders			
VI	Describe the bio-psychosocial therapies and explain the role of the nurse.	**Bio-psycho and social therapies** a. Psychopharmacology—definition, classification of drugs antipsychotic, antidepressant, antimanic, antianxiety agents, antiparkinsons b. Psychosocial therapies—individual therapies, group therapy, behavior therapy, occupational therapy, family therapy, milieu therapy c. Role of nurse in these therapies d. Somatic therapy—electro-convulsive therapy, insulin therapy e. Role of nurse in these therapies	12	Lecture-cum-discussions Seminar Videos Demonstration Field visits—rehabilitation center, day-care centers Role plays	Short answers Essay types Return demonstration Quiz Drug study
VII	Describe the concept of preventive community mental health services. Enumerate the nurse's role in national mental health program	**Community mental health** a. Concept, importance, scope b. Attitudes, stigma and discrimination related to the mentally ill c. Prevention of mental illness (preventive psychiatry) during childhood, adolescent, adult hood and old age d. Community mental health services e. Role of nurse in national mental health program and psychiatric care in community	5	Lecture-cum-discussions Role play Videos	Short answers Essay type Assignment

Unit	Learning objectives	Content	Hours	Teaching learning activities	Methods of assessment
VIII	Explain different psychiatric emergencies and their management. Demonstrate skills in crisis intervention.	**Psychiatric emergencies and crisis intervention** a. Types of psychiatric emergencies: Over active, under active patient, violent behavior b. Suicide, adverse drug reactions, withdrawal symptoms, acute psychosis, etc. c. Crisis and its intervention: AIDS, adolescent crisis	5	Lecture-cum-discussion Videos Role plays Demonstration	Short answers Objective type Essay type
IX	Describe the legal aspects to be kept in mind in the care of mentally ill patients.	**Forensic psychiatry/legal aspects** a. India Lunatic Act 1912 b. Narcotic Drugs and Psychotropic Act 1965, 1985 c. Mental Health Act 1987, 2014 d. Admission and discharge procedures e. Standards of psychiatric nursing practice f. Rights of mentally ill patients g. Legal responsibilities in the care of mentally ill patients	5	Lecture-cum-discussion Demonstration	Short answers Essay type Objective quiz

Introduction

CHAPTER OUTLINE

- ❑ Concepts of Mental Health and Mental Illness
- ❑ Misconceptions Related to Mental Illness
- ❑ Principles of Mental Health Nursing
- ❑ Definitions of Terms Used in Psychiatry
- ❑ Review of Defense Mechanisms
- ❑ Mental Health Team/Multidisciplinary Team

Health is a state of complete physical, mental and social well-being and not merely the absence of disease. Hence, mental health is an integral and essential component of health. It is the foundation for both individual well-being and effective functioning in a community. The World Health Organization says, "There is no health without mental health". Mental health is a basic human right which is crucial to personal, community and socio-economic development.

CONCEPTS OF MENTAL HEALTH AND MENTAL ILLNESS

Mental health is a state of mental well-being that enables people to cope with the stresses of life, realize their abilities, learn well and work well, and contribute to their community. It is related to promotion of mental well-being, prevention of mental disorders, treatment and rehabilitation of people affected by mental disorders.

Mental illness is maladjustment in living. It produces disharmony in a person's ability to meet human needs comfortably or effectively and function within a culture. A mentally ill person loses his ability to respond according to the expectation he has for himself and the demands that society has for him. In general, an individual may be considered to be mentally ill if:

- ❖ The person's behavior is causing distress and suffering to self and/or others.
- ❖ The person's behavior is causing disturbance in his day-to-day activities, job and inter-personal relationships.

DEFINITIONS OF MENTAL HEALTH

- ❖ Mental health is, "An adjustment of human beings to the world and to each other with a maximum of effectiveness and happiness."
  —**Karl Menninger, 1947**

- ❖ Mental health is, "Simultaneous success at working, loving and creating with the capacity for mature and flexible resolution of conflicts between instincts, conscience, important other people and reality."
  —**American Psychiatric Association, 1980**

- ❖ Mental health is a state of well-being in which an individual realizes his or her own abilities, can cope with the normal stresses of life, can work productively and is able to make a contribution to his or her community.
  —**World Health Organization, 2001**

- ❖ Mental health is the ability to adapt and self-manage. —**Huber et al., 2011**

Thus, mental health would include not only the absence of diagnostic labels such as schizophrenia and obsessive-compulsive disorder, but also the ability to cope with the stressors of daily living, freedom from anxieties and generally a positive outlook towards life's vicissitudes and to cope with those.

CRITERIA FOR MENTAL HEALTH

The criteria for mental health include (**Figure 1.1**):

- ❖ **Ability to accept self:** A mentally healthy individual feels comfortable about himself. He feels reasonably secure and adequately accepts his shortcomings. He also feels worthwhile and important.
- ❖ **Positive self-respect:** A mentally healthy individual has an objective view of self besides having the knowledge and acceptance of his strengths and limitations.
- ❖ **Social acceptance:** A mentally healthy individual has the ability to achieve a satisfactory role within the group and society. He is able to love and accept the love of others, and have friendships that are satisfying and lasting. He is able to feel as a part of a group without being submerged by it.
- ❖ **Ability to fulfill life's tasks:** A mentally healthy individual is able to think for himself, set reasonable goals and take his own decisions. He does something about the problems as they arise. He shoulders his daily responsibilities and is not bowled over by his own emotions of fear, anger, love or guilt.
- ❖ **Capacity to feel right towards others:** A mentally healthy individual shows understanding of other people's problems and motives. He enjoys good mental health and is able to exhibit sincere interest in other's welfare. He takes responsibility for his neighbors and fellow members, has the capacity for empathy and social sensitivity, a respect and concern for the wants and needs of others.

- ❖ **Adequate contact with reality:** A mentally healthy individual has an undistorted perception of the environment. He lives in a world of reality rather than fantasy.
- ❖ **Control of thoughts and imagination:** A mentally healthy individual has the ability to manage his thoughts and imagination in an appropriate way. He shows emotional maturity in his behavior and develops a capacity to tolerate frustration and disappointments in his daily life.
- ❖ **Efficiency in work/play:** A mentally healthy individual achieves tasks associated with each level of development successfully.
- ❖ **Healthy emotional life:** A mentally healthy individual has developed a philosophy of life that gives meaning and purpose to his daily activities, has a variety of interests and generally lives a well-balanced life of work, rest and recreation. He maintains anxiety at a manageable level in response to stressful situation.

Indicators of Mental Health

Jahoda (1958) has identified six indicators of mental health (**Figure 1.2**):

1. **A positive attitude towards self:** This includes an objective view of self including knowledge and acceptance of strengths and limitations. The individual feels a strong sense of personal identity and security within the environment.
2. **Growth, development and the ability for self-actualization:** This indicator correlates with whether the individual successfully achieves the tasks associated with each level of development or not.
3. **Integration:** It includes the ability to adaptively respond to the environment and the development of a philosophy of life both of which help the individual maintain anxiety at a manageable level in response to stressful situations.

1. Ability to accept self
2. Positive self-respect
3. Social acceptance
4. Ability to fulfill life's tasks
5. Capacity to feel right towards others
6. Adequate contact with reality
7. Control of thoughts and imagination
8. Efficiency in work/play
9. Healthy emotional life

Figure 1.1: Criteria for mental health

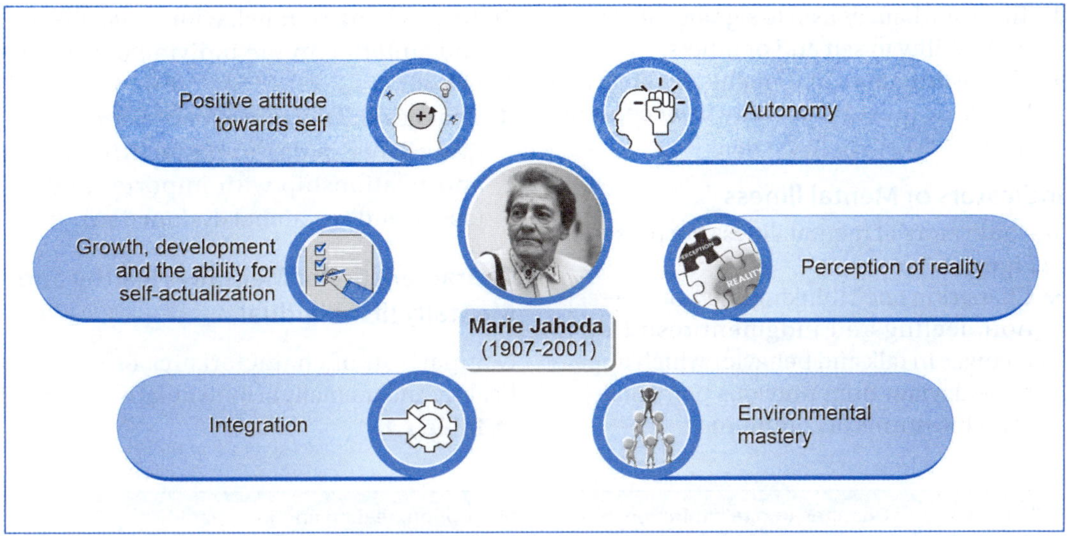

Figure 1.2: Indicators of mental health

4. **Autonomy:** It refers to the individual's ability to perform in an independent and self-directed manner wherein the individual makes choices and accepts responsibility for the outcomes.
5. **Perception of reality:** It includes perception of the environment without distortion, as well as the capacity for empathy and social sensitivity—a respect and concern for the wants and needs of others.
6. **Environmental mastery:** This indicator suggests that the individual has achieved a satisfactory role within the group, society or environment. He is able to love and accept the love of others.

Definitions of Mental Illness

❖ Mental and behavioral disorders are understood as clinically significant conditions characterized by alterations in thinking, mood (emotions) or behavior associated with personal distress and/or impaired functioning.   **—WHO, 2001**
❖ Mental illness or mental disorder is an illness or syndrome with psychological or behavioral manifestations and/or impairment in functioning as a result of a social, psychological, genetic, physical/chemical or biological disturbance.
         —American Psychiatric Association

❖ A mental disorder is a syndrome characterized by clinically significant disturbance in an individual's cognition, emotion regulation or behavior that reflects a dysfunction in the psychological, biological or development processes underlying mental functioning.
         —Diagnostic and Statistical Manual of Mental Disorders V, 2013

❖ Mental illness is maladaptive responses to stressors from the internal or external environment, evidenced by thoughts, feelings and behaviors that are incongruent with the local and cultural norms and interfere with the individual's social, occupational and/or physical functioning.
         —Morgan and Townsend, 2021

Criteria for Mental Illness

According to the American Psychiatric Association (APA) 2013, a psychological disorder is a condition that is said to meet following criteria:
1. There are significant disturbances in thoughts, feelings and behavior.
2. The disturbances reflect some kind of biological, psychological or developmental dysfunction.

3. The disturbances lead to significant distress or disability to self and or others.
4. The disturbances in thoughts, feelings and behavior must be socially unacceptable responses to certain events.

Indicators of Mental Illness

The indicators of mental illness are presented in **Figure 1.3.**

❖ Changes in one's thinking, memory, perception, feeling and judgment resulting in changes in talk and behavior which appear to be deviant from previous personality or from the norms of community.

❖ These changes in behavior cause distress and suffering to the individual or others or both.

❖ Changes and the consequent distress cause disturbance in day-to-day activities, work and relationship with important others (social and vocational dysfunction).

Characteristics of Mentally Healthy and Mentally Ill Individual

Comparison of characteristics of mentally healthy and mentally ill individual is presented in **Table 1.1**.

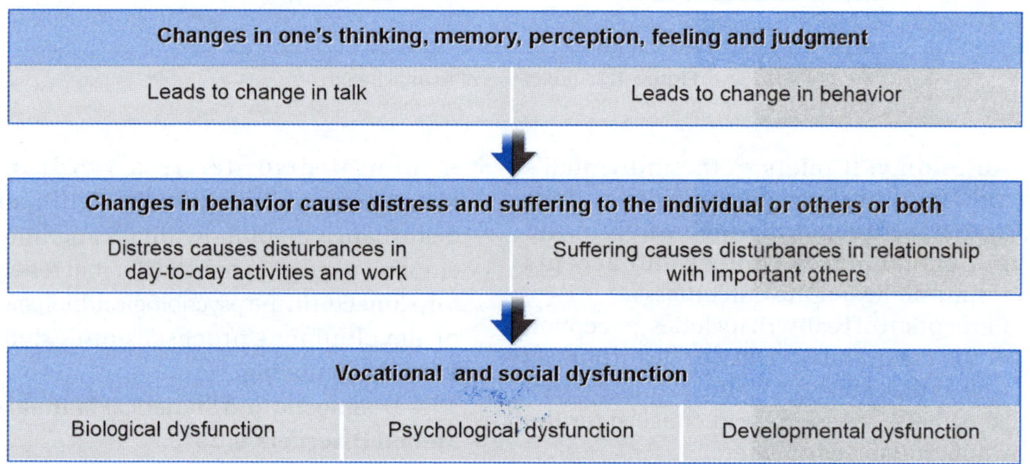

Figure 1.3: Indicators of mental illness

TABLE 1.1: Characteristics of mentally healthy and mentally ill individual	
Mentally healthy	**Mentally ill**
Able to cope with stress. Has the ability to make adjustments. Uses adaptive coping strategies and stress reduction strategies like problem solving and cognitive restructuring, etc.	Unable to cope with stress. Uses maladaptive coping strategies like substance abuse
Experiences satisfaction and stability in relationships. Can rely on social support	Shows pattern of unstable relationships. Passively allows others to assume responsibility for major areas of life. Has chronic feeling of emptiness
Able to form close and lasting relationships	Unable to establish meaningful relationships
Has a sense of personal worth, feels worthwhile, important, has reasonable level of self-confidence	Does not recognize capabilities because of poor self-confidence
Solves his problems largely by his own effort	Exhibits dependency needs because of feelings of inadequacy
Makes his own decisions	Displays poor judgment
Has a sense of responsibility	Unable to accept responsibility for actions

Contd…

Contd...

Mentally healthy	Mentally ill
Can give and accept love, able to form lasting relationships	Unable to establish a meaningful relationship
Lives in a world of reality rather than fantasy	Unable to perceive reality
Shows emotional maturity in his behavior and develops a capacity to tolerate frustration and disappointments in his daily life	Shows immature behavior, avoids problems rather than coping with them
Optimistic	Pessimistic
Has variety of interests and generally lives a well-balanced life of work, rest and recreation	Exhibits disorganized and unacceptable behavior
Can do well in task attempted. Optimum use of his capabilities	Decline in work output or academic performance

MISCONCEPTIONS RELATED TO MENTAL ILLNESS

Beliefs about mental illness have been characterized by superstition, ignorance and fear. Although time and again advances in scientific understanding of mental illness have dispelled many false ideas, there remain a number of popular misconceptions. Some of the myths and facts are described below:

❖ **Myth:** Mental illness is caused by a supernatural power and is the result of a curse or possession by evil spirit: Many people do not consider mental illness as an illness but a possession by spirits or a curse that has befallen on the patient or family because of past sins or misdeeds in previous life.

❖ **Fact:** Mental illnesses are not due to possession by evil spirit, or due to black magic or due to curse or punishment for sins. These disorders like any medical illness arise from chemical imbalance in the brain which require medical treatment.

❖ **Myth:** Mentally ill people show bizarre behavior and are dangerous: Patients in mental hospitals and clinics are often picturized as a weird lot who spend their time exhibiting bizarre behavior like twisting of hands, etc. People who have or had a mental illness are viewed with suspicion and as dangerous persons.

❖ **Fact:** Mentally ill individuals are confused, frightened and in despair. They are not violent, bizarre or dangerous. Very few patients show violence in the acute phase which is treatable with proper medication.

❖ **Myth:** Mental illness is something to be ashamed of: This idea arouses an unsympathetic, cruel attitude towards a mentally ill person. This is the reason why many people hide mental illness in the family.

❖ **Fact:** Early detection and prompt treatment for mental illnesses results in better improvement in mentally ill patients enabling them to lead socially productive lives. There is no reason to hide mental illness if it is treated well.

❖ **Myth:** Mental illness is not curable: People object to have normal relationship with mentally ill people or offer them employment even after being cured or even to accept them as neighbors.

❖ **Fact:** About 80% of the mental illnesses are fully curable and preventable. Excluding schizophrenia, all other mental illnesses can be easily controlled and prevented through proper medications and psychological therapies.

❖ **Myth:** Mental illness is contagious: The fear that it is contagious is the main false notion which leads people to view suspiciously or object to marital relations with a person belonging to the household of the mentally ill.

❖ **Fact:** Mental illnesses do not spread through contact of any form. Individual genetic vulnerability or predisposition and precipitating factors play an important role in disease occurrence. Some of the mental illnesses are chronic non-communicable illnesses just like diabetes, hypertension, heart diseases.

❖ **Myth:** Mental illness is hereditary: It is not a rule that children of mentally ill patients will become mentally ill.

❖ **Fact:** The role of genetic factors is well established only in some psychiatric illnesses (for example, schizophrenia, mania and depression). It is also not true that if a family member is suffering from schizophrenia the other members will always develop the same illness. The chances though are more likely, factors such as personality and environment play an equally important role.

❖ **Myth:** Marriage can cure mental illness.

❖ **Fact:** A mentally ill person can get worse if he gets married when he is ill, as marriage can become an additional stress. A patient who has recovered can get married and live a normal life like any other person.

❖ **Myth:** Mental hospitals are places where only dangerous mentally ill individuals are treated and restraint is a major form of treatment: People hesitate to take their relatives to mental hospitals for treatment because of fear. Further, as ex-patient of a mental hospital, the individual and his family members are often isolated. Therefore, people seek help from mental hospitals only as a last resort.

❖ **Fact:** Mentally ill individuals are treated humanely in mental hospitals with a combination of medicines and psychosocial interventions. In certain instances electro-convulsive therapy (shock treatment) is given. It is a safe procedure where the brain is stimulated using a brief current. Patient is not aware of the procedure as it is given under general anesthesia.

❖ **Myth:** Mentally ill are unproductive and burden to family.

❖ **Fact:** With proper medications, rehabilitation and supportive environment many mentally ill individuals can return to a normal and productive life.

❖ **Myth:** Mental illness is a weakness of character. If he wishes he can control it.

❖ **Fact:** Mental illnesses are not due to weakness of character. It is not possible to overcome them with will power as the symptoms are beyond one's control.

PRINCIPLES OF MENTAL HEALTH NURSING

The following principles are general in nature and form guidelines for emotional care of a patient. These principles are based on the concept that each individual has an intrinsic worth and dignity and has potentialities to grow. These are guidelines for nurses to provide quality care to psychiatric patients **(Figure 1.4)**.

1. Patient is Accepted Exactly as He is

Accepting means being non-judgmental. Acceptance conveys the feeling of being loved and cared. It does not mean complete permissiveness but setting of positive behaviors to convey to him the respect as an individual human being. A nurse should be able to convey to the patient that she may not approve everything he does while at the same time he will not be judged or rejected because of his behavior. Acceptance is expressed in the following ways:

a. Being Non-judgmental and Non-punitive

The patient's behavior is not judged as right or wrong, good or bad. Patient is not punished for his undesirable behavior. All direct (chaining, restraining, putting him in a separate room) and indirect (ignoring his presence or withdrawing attention) methods of punishment must be avoided. A nurse who shows acceptance does not reject the patient even when he behaves contrary to her expectations.

b. Being Sincerely Interested in the Patient

Being sincerely interested in another individual means considering the other individual's interest. This can be demonstrated by:

❖ Studying patient's behavior pattern

❖ Allowing him to make his own choices and decisions as far as possible

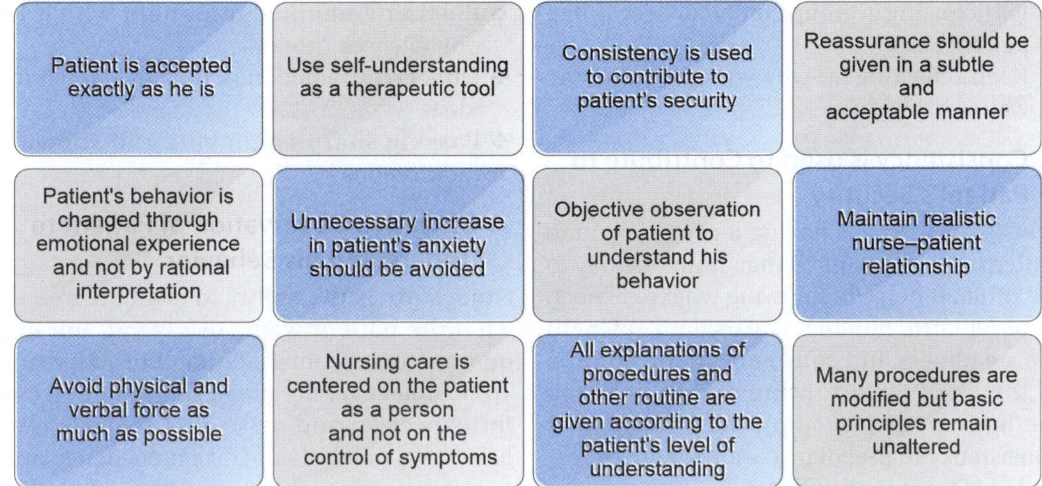

Figure 1.4: General principles of mental health nursing

❖ Being aware of his likes and dislikes
❖ Being honest with him
❖ Taking time and energy to listen to what he is saying
❖ Avoiding sensitive subjects and issues

c. Recognizing and Reflecting on Feelings which Patient may Express

When patient talks it is not the content that is important to note but the feeling behind the conversation which is to be recognized and reflected.

d. Talking with a Purpose

The nurse's conversation with a patient must revolve around his needs, wants and interests. Indirect approaches like reflection, open-ended questions, focusing on a point, presenting reality are more effective when the problems are not obvious. Avoid evaluative, hostile, probing questions and use understanding responses which may help the patient to explore his feelings.

e. Listening

Listening is an active process. The nurse should take time and energy to listen to what the patient is saying. She must be a sympathetic listener and show genuine interest.

f. Permitting Patient to Express Strongly-held Feelings

Strong emotions bottled up are potentially explosive and dangerous. It is better to permit the patient to express his strong feelings without disapproval or punishment. Expression of negative feelings (anxiety, fear, hostility and anger) may be encouraged in a verbal or symbolic manner. The nurse must accept the expression of patient's strong negative feelings quietly and calmly.

2. Use Self-understanding as a Therapeutic Tool

A psychiatric nurse should have a realistic self-concept and be able to recognize one's own feelings, attitudes and responses. Her ability to be aware of and accept her own strengths and limitations should help her see the strengths and limitations in other people too. Self-understanding helps her to be assertive in life situations without being aggressive and feeling guilty. Some of the self-understanding methods are:

❖ Exchanging personal experiences freely and honestly with colleagues
❖ Discussing own personal reactions with an experienced person

- ❖ Participating in group conference regarding patient care
- ❖ Keep reflecting on why you feel or act the way you do

3. Consistency is used to Contribute to Patient's Security

Consistency means having a certain routine pattern that does not change from one day to the other. It helps in knowing what to expect. In psychiatric nursing, consistency refers to the steadiness and constancy in the attitude of the staff, ward routine and in defining the limitations placed on the patient. This consistency in psychiatric wards reduces fear and anxiety among patients.

4. Reassurance should be given in a Subtle and Acceptable Manner

Reassurance is building patient's confidence. To give reassurance, the nurse needs to understand and analyze the situation as to how it appears to the patient. False reassurance can also reflect a lack of interest and understanding or unwillingness on the part of the nurse to empathize with the patient's life situation.

5. Patient's Behavior is Changed through Emotional Experience and not by Rational Interpretation

Major focus in psychiatry is on feelings and not on the intellectual aspect. Advising or rationalizing with patients is not effective in changing behavior. Role-play and socio-drama are a few avenues of providing corrective emotional experiences to a patient and facilitating insight into his own behavior. Such experiences can truly bring about the desired behavioral changes.

6. Unnecessary Rise in Patient's Anxiety should be Avoided

The following approaches may increase patient's anxiety and should therefore be avoided:

- ❖ Showing nurse's own anxiety
- ❖ Showing attention to patient's deficits
- ❖ Making the patient face repeated failures

- ❖ Placing demands on patient which he obviously cannot meet
- ❖ Direct contradiction of patient's psychotic ideas
- ❖ Passing sharp comments and showing indifference

7. Objective Observation of Patient to Understand his Behavior

Objectivity is the ability to evaluate exactly what the patient wants to say and not mix up one's own feelings, opinion or judgment. To be objective, the nurse should indulge in introspection and make sure that her own emotional needs do not take precedence over patient's needs.

8. Maintain Realistic Nurse–Patient Relationship

Realistic or professional relationship focuses upon the personal and emotional needs of the patient and not on nurse's needs. To maintain a professional relationship the nurse should have a realistic self-concept and should be able to empathize and understand the feelings of the patient and the meaning of his behavior.

9. Avoid Physical and Verbal Force as Much as Possible

All methods of punishment must be avoided. If the nurse is an expert in predicting patient behavior, she can mostly prevent the onset of undesirable behavior.

10. Nursing Care is Centered on the Patient as a Person and not on the Control of Symptoms

Analysis and study of symptoms is necessary to reveal their meaning and significance to the patient. Two patients exhibiting same symptoms may express two different needs.

11. All Explanations of Procedures and Other Routines are given According to the Patient's Level of Understanding

The extent of explanation that can be given to a patient depends on his span of attention, level of anxiety and level of ability to decide. But explanation should never be withheld on the basis that psychiatric patients are not having any contact with reality or have no ability to understand.

12. Many Procedures are Modified but Basic Principles Remain Unaltered

In the field of psychiatric nursing, many methods are adapted to the individual needs of patients though underlying nursing scientific principles remain the same. Some nursing principles to be kept in mind are: safety, comfort, privacy, maintaining therapeutic effectiveness, economy of time, energy and material.

DEFINITIONS AND TERMS USED IN PSYCHIATRY

Hallucination: A false sensory perception in the absence of an actual external stimulus. Hallucinations may be described in terms of their sensory modality as visual, auditory, olfactory, gustatory, tactile.

Delusion: A false, unshakeable belief which is not amenable to reasoning and is not in keeping with the patient's socio-cultural and educational background.

Delirium: State of mental confusion and excitement that happens in a short period of time and is characterized by disorientation for time and place usually with illusions and hallucinations.

Circumstantiality: A pattern of communication that is demonstrated by the speaker's inclusion of many irrelevant and unnecessary details in his speech before he is able to come to the point.

Amnesia: Pathological impairment of memory.

Compulsion: Pathological need to act on an impulse that, if resisted, produces anxiety; repetitive behavior in response to an obsession or performed according to certain rules, with no true end in itself other than to prevent something from occurring in the future (the patient fears something bad will occur in future if he does not indulge in such behaviors).

Dementia: Broad impairment of intellectual function that usually is progressive and interferes with normal social and occupational activities.

Euphoria: Excessive feeling of happiness or elation.

Flight of ideas: Rapid shift between topics that are unrelated to each other. The client's thoughts and conversation move quickly from one topic to another so that one train of thought is not completed before another appears. These rapidly changing topics are understandable because the links between them are normal, a point that differentiates them from loosening of associations. Flight of ideas is characteristic of mania.

Illusion: The misinterpretation of a real, external sensory experience. It is mental misperception of actual sensory stimuli.

Mental health: The successful adaptation to stressors from the internal or external environment.

Mental illness: Maladaptive responses to stressors from the internal or external environment, evidenced by thoughts, feelings, and behaviors that are incongruent with the local and cultural norms, and interfere with the individual's social, occupational, and/or physical functioning.

Mental retardation: Intellectual functioning significantly below average with IQ of 70 or below.

Obsession: Pathological persistence of an irresistible thought or feeling that cannot be eliminated from consciousness by logical effort; associated with anxiety.

Panic attack: Intense feeling of fear or terror that occurs suddenly and intermittently without warning.

(A detailed list of terms used in psychiatry are presented in Glossary)

REVIEW OF DEFENSE MECHANISMS

Coping is a way one adapts to a stressor psychologically, physically and behaviorally. The ego usually copes with anxiety through rational means. When anxiety is too painful, the individual copes by using defense mechanisms to protect the ego and diminish the anxiety.

Defense mechanisms are methods of attempting to protect self and cope with basic drives or emotionally painful thoughts, feelings or events. The purpose of defense mechanisms is to reduce or eliminate anxiety. They can be helpful when used in very small doses, and if overused become ineffective leading to breakdown of the personality. Most defense mechanisms operate at the unconscious level of awareness. The commonly used defense mechanisms are presented in **Table 1.2**.

TABLE 1.2: Commonly used defense mechanisms

Defense mechanism and description	Example	Overuse may lead to
Repression: Unconscious and involuntary forgetting of painful ideas, events and conflicts	Forgetting a loved one's birthday after a fight	Conscious perception of instincts and blockage of feelings
Denial: Unconscious refusal to admit an unacceptable idea or behavior	Mother of a child who is fatally ill though fully informed of the diagnosis and the expected outcome refuses to admit it. It is because she cannot tolerate the pain that acknowledging the reality would cause	Repression, dissociative disorders
Displacement: Unconscious discharging of pent-up feelings to a less threatening object	A husband yells at his wife after a bad day at work	Loss of friends and relationships, confusion in communication
Reaction formation: Replacement of unacceptable feelings with their exact opposites	A boy who is jealous and hates his elder brother shows him exaggerated respect and affection	Failure in resolving internal conflict
Rationalization: Justification of failures and offering socially approved reasons for socially unacceptable behavior	A student complains about the unfavorable hostel atmosphere for his failure in the examination	Self-deception
Sublimation: Conscious or unconscious channeling of instinctual drives into acceptable activities	Aggressiveness being transformed to competitiveness in business or sports	Channeling of instincts rather than being blocked or diverted
Compensation: Conscious covering up for a weakness by over emphasizing or making up a desirable trait	A student who fails in his studies compensates for it by becoming the college champion in athletics	Modest instinctual satisfaction
Projection: Unconscious (or conscious) blaming of someone else for one's difficulties	A surgeon blames the theater nurse for an unsuccessful operation. Here the surgeon blames the theater nurse for his own mistake using the projection mechanism	Failure in taking personal responsibility; building up of delusional tendencies

Contd...

Contd…

Defense mechanism and description	Example	Overuse may lead to
Intellectualization: Undue emphasis on the inanimate to avoid intimacy with people; increased attention on external reality to avoid expression of inner feelings; excessive stress on irrelevant details to avoid perceiving the whole	Person shows no emotional expression when discussing a serious car accident	Limiting of affective expression on experience
Undoing: Reversing or undoing a thought or feeling by performing an action that signifies an opposite feeling than original thought or feeling	Buying a gift for someone for whom there is a feeling of dislike	Sending a double message
Regression: Reverting to an older, less mature way of handling stresses and feelings	An adult throwing a temper tantrum when he does not get his own way	Interference with progression and development of personality
Dissociation: Unconscious separation of painful feelings and emotions from an unacceptable idea, situation or object	Amnesia preventing recall of previous days autoaccident. Adult remembering nothing of childhood sexual abuse	Dissociative disorders
Conversion: Unconscious expression of intrapsychic conflict symbolically through physical symptoms	Student awakening with a migraine headache in the morning of a final examination and feeling too ill to take the exam	Inability in dealing with anxiety which may lead to actual physical disorders such as gastric ulcers
Suppression: Voluntary rejection of unacceptable thoughts or feelings from conscious awareness	Student failing in an examination not forthcoming about his marks	Acknowledging the discomfort though not willingly
Substitution: Unconscious replacement of unacceptable impulses, attitudes, needs or emotions with those that are more acceptable	Student nurse taking up teaching as she is unable to master clinical competencies	Acknowledging the discomfort though not willingly
Isolation: Attempt to avoid a painful thought or feeling by objectifying and emotionally detaching oneself from the feeling	Acting aloof and indifferent towards someone who is disliked	Loss of ability in dealing with true feelings and increased stress

Implications

❖ Defense mechanisms enable a person to resolve conflicts. They are essential to the maintenance of normal equilibrium.

❖ Difficulties occur only if the defense mechanisms are inadequate to deal with anxiety or inappropriate to the situation in which they are used.

❖ Many mental mechanisms are a means of compromising with forbidden desires, feeling of guilt, etc.

❖ Mental mechanisms when used moderately are harmless, protect the ego and help face conflicts and frustrations easily. They also help to relieve tensions and make the person feel comfortable.

❖ Excessive and persistent use of these defense mechanisms is harmful. They do not solve the problems but only relieve the related anxiety. Too much dependence makes us incapable of facing problems. For example, if a student is unable to face the examination and withdraws from taking it, he may experience greater difficulty in the next attempt. It would thus be better to face the problems than resorting to such mechanisms.

❖ Many a times more than one mechanism may operate in the process of adjusting to the situation.

Relevance to nursing practice: The nurse must recognize and understand maladaptive defense mechanisms that patients use. The nurse has to carefully point out these mechanisms and work with patients to encourage adaptive mechanisms.

MENTAL HEALTH TEAM OR MULTIDISCIPLINARY TEAM

Effective mental health care requires a high performing interprofessional team. Multidisciplinary approach refers to collaboration between members of different disciplines who provide specific services to the patient. The multidisciplinary team/mental health team is made up of a group of people each of whom possesses particular skills and expertise. Members of the multidisciplinary team include the following **(Figure 1.5)**:

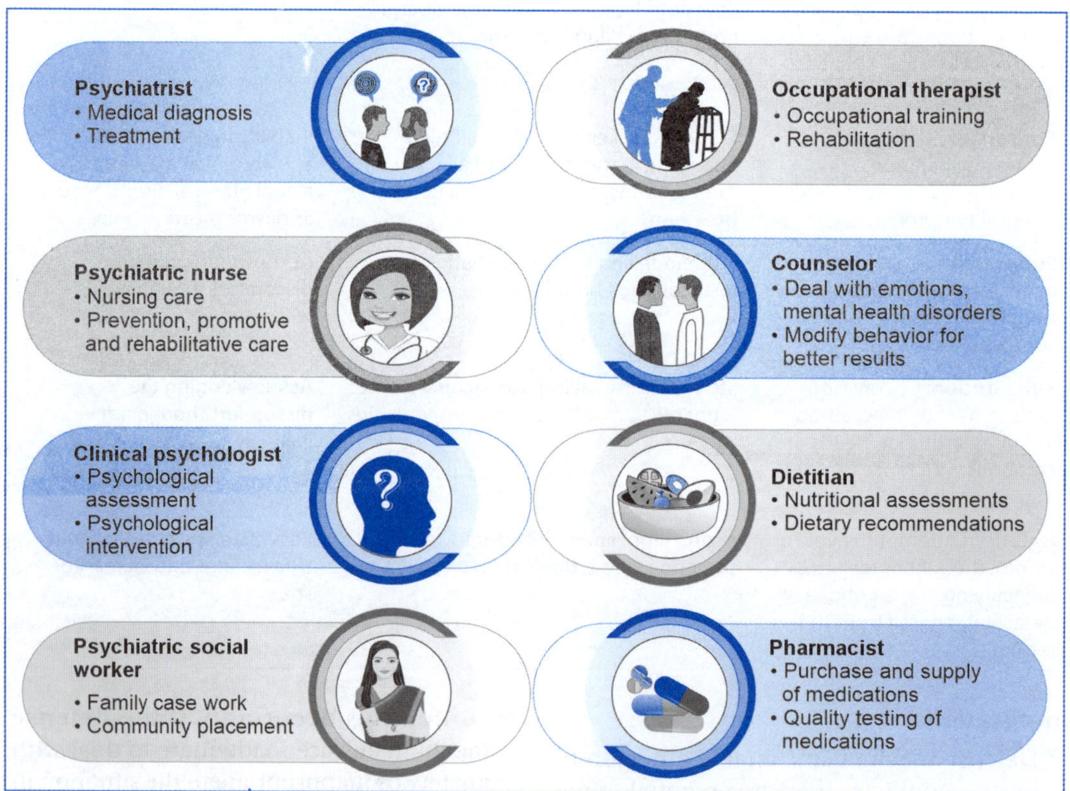

Figure 1.5: Mental health team

A **psychiatrist** is a medical doctor with special training in psychiatry. He is accountable for the medical diagnosis and treatment of the patient. Other important functions are:

* Admitting patient into acute care setting
* Prescribing and monitoring psycho-pharmacologic agents
* Administering electroconvulsive therapy
* Conducting individual and family therapy
* Participating in interdisciplinary team meetings
* Owing to their legal power to prescribe and write orders, psychiatrists often function as leaders of the team

A **psychiatric nurse** is a registered nurse with specialized training in the care of psychiatric patients; she may have a Diploma, MSc, MPhil or PhD in psychiatric nursing. She is accountable for the bio-psychosocial nursing care of patients and their milieu. Other functions include:

* Providing comprehensive, evidence-based nursing care
* Administering and monitoring medications
* Assisting in numerous psychiatric and physical treatments
* Participating in interdisciplinary team meetings
* Teaching patients and families
* Taking responsibility for patients' records
* Acting as patient's advocate
* Interacting with patients' significant others

A **clinical psychologist** should have a Master's Degree in Psychology or PhD in clinical psychology with specialized training in mental health settings. Psychologists conduct cognitive, academic and personality testing, interpret psychological tests and implement psychological therapies besides offering direct services such as individual, family or marital therapies.

A **psychiatric social worker** should have a Master's Degree in Social Work or PhD degree with specialized training in mental health settings. He is accountable for family case work and community placement of patients. He assesses the individual, family and community support system, helps in discharge planning, counseling for rehabilitation and job placement. He should also be aware of state laws and legal rights of the patient and protect them. He conducts individual, family and group therapy sessions and emphasizes intervention with the patient in social environment in which he will live.

An **occupational therapist or an activity therapist** has specialized training, is accountable for occupational, activity programs and rehabilitation of the patient. He assists the patients to gain skills that help them cope more effectively, gain or retain employment and use their leisure time.

A **counselor** has a master's in clinical/counseling psychology. He helps the individuals and families deal with difficult emotions, mental health disorders and trauma. He coaches them to manage their stress, redirect disturbing emotions and set goals for themselves besides helping them to modify their behaviors for better results.

A **dietitian** with specialized training in food and nutrition helps in menu planning and promotion of healthy eating, and is accountable for nutritional assessments, dietary recommendation and nutritional education.

A **pharmacist** is responsible for monitoring the supply of all medicines used in the psychiatric hospital and is in-charge of purchasing, dispensing and quality testing of medication stock.

Each member of the multidisciplinary team needs to have an understanding of other member's roles in meeting the needs of patients. However, harmonious functioning of the multidisciplinary team is dependent on the nurse's ability to be an effective communicator and to have an understanding of the roles and functions of other team members.

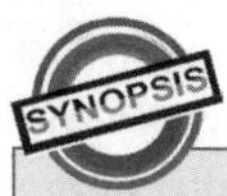

- Mental health is an integral and essential component of health. There is no health without mental health.
- Mental health is a state of mental well-being that enables people to cope with the stresses of life, realize their abilities, learn well and work well, and contribute to their community.
- Mental illness is maladjustment in living. It produces disharmony in a person's ability to meet human needs comfortably or effectively and function within a culture.
- The criteria for mental health include: ability to accept self, positive self-respect, social acceptance, ability to fulfill life's tasks, capacity to feel right towards others, adequate contact with reality, control of thoughts and imagination, efficiency in work/play and emotional healthy life.
- Jahoda has identified six indicators of mental health: positive attitude towards self, growth, development and the ability for self-actualization, integration, autonomy, perception of reality, environmental mastery.
- The indicators of mental illness are changes in one's thinking, memory, perception, feeling and judgment. These changes cause distress and disturbance in day-to-day activities and are also distressing to others.
- Beliefs about mental illness have been characterized by superstitions, ignorance and fear.
- General principles form guidelines for emotional care of a patient. These are: patient is accepted exactly as he is, use self-understanding as a therapeutic tool, consistency is used to contribute to patient's security, reassurance should be given in a subtle and acceptable manner, patient's behavior is changed through emotional experience and not by rational interpretation, unnecessary increase in patient's anxiety should be avoided, objective observation of patient to understand his behavior, maintain realistic nurse–patient relationship, avoid physical and verbal force as much as possible, nursing care is centered on the patient as a person and not on the control of symptoms, all explanations of procedures and other routine are given according to the patient's level of understanding, many procedures are modified but basic principles remain unaltered.
- The ego usually copes with anxiety through rational means. When anxiety is too painful, the individual copes by using defense mechanisms to protect the ego and diminish anxiety.
- Defense mechanisms are methods of attempting to protect self and cope with basic drives or emotionally painful thoughts, feelings or events.
- Mental mechanisms when used moderately protect the ego, help face conflicts and frustrations easily and are harmless.
- The harmonious functioning of the multidisciplinary team is dependent on the nurse's ability to be an effective communicator and to have an understanding of the roles and functions of other team members.

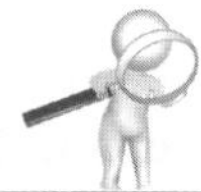

REVIEW QUESTIONS

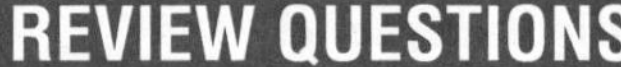

Long Essays

1. What is the meaning of mental health? Explain criteria for mental health? List the 6 indicators of mental health stated by Jahoda.
2. What is the meaning of mental illness? Explain criteria for mental illness? List three indicators of mental illness.
3. Explain commonly used defense mechanisms with examples.
4. Explain general principles of psychiatric nursing.

Short Essays

1. Describe characteristics of mentally healthy and mentally ill individual.
2. Explain misconceptions related to mental illness.
3. List the multidisciplinary team members in psychiatry. Describe role of nurse in multidisciplinary team.
4. Describe in detail on principles of mental health nursing.

Short Answers

1. Criteria for mental health
2. Characteristics of a mentally healthy person
3. List defense mechanisms
4. List multidisciplinary team members

Give the Meaning of the Following

Mental illness, mental health, defense mechanisms, repression, denial, displacement, projection, regression, suppression, psychiatrist, psychiatric nurse.

Fill in the Blanks

1. Unconscious refusal to admit an unacceptable idea or behavior is called __________.
2. Unconscious blaming of someone else for one's difficulties is termed as __________.
3. Unconscious replacement of unacceptable impulses, attitudes, needs or emotions with those that are more acceptable is termed as __________.
4. __________ is a medical doctor with special training in psychiatry.
5. __________ refers to the individual's ability to perform in an independent and self-directed manner.

State the Following Statements are True or False

1. When a person is suffering with mental illness there are significant disturbances in thoughts, feelings and behavior.
2. Mentally healthy person uses maladaptive coping strategies to deal with stress.
3. Mentally healthy person makes his own decisions.
4. Mental illnesses are caused by super natural power.
5. Listening is a passive process.

Multiple Choice Questions

1. **Which of the following is a criterion for mental health?**
   a. Efficiency in work and play
   b. Disturbance in day-to-day activity
   c. Ability to perform activities independently
   d. Personal insecurity
2. **Which of the following is an important characteristic of a mentally healthy person?**
   a. Ability to perform activities independently
   b. Ability to make adjustments
   c. Feeling secure
   d. Changes in behavior

3. **Which of the following is an appropriate statement for the principle that 'patient is accepted exactly as he is':**
   a. Objective observation of patient behavior
   b. Explaining all the procedures to patient according to his level of understanding
   c. Maintaining realistic nurse-patient relationship
   d. Being non-judgmental and non-punitive

4. **One of the general principles of psychiatric nursing is:**
   a. Reassuring the patient
   b. Use self-understanding as a therapeutic tool
   c. Repeated talking
   d. Judgment of patient symptoms

5. **Which among the following is an example of displacement?**
   a. Discharging pent up feelings to a less threatening object
   b. Replacing unacceptable feelings with exactly opposite feelings
   c. Blaming someone else for one's difficulties
   d. Forgetting painful ideas/conflicts

6. **A student failed in her psychology exam and spent the entire evening criticizing the teacher and the institution. This behavior is an example of:**
   a. Rationalization
   b. Compensation
   c. Projection
   d. Displacement

ANSWER KEY

Fill in the Blanks				
1. Denial	2. Projection	3. Substitution,	4. Psychiatrist	5. Autonomy

State the Following Statements are True or False				
1. True	2. False	3. True	4. False	5. True

Multiple Choice Questions					
1. a	2. b	3. d	4. b	5. a	6. c

History of Psychiatry

Mental health nursing also known as psychiatric nursing is a specialized field of nursing practice that deals with the care of individuals with mental health disorder. It helps them to recover and improve their quality of life. Mental health nurses provide care for individuals, families, groups and communities to promote mental health. They work in hospitals, clinics, counseling centers, long-term care centers, half way homes, day care centers and community centers. Patients often range in age from children through adolescence to adulthood. Thus, psychiatric nursing deals with the promotion of mental health, prevention of mental illness, care and rehabilitation of mentally ill individuals both in hospital and community.

HISTORY OF PSYCHIATRY

The occurrence of mental illnesses has been identified and documented since ancient times. Evolution of mental health services and treatment can be described under the following headings **(Figure 2.1)**:

Early Civilization

Historically, mental illness was viewed as a demonic possession, the influence of ancestral spirits, the result of violating a taboo or neglecting a cultural ritual and spiritual condemnation. As a consequence, the mentally ill were often starved, beaten,

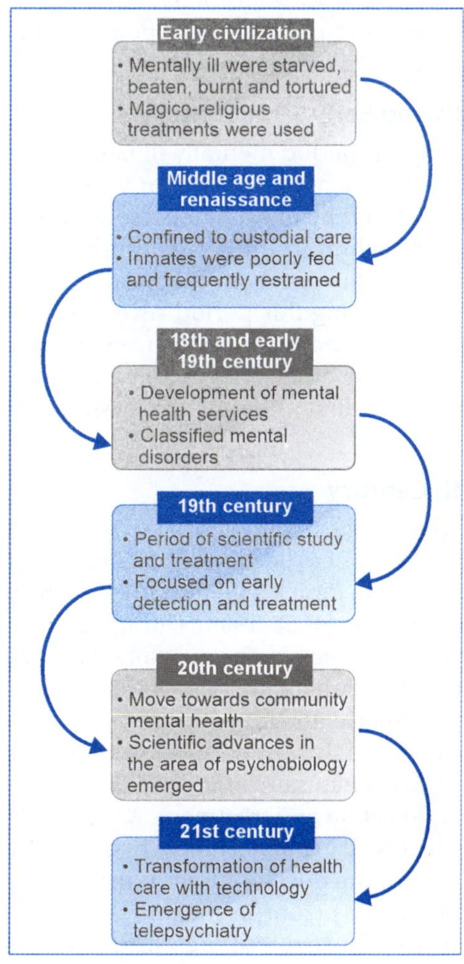

Figure 2.1: Evolution of mental health services and treatment

burnt, amputated and tortured so as to make the body an unsuitable place for the demon. The therapists were priests who used magico-religious treatment. Early civilization such as the Greek and Roman cultures developed the ideas of body humors—blood, black bile, yellow bile and phlegm, which could influence emotional stability. Hippocrates believed that black bile causes melancholy and that bloodletting could remove this excess.

Middle Age and Renaissance

During this period mentally ill were excluded from community life and confined to institutions. They were treated as criminals and punished for their behaviors. Care was custodial and inmates were poorly fed and clothed and were frequently restrained.

18th and Early 19th Century

During this period mentally ill patients were committed to asylum. Care for these people was provided by untrained persons. The first lunatic asylum in India was established in Mumbai in the year 1745, followed by Kolkata in 1784. During this period several theories were developed regarding causes of mental illness. In the nineteenth century, physicians began their first attempts to classify mental disorders.

19th Century

The period of scientific study and treatment of mental disorders began with Sigmund Freud (1856–1939), Emil Krepeline (1856–1926) and Eugen Bleuler (1857–1939). During this period methods of caring for the mentally ill was more humane and mental illnesses were regarded as psychiatric disorders. Modern psychiatry understands mental illnesses based on concepts of natural science and is focused on early detection and treatment. A great leap in the treatment of mental illness began in about 1950 with the development of psychotropic drugs such as chlorpromazine and lithium. With psychotropic drugs more patients became treatable resulting in restraints being removed. Various somatic therapies like insulin shock therapy (1927), psychosurgery (1936), and ECT (1938) were also developed.

20th Century

During 1960 AD–2000 AD focus shifted from hospital-based care to community care. There was a slow and steady reduction of beds in custodial institutions followed by a growth in general hospital psychiatric units and outpatient services. Deinstitutionalization, a deliberate shift from institutional care in state hospitals to community facilities was observed. The first general hospital psychiatric units were set up at the RG Kar medical college, Kolkata in 1933. It was followed by similar set ups in Mumbai, 1938 and Patna, 1939.

In 1964, as a part of the comprehensive rural health services project (CRHSP) in Ballabgarh, weekly community mental health services were started by the All India Institute of Medical Sciences, New Delhi. World Health Organization (WHO) funded the project at Raipur Rani in Haryana under the aegis of Postgraduate Institute of Medical Education and Research (PGIMER), Chandigarh and at Sakalwara, Karnataka under the aegis of National Institute of Mental Health and Neurosciences (NIMHANS), Bengaluru.

During 1980s, scientific advances in the area of psychobiology, brain imaging techniques, knowledge about neurotransmitters and neuronal receptors, molecular genetics related to psychiatry, etc., emerged.

21st Century

The last two decades have seen an explosion in the knowledge base of neurosciences, epidemiology and therapeutics. There has also been a parallel growth in interdisciplinary linkages that support socially and culturally integrated approaches appropriate to mental health services. Telemedicine has been successfully integrated into psychiatric facilities and now reaching rural and other remote areas.

Some Important Milestones

❖ **580–510 BC:** Pythagoras developed the concept of brain being the seat of intellectual activity.

- ❖ **460–370 BC:** Hippocrates described mental illness as hysteria, mania and depression.
- ❖ **427–347 BC:** Plato identified the relationship between mind and body.
- ❖ Asciepiades referred to as the Father of Psychiatry made use of simple hygienic measures such as diet, bath, massage in place of mechanical restraints.
- ❖ The Greeks were the first to study mental illness scientifically and separate the study of mind from religion. Aristotle, a Greek philosopher, emphasized the release of repressed emotions for the effective treatment of mental illness. He suggested catharsis and music therapy for patients with melancholia.
- ❖ During middle ages, the mentally ill were not considered as outcasts but as people to be helped. One of the great figures during this time was St. Augustine who believed that although God acted directly in human affairs people were responsible for their own actions.
- ❖ **Renaissance in Europe (1300–1600 AD):** This period represented the saddest chapter in the history of psychiatry when it was believed that demons were the cause of hallucinations, delusions and sexual activity and the treatment was torture and even death.
- ❖ **1773:** The first mental hospital in the US was built in Williamsburg, Virginia.
- ❖ **1793:** Philippe Pinel removed the chains from mentally ill patients confined in Bicetre, a hospital outside Paris thereby bringing the first revolution in psychiatry. He is considered the 'Father of Modern Psychiatry'.
- ❖ **1812:** The first American textbook in psychiatry was written by Benjamin Rush, who is referred to as the Father of American Psychiatry.
- ❖ **1903:** Emil Kraepelin differentiated between dementia praecox and manic depression.
- ❖ **1908:** Clifford Beers, an ex-patient of a mental hospital wrote the book, 'The Mind That Found Itself' based on his bitter experiences in the hospital. He founded the American Mental Health Association which made a major contribution towards the improvement of conditions in mental hospitals.
- ❖ **1912:** Eugen Bleuler, a Swiss psychiatrist coined the term 'schizophrenia'.
- ❖ **1912:** The Indian Lunacy Act was passed.
- ❖ **1927:** Insulin shock treatment was introduced for schizophrenia.
- ❖ **1936:** Frontal lobotomy was advocated for the management of psychiatric disorders.
- ❖ **1938:** Electroconvulsive therapy (ECT) was used for the treatment of psychoses.
- ❖ **1939:** Development of psychoanalytical theory by Sigmund Freud led to new concepts in the treatment of mental illness.
- ❖ **1946:** Bhore Committee presented the situation with regard to mental health services. Based on its recommendations, five mental hospitals were set up at Amritsar (1947), Hyderabad (1953), Srinagar (1958), Jamnagar (1960) and Delhi (1966). An All India Institute of Mental Health was also set up at Bengaluru (currently known as National Institute of Mental Health and Neurosciences or NIMHANS).
- ❖ **1949:** Lithium was first used for the treatment of mania.
- ❖ **1952:** Chlorpromazine was introduced which brought about a revolution in psychopharmacology and changed the whole picture of mental health care.
- ❖ **1958:** The Indian Journal of Psychiatry started in 1958. The journal got indexed in national Library of Medicine.
- ❖ **1960:** Central Institute of Psychiatry (CIP), Ranchi and Madras Mental Hospital started offering special services such as geriatric, epileptic, neuropsychiatric services, child and adolescent clinics.
- ❖ **1960:** Concept of day hospitals and alternative accommodations were explored for mentally ill patients.
- ❖ **1963:** The 'Community Mental Health Centers' Act was passed.
- ❖ **1909–1978:** Dr Vidya Sagar devoted 35 long years of his life in the service of patients with mental illness. He was a

pioneer in community psychiatry. His most important contribution to psychiatry was the involvement of family in the care of patients with psychiatric illness.

- ❖ **1970s:** Slow and steady reduction of beds in custodial institutions, growth in General Hospital Psychiatric Units and outpatient services was seen.
- ❖ **1978:** The Alma-Ata declaration of "Health for All by 2000 AD" posed a major challenge to Indian mental health professionals. In order to achieve mental health for all (as a part of the achievement of Health for All by 2000 AD), in 1980 the Government of India called for experts in the field for assessing mental health needs of the people and recommended steps for providing mental health care.
- ❖ **1981:** Community psychiatric centers were set up to experiment with primary mental health care approach at Raipur Rani, Chandigarh and Sakalwara, Bengaluru.
- ❖ **1982:** Focus shifted to community-based care which became the basis for setting up the National Mental Health Program.
- ❖ **1987:** The Indian Mental Health Act was passed.
- ❖ **1990:** The Government of India formed an Action Group at Delhi to pool the opinion of mental health experts about the National Mental Health Program (NMHP).
- ❖ During 1990, National Institute of Mental Health and Neurosciences (NIMHANS), Bengaluru took the leadership in orienting healthcare professionals about the mental health programs of our country. A number of innovative approaches for the treatment and rehabilitation of mental illness were initiated, the most important ones being:
  - ○ Integration of mental healthcare with general healthcare.
  - ○ Establishment of school mental health programs.
  - ○ Promotion of child mental health through the involvement of Anganwadis [Integrated Child Development Services (ICDS) Program].
  - ○ Initiation of crisis intervention for suicide prevention.
  - ○ Establishment of Halfway homes for mentally ill individuals for social skills training and vocational training.
  - ○ Education and involvement of the general public through the activities of non-governmental organizations.
  - ○ Development of media materials for public education.
  - ○ Training for non-professionals to work with mentally ill individuals.
- ❖ **1995:** Person with Disability Act was passed to protect the rights of persons with mental illness and mainstreaming them into the society.
- ❖ **1997:** National Human Rights Commission prepared a plan of action for improving the conditions prevailing in mental hospitals of the country and enhancing awareness of the rights of those with mental disability.
- ❖ **1996-97:** The district mental health program started, emphasized on treatment and care at the primary health care level.
- ❖ **2001:** Current situation analysis (CSA) was done to evolve a comprehensive plan of action to energize the NMHP.
- ❖ **2001:** Advanced Center for Ayurveda in Mental Health and Neurosciences at the National Institute of Mental Health and Neurosciences (NIMHANS) initiated research studies in areas like epilepsy, mental retardation, schizophrenia, etc. The Advanced Center for Yoga Therapy and Research at NIMHANS started intervening in psychiatric disorders through yogic approach.
- ❖ **2001:** The National Human Rights Commission of India is mandated under section 12 of the protection of Human Rights Act 1993 to visit Government run mental hospitals to study the living conditions of inmates and make recommendations thereon.
- ❖ **2001:** On 6th Aug 2001, 27 mentally ill people died as they were tied to their beds when fire engulfed the thatched roof of the Moideen Badusha Mental Home at Erwadi,

Tamil Nadu State. Following this tragedy, the National Human Rights Commission of India (NHRC) advised all the chief ministers to submit a certificate stating no person with mental illness is kept chained in either Government or private institution. The Erwadi incident opened the eyes of the Government which in turn took lots of affirmative actions to improve mental health sector in the country. It included district wise survey of all registered and unregistered bodies purporting to offer mental health care and granting of licenses only on meeting the set standards.

❖ **2001:** Government implemented the District Mental Health Program. It focused on treatment availability at primary level, community awareness and renovation and construction of hospitals for improving mental health services in the State. It also covered training components for human resource development in the field of mental health.

❖ **2002:** National Survey of Mental Health Resources carried out by the Directorate General of Health Services, Ministry of Health and Family Welfare.

❖ **2007:** Under the Eleventh five-year plan, Centers of Excellence in the field of mental health were established to upgrade and strengthen identified existing mental health hospitals for addressing acute manpower gap and provision of state-of-the-art mental healthcare facilities in the long run. During this period, 11 mental health institutes were funded for developing as Centers of Excellence in Mental Health.

❖ **2008:** WHO Mental Health Gap Action Program was launched which aimed at scaling up services for mental, neurological and substance use disorders for countries especially with low and middle income.

❖ **2013:** World Health Organization launched the Mental Health Action Plan 2013–2020 on 7th October, 2013. The action plan identified the important role of mental health in achieving health for all people. It stressed the prevention of mental illness and aimed to achieve equity through universal health coverage.

❖ **2013:** Under the Twelfth five year plan the Government of India integrated different components of National Mental Health Program with the components of National Rural Health Mission namely school health, reproductive child health and adolescent friendly clinics to reach out to the community in a more effective manner.

❖ **2013:** Under central sector, the Ministry of Social Justice and Empowerment launched Deendayal Disabled Rehabilitation Scheme (DDRS) and provided financial assistance to Non-Governmental Organizations (NGOs) for providing various services to persons with disabilities and mental retardation including special schools, half way homes, etc. The National Trust for the Welfare of Persons with autism, cerebral palsy, mental retardation and multiple disabilities implemented various other schemes for the rehabilitation of such individuals.

❖ **2014:** National Mental Health Policy was duly considered by the Ministry of Health and Family Welfare, Government of India. This Policy was in accordance with the intent of World Health Assembly resolution and incorporated an integrated, participatory rights and evidence-based approach.

❖ **2017:** The Mental Health Care Act was passed on April 7, 2017 and enforced on May 29, 2018. This law provided for and regulated mental health care and treatment in India. It abolished the Mental Health Act 1987.

❖ **2020:** India experienced the effects of global COVID-19 pandemic which amplified mental health issues such as anxiety, depression, stress, insomnia, denial, anger and fear. The Government developed Comprehensive Training Modules for Healthcare Providers to deal with post COVID mental health issues to equip doctors, nurses, paramedical healthcare workers, community health workers and other frontline workers with knowledge and skills so as to provide psychosocial support to those affected by post COVID mental health issues.

❖ **2021:** In the ongoing Coronavirus disease (COVID) pandemic, travel restriction and reduced in-person interaction provided a huge impetus to telepsychiatry. Recent advancements in technology helped to improve clinical care in psychiatry.

❖ **2022:** Tele mental health assistance and networking across states (Tele-MANAS) initiative was launched by Ministry of Health and Family Welfare during October 2022. It aimed to provide free tele-mental health services all over the country round the clock particularly catering to people in remote or underserved areas.

World Mental Health Day is observed on 10th October every year with an overall objective of raising awareness on mental health issues around the world and mobilizing efforts in support of mental health.

HISTORY OF PSYCHIATRIC NURSING

Prior to 1860, psychiatric nursing was almost non-existent as custodial care was emphasized in psychiatric hospitals with untrained people being involved in providing care **(Figure 2.2)**.

During 18th Century

❖ In 1873, Linda Richards developed better nursing care in psychiatric hospitals and organized nursing services and educational programs in state mental hospitals. It is for these initiatives that she is recognized as the first professionally-trained American psychiatric nurse.

❖ In 1882, the first school to prepare nurses to care for mentally ill at McLean Hospital in Weverly, Massachusetts was started. The care was primarily custodial. Nurses were prepared in this school to attend to the physical needs, administer medications, meet the nutritional and hygienic needs and monitor ward activities. During this period nurses adopted medical surgical nursing principles to care for patients with psychiatric disorders.

❖ In the United States, Dorothea Dix (1802–1887) an activist, provided nursing care to soldiers during the civil war and reformed the treatment of the mentally ill. She advocated for humane treatment as well as safe and comfortable environments.

❖ Major advancement in psychiatric nursing occurred after World War II because of the emergence of services related to psychiatric problems. During the world war nurses attended to the physical as well as psychological needs of the soldiers.

19th Century

❖ The role of psychiatric nursing began to emerge in the early 1950s. This development was significantly influenced by use of psychotropic drugs.

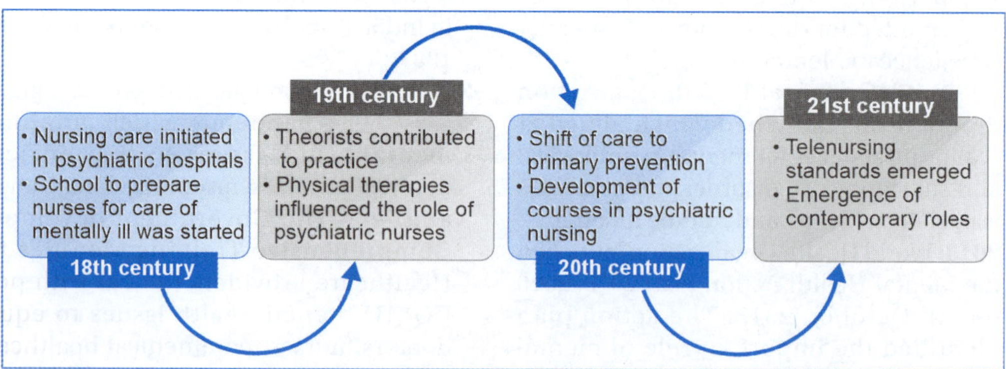

Figure 2.2: Evolution of psychiatric nursing

- ❖ Another important factor in the development of psychiatric nursing was the emergence of various somatic therapies like insulin shock therapy (1927), psychosurgery (1936), and ECT (1938). These therapies required the medical surgical skills and psychological skills of the nurses.
- ❖ Two early nursing theorists Hildegard Peplau (1952) and June Mellow (1968) contributed immensely to the shaping and practice of psychiatric nursing. Peplau published interpersonal relations in nursing wherein she described the therapeutic nurse patient relationship, its phases and tasks. It is the foundation of psychiatric nursing practice being followed today. Mellow's work, 'Nursing therapy' described her approach focusing on patient's psychosocial needs and strengths. In 1954, the first graduate level nursing program was developed by Peplau at Rutgers university to train clinical nurse specialists in the field of psychiatric nursing. For her significant contributions to the specialty, Hildegard Peplau is considered the founder of psychiatric-mental health nursing theory and professional practice. She is often referred to as the 'mother' of psychiatric nursing and in an authorized biography by Callaway (2002) as the 'psychiatric nurse of the century'.

20th Century

- ❖ In the 1960s, the focus of psychiatric nursing began to shift to primary prevention and implementation of care and consultation in the community. The Community Mental Health Centres Act facilitated the expansion of psychiatric mental health.
- ❖ Gerald Caplan concept of preventive psychiatry gave role expansion to psychiatric nurses. It gave a concept of family involvement in psychiatric nursing care and home care nursing.
- ❖ Psychiatric nursing subject was included in the curriculum of various nursing courses. Psychiatric nursing sub specialty emerged in master's program.

21st Century

Over the years, the role of a professional psychiatric nurse has grown in complexity. In contemporary psychiatric nursing practice, the role includes parameters of clinical competence, patient advocacy, fiscal responsibility, professional collaboration, social accountability, legal and ethical obligations. Digital revolution expanded the scope of psychiatric nurses to provide digital services to mentally ill patients as well.

Some Important Milestones

1840s: Florence Nightingale made an attempt to meet the needs of psychiatric patients with proper hygiene, better food, light and ventilation and use of drugs to chemically restrain violent and aggressive patients.

1873: Linda Richards graduated from the New England Hospital for women and Children in Boston. She was the first nurse to graduate from the one-year course who went on to develop 12 training schools in the USA.

1882: First school to prepare nurses to care for the mentally ill was opened at McLean Hospital in Waverly.

1913: Johns Hopkins became the first school of nursing to include a fully developed course for psychiatric nursing in the curriculum.

1920: The first psychiatric nursing text book, 'Nursing Mental Diseases' by Harriet Bailey was published.

1921: Short training courses of 3–6 months were conducted in Ranchi.

1943: The Chennai Government organized a three-month psychiatric nursing course for male nursing students.

1946: Health Survey Committee's report recommended preparation of nursing personnel in psychiatric nursing also. Training commenced in existing institutions like mental hospitals of Bengaluru and Ranchi.

1952: Dr Hildegard Peplau defined the therapeutic roles of psychiatric nurse. She described the skills and roles of the psychiatric nurse in her book 'Interpersonal Relations in Nursing'. It was the first systematic theoretical framework developed for psychiatric nursing.

1953: Maxwell Jones introduced therapeutic community.

1953–54: The urgent need for nurses trained in psychiatric care was felt by the Government of India.

1954: Nur Manzil Mental Health Centre, Lucknow introduced psychiatric nursing orientation courses with a duration of 4–6 weeks.

1956: One-year post-certificate course in psychiatric nursing was started at NIMHANS, Bengaluru.

1958: All the wards at the Agra Mental Hospital were ordered to be kept open and all ward locks removed from the charge of the ward attendant. Nurses took an active role in patient care and handled their newer responsibilities with great consciousness and devotion. It was observed that nursing staff have better opportunities to judge the behavior of the patient besides more interpersonal contacts between patients and staff.

1960: The focus began to shift to primary prevention and implementing care and consultation in the community.

1963: Journal of Psychiatric Nursing and Mental Health Services was published.
Mysore Government started a nine-month course in psychiatric nursing for male nursing students, in lieu of midwifery.

1964: Mudaliar committee felt the need for preparing a large number of psychiatric nurses and recommended inclusion of psychiatry in the nursing curriculum (as per International Council of Nursing).

1965: The Indian Nursing Council included psychiatric nursing as a compulsory course in the BSc Nursing program.

1967: The Trained Nurses Association of India (TNAI) formed a separate committee for improving the perception of psychiatric nursing as well as to set guidelines for nursing teachers to conduct theory classes and clinical training in psychiatric nursing.

1972: American Nurses Association published Standards of Psychiatric Mental Health Nursing Practice to improve quality care—Recent revision 2014.

1975: Psychiatric Nursing was offered as an elective subject in MSc Nursing at the Rajkumari Amrit Kaur College of Nursing, New Delhi. Now various colleges offer psychiatric nursing as an elective subject in MSc Nursing.

1980: Scientific advances in the area of psychobiology contributed to the shift from psychodynamic models to more balanced psychobiological models of psychiatric nursing care.

1986: The Indian Nursing Council (INC) made psychiatric nursing a component of General Nursing and Midwifery course. American Psychiatric Nurses Association was established.

1990: This period is called the "Decade of the Brain". During this period dramatic increase in the number of psychiatric medications on the market resulted in shorter hospitalization. This led to the inclusion of more content on psychopharmacology and pathophysiology of psychiatric disorders in nursing curriculum.

1990: During these years integration of neurosciences into holistic bio-psychosocial practice of psychiatric nursing occurred. Advances in understanding the inter-relationships of brain, behavior, emotions and cognition offered many new opportunities for psychiatric nurses. International Council of Nurses declared1990 as the year of mental health nursing.

1991: Indian Society of Psychiatric Nurses established at NIMHANS, Bengaluru.

1995: Journal of American Psychiatric Nurses Association was established.

2003: American Nurses Association began certifying psychiatric mental health practitioners.

2010: ISPN published journal titled Indian Journal of Psychiatric Nurses.

2019: Indian Nursing Council published practice standards for psychiatric mental health nursing.

2020: National Institute of Mental Health and Neurosciences developed telenursing practice standards.

2021: Indian Nursing Council revised Mental health Nursing curriculum for Basic BSc Nursing students.

2022: Nurses in mental health settings began using telehealth technology to conduct assessments, provide counseling and therapy, and monitor medication use.

2023: Indian Nursing Council believes there is a great need to establish a postgraduate program titled Nurse Practitioner in Psychiatric Mental Health (NPMH) to provide comprehensive quality care to persons with mental illness and their families and meet the challenges and demands of mental health care needs in India. It is reflected in the National Health Policy (NHP, 2017).

Indian Society of Psychiatric Nurses

The Indian Society of Psychiatric Nurses (ISPN) was founded in 1991 at NMHANS, Bangalore under the guidance of Dr K Reddemma with a motive to enhance advanced knowledge and skills in the field of psychiatric nursing, to provide a platform for discussion and deliberation on evidence-based practice, to create awareness and translate the research findings to practice. ISPN is publishing its own journal called the 'Indian Journal of Psychiatric Nurses.'

SCOPE OF MENTAL HEALTH NURSING

According to Dery, et al., 2017, scope of nursing practice refers to the range of functions and responsibilities that have been legally assigned to registered nurses and for which they have the education, knowledge and skills.

Psychiatric mental health nursing is a specialized area of nursing practice which uses nursing, neurobiological and psychosocial theories and research evidence as its science and purposeful use of self as its art to promote mental health through the assessment, diagnosis and treatment of human responses to mental health problems and psychiatric disorders.

Psychiatric nurses provide patient centered comprehensive psychiatric care in a variety of settings across the entire continuum of care. The continuum of care levels span from illness to wellness states. The primary goal of a continuum of care is to provide treatment that allows the patient to achieve the highest level of functioning in the least restrictive environment.

The essential components of psychiatric nursing practice include promotion of mental health, prevention of mental health problems, care and treatment of persons with psychiatric disorders and rehabilitation of mentally ill individuals.

Areas of concern for a psychiatric nurse include a wide range of actual or potential mental health problems such as:

❖ Promotion of well-being, mental and physical health
❖ Prevention of mental illnesses
❖ Emotional stress or crisis related to illness, pain, disability and loss
❖ Impaired ability to function related to mental health problems

- Alteration in thinking, perceiving and communicating due to mental health problems
- Behavioral and mental states that indicate potential danger to self or others
- Self-concept and body image changes, developmental issues, life process changes, physical symptoms that occur due to psychological changes
- Psychological symptoms that occur along with altered physiological status
- Side effects or complications associated with psychopharmacological interventions and other treatment modalities
- Alcohol and substance abuse and dependence problems
- Interpersonal, organizational or other environmental circumstances and their effects on mental well-being of the individual, family and community

Today, the scope of mental health nursing is not restricted within the confines of bedside nursing care. A mental health nurse needs to be skilled and clinically competent; sensitive to the social environment, advocacy needs of patients and their families and be aware of the legal and ethical dilemmas as well. The career for psychiatric nurses is long and wide. The scope of psychiatric nursing can be discussed under the following headings:

- Contemporary roles of psychiatric nurse
- Focused areas of psychiatric nursing practice
- Trends, issues and challenges in psychiatric nursing

Contemporary Roles of Psychiatric Nurse

Although psychiatric nurses have traditionally worked on inpatient psychiatric units they have continued to expand their role into the community **(Figure 2.3)**.

There are two levels of psychiatric mental health nurses: The generalist (registered psychiatric nurse) and the specialist (CNS). The scope and roles of both the generalist and the specialist are guided by nurse practice acts and standards of care.

1. Mental Health Generalist

A psychiatric mental health generalist nurse is a licensed registered nurse responsible for delivering primary mental health care. It incorporates both physical and mental health care. While exercising holistic approach to practice, a generalist also performs psychiatric nursing in prevention programs, community and day treatment centers, psychiatric rehabilitation facilities, homeless shelters and many other settings.

2. Psychiatric Clinical Nurse Specialist

Psychiatric clinical nurse specialist (CNS) or nurse practitioner holds a master's or doctoral degree in psychiatric mental health nursing. CNS is an advanced practice nurse who is usually a primary health care provider, functions autonomously, often works in a semi-isolated situation, has medication prescription privileges (depending on individual state laws), manages the overall care of people with emotional and psychiatric problems, and usually has a consultative arrangement with a psychiatrist.

3. Community Mental Health Nurse

Community mental health nursing (CMHN) is the application of knowledge of psychiatric nursing in preventing mental illness, promoting and maintaining mental health of the people. It includes early diagnosis, appropriate referrals, care and rehabilitation of mentally ill people. The central role of community mental health nurse is to assist people suffering from mental illness to achieve and maintain their highest level of function and independence within the community.

4. Psychiatric Home Care Nurse

Home health care is one of the aspects of community health nursing. Psychiatric home care nurses provide care on a visiting basis to people needing assistance. These nurses provide comprehensive care including psychiatric and physical assessment, direct nursing care, behavioral management, crisis intervention, psychoeducation, in-home detoxification, medication management,

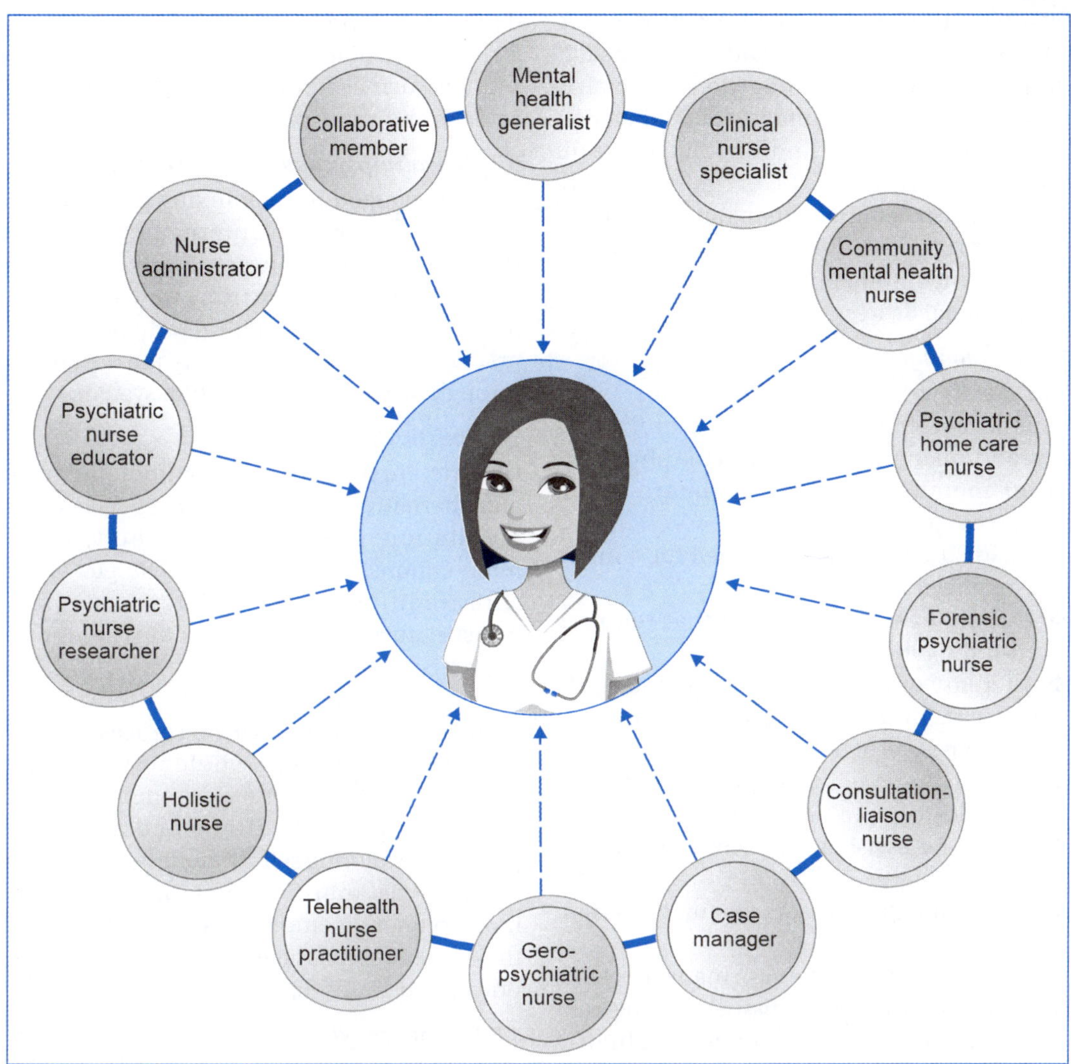

Figure 2.3: Contemporary roles of psychiatric nurse

case management and consultation with colleagues.

5. Forensic Psychiatric Nurse

Forensic nursing is an expanded scope of practice and a growing specialty in countries like the UK, Australia, Germany, Japan and Canada. A forensic psychiatric nurse works with individuals who have mental health needs and have entered the legal system. The special responsibilities of forensic psychiatric nurse are forensic evaluation for legal sanity, assessment of potential for violence, parole/

probation considerations, assessment of racial/cultural factors during crime, sexual predator screening and assessment, competency therapy, formal written reports to court, review of police reports, on-scene consultation to law enforcement.

6. Psychiatric Consultation–Liaison Nurse

Psychiatric Consultation–Liaison Nurse (PCLN) has arisen in response to the increased recognition of the importance of psycho-physiological inter-relationships and their impact on physical illness, recovery and wellness. It is an advanced practice nurse who practices psychiatric and mental health nursing in a medical setting/non-psychiatric setting providing consultation and education to patients, families, and health care team and the community. PCLN may provide assessment, recommendations and supportive therapy to patients who are anxious, depressed or experiencing other psychological problems or emotional distress.

7. Case Manager

Nurse case managers act as advocates for patients and their families by co-ordinating care and linking the patient with the physician, other members of the healthcare team, resources and the payers.

Factors that indicate the need for a nurse case manager are:

- ❖ A complex treatment plan that requires co-ordination
- ❖ An injury or illness that may permanently prevent the patient from returning to a previous level of health
- ❖ Pre-existing medical condition that may complicate or prolong recovery
- ❖ A need for assistance in accessing health-care resources
- ❖ Environmental stressors that may interfere with recovery

In the community, the case manager works with patients on a variety of issues ranging from accessing needed medical and psychiatric services to carrying out tasks of daily living such as using public transportation, managing money and buying groceries.

Case management can be provided by an individual or a team. It may include both face-to-face and telephone contact with the patient as well as contact with other service providers.

One of the most valuable assets case managers possess is their ability to synthesize patient data and act as conduits between patients and the health care system.

8. Geropsychiatric Nurse

Geropsychiatric nurse is specialized in caring for older adults with a diagnosis of emotional and behavioral disorders such as depression, dementia, chronic schizophrenia, delirium, etc. They are employed in various health care settings such as home care, ambulatory care settings and acute care settings.

9. Telehealth-psychiatric Nurse Practitioner

Nurses engaged in telenursing practice use technologies such as internet, computers, telephones, digital assessment tools and telemonitoring equipment to deliver nursing care. A telehealth-psychiatric nurse practitioner supports mental health of patients through online communication system.

10. Holistic Nurse

Holistic nursing integrates complementary and alternative modalities such as relaxation, meditation, guided imagery, body mind interventions, biofeedback, reikhi, etc. along with traditional nursing interventions. A holistic nurse uses theories of wholeness, expertise, caring and intuition. In CAM therapies, patients become therapeutic partners in a mutually evolving process toward healing, balance and wholeness. Holistic nurses conduct holistic assessments, select appropriate interventions and assist the patient in exploring self-awareness, spirituality and personal transformation in healing. The most frequently employed therapies used by the nurses are massage, music, exercise, diet, prayer and counseling.

11. Psychiatric Nurse Researcher

Nurse researchers are scientists who seek to find answers to questions through methodical observations and experimentation. They design studies, conduct research and disseminate findings at professional meets and in peer reviewed journals. They are doctorally or post-doctorally prepared persons who initiate or participate in all phases of the research process. They work in a variety of settings.

12. Psychiatric Nurse Educator

The psychiatric nurse educator works in educational institutions, staff development department of healthcare agencies, patient education department (teach the mentally ill patients and their families about care to be provided at home). Another function of nurse educator is planning and changing the curriculum according to the needs of society and learner.

13. Nurse Administrator/Manager

A nurse manager works less directly with patients but has the responsibility to provide nursing leadership to ensure that an appropriate therapeutic milieu is maintained. Besides representing nursing views to senior managers, key responsibility also includes support and development of nurses. Nurse manager plays an important role in negotiating and allocating nursing resources within clinical directorates. Individuals who assume a nurse executive role typically hold a master's degree. They serve at all management levels in health care organizations and in the community.

14. Psychiatric Nurse as Collaborative Member of the Interdisciplinary Team

Collaboration implies a commitment to common goals with shared responsibility for the outcome of care. It also implies helping to facilitate the mental health of the patient, family or community within the context of the treatment team. Nurses bring their own specialized knowledge to the treatment process thereby enhancing information about the patient's assessment, treatment needs and progress. Seven characteristics of effective collaboration include: trust, respect, commitment, co-operation, co-ordination, communication and flexibility.

The new opportunities for psychiatric nursing practice emerging throughout the continuum of mental health care are exciting for the specialty. They allow psychiatric nurses to demonstrate their flexibility, accountability, and self-direction as they move forward into these expanding areas of practice. The expansion of mental health treatment settings is providing psychiatric nurses with the opportunity to implement primary, secondary and tertiary prevention functions from a holistic, biopsychosocial perspective thus expanding their base of practice to better meet the mental health needs of individuals, families, groups and communities.

Focused Areas of Psychiatric Nursing Practice

Areas of focus within psychiatric nursing have emerged based on current and anticipated societal needs. These areas of focus include adult, child-adolescent, geriatric, developmental disability, forensic, addiction, community and family psychiatry.

Clinical practice settings for psychiatric nurses include psychiatric emergency services, crisis intervention centers, acute inpatient care, chronic inpatient care, rehabilitation centers, outpatient department, day care centers, partial hospitalization centers, child-adolescent psychiatry centers, family therapy units, psychotherapy units, home settings, community based centers, telenursing, hospice care centers, medical inpatient wards, industrial medical centers, forensic psychiatric wards and private practice.

Trends and Challenges in Psychiatric Nursing

Newer trends in the health care system affect the roles of a psychiatric–mental health nurse. She faces various challenges because of changes in the patient care approach.

Factors affecting the role of a psychiatric nurse are trends in health care, economic issues, changes in illness orientation, changes in care delivery, information technology, consumer empowerment, deinstitutionalization, physician shortage and gaps in service, demographic changes, changes in needs of the patients **(Table 2.1)**.

Educational Programs for the Psychiatric Nurse

❖ Diploma in Psychiatric Nursing (The first program was offered in1956 at NIMHANS, Bengaluru)
❖ MSc in Psychiatric Nursing (The first program was offered in 1976 at Rajkumari Amrit Kaur College of Nursing, New Delhi)

TABLE 2.1: Factors affecting role of a psychiatric nurse

Factors	Description
Trends in health care	Increased mental health problems, provision for quality and comprehensive services, multidisciplinary team approach, providing continuity of care, care provided in alternative settings
Economic issues	Industrialization, urbanization, raised standard of living
Changes in illness orientation	Shift from illness to prevention (modification of style), specific to holistic, quantity of care to quality of care
Changes in care delivery	Care delivery is shifted from institutional services to community services, genetic services to counseling services, nurse-patient relationship to nurse-patient partnership
Information technology	Telenursing, telemedicine, mass media, electronic systems, nursing informatics
Consumer empowerment	Increased consumer awareness, awareness of the community in early detection and treatment of mental illness as well as proper utilization of available psychiatric hospitals, demanding quality healthcare services at affordable cost with less restrictive and more humane rates
Deinstitutionalization	Bringing mental health patients out of the hospital and shifting care to community
Physician shortage and gaps in service	Physician shortage may provide an opportunity for new roles such as functioning as a nurse practitioner. With respect to gaps in services, nurses always meet the needs of people for whom services are not available such as home visiting nurse
Demographic changes	Increasing number of the elderly group, increased number of nuclear families
Changes in needs of the patients	Wanting a more holistic orientation in health care

❖ MPhil in Psychiatric Nursing (The first program was offered in 1990 at MG University, Kottayam)
❖ Doctorate in Psychiatric Nursing
❖ Short-term training programs for both degree and diploma holders in nursing

Standards of Mental Health Nursing

The development of standards for nursing practice is a beginning step towards the attainment of quality nursing care. The adoption of standards helps to clarify nurses' areas of accountability and provide a basis for evaluation of practice. These standards are therefore a means for improving the quality of care for mentally ill people.

Development of Code of Ethics

This is very important for a psychiatric nurse as she takes up independent roles in psycho-therapy, behavior therapy, cognitive therapy, individual therapy, group therapy, maintains patient's confidentiality, protects his rights and acts as patient's advocate.

Legal Aspects in Psychiatric Nursing

Knowledge of legal boundaries governing psychiatric nursing practice is necessary to protect the public, the patient, and the nurse. The practice of psychiatric nursing is influenced by law particularly in its concern for the rights of patients and the quality of care they receive.

The patient's right to refuse a particular treatment, protection from confinement, intentional torts, informed consent, confidentiality, and record keeping are a few legal issues in which the nurse has to participate and gain quality knowledge.

Promotion of Research in Mental Health Nursing
The nurse contributes to nursing and the mental health field through innovations in theory and practice and participation in research.

Cost Effective Nursing Care
Studies need to be conducted to find out the viability in terms of cost involved in training a nurse and the quality of output in terms of nursing care rendered by her.

Focus of Care
A psychiatric nurse has to focus care on certain target groups like the elderly, children, women, youth, mentally retarded and chronic mentally ill.

Challenges in Psychiatric Nursing
❖ Knowledge development, dissemination and application
❖ Overcoming stigma
❖ Healthcare delivery system issues
❖ Impact of technology

NATIONAL MENTAL HEALTH PROGRAM

The Government of India launched the National Mental Health Program (NMHP) in 1982 keeping in view the heavy burden of mental illness in the community and the absolute inadequacy of mental health care infrastructure in the country to deal with it. India is the first among the developing countries to formulate the National Mental Health Program.

Aims

1. Prevention and treatment of mental neuro-logical disorders and their associated disabilities.
2. Use of mental health technology to improve general health services.
3. Application of mental health principles in total national development to improve quality of life.

Objectives

1. To ensure availability and accessibility of minimum mental health care for all in the foreseeable future, particularly to the most vulnerable and underprivileged sections of the population.
2. To encourage application of mental health knowledge in general healthcare and social development.
3. To promote community participation in the mental health services development and to stimulate efforts towards self-help in the community.

Strategies

1. Integration of mental health with primary health care through the NMHP.
2. Provision of tertiary care institutions for treatment of mental disorders.
3. Eradicating stigmatization of mentally ill patients and protecting their rights through regulatory institutions like the Central Mental Health Authority and State Mental Health Authority.

Approaches

1. Integration of mental healthcare services with the existing general health services.
2. Utilization of the existing infrastructure of health services and delivering the minimum mental healthcare services.
3. Provision of appropriate task-oriented training to the existing health staff.
4. Linkage of mental health services with the existing community development program.

Components

The components of National Mental Health Program are listed in **Figure 2.4**.

1. Treatment: Multiple levels
a. Village and Sub-center Level Multipurpose Workers (MPW) and Health Supervisors (HS) under the supervision of Medical Officer (MO) to be trained for:
   ○ Management of psychiatric emergencies
   ○ Administration and supervision of maintenance treatment for chronic psychiatric disorders

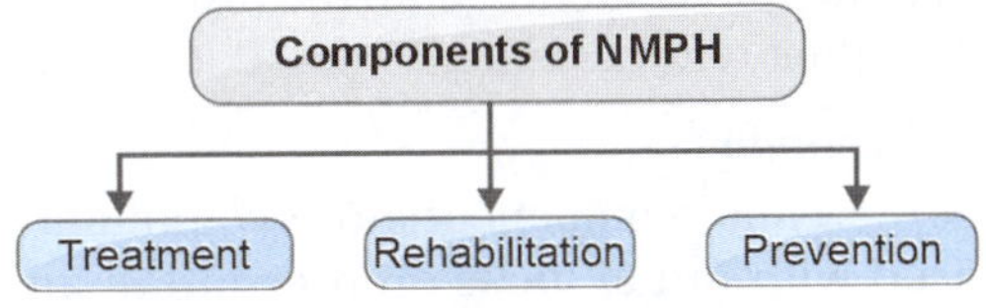

Figure 2.4: Components of NMHP

- Diagnosis and management of grand mal epilepsy, especially in children
- Liaison with local school teachers and parents regarding mental retardation and behavioral problems in children
- Counseling problems related to alcohol and drug abuse

b. **MO of Primary Health Center (PHC) aided by HS, to be trained for:**
- Supervision of MPW's performance
- Elementary diagnosis
- Treatment of functional psychosis
- Treatment of uncomplicated cases of psychiatric disorders associated with physical diseases
- Management of uncomplicated psychosocial problems
- Epidemiological surveillance of mental morbidity

c. **District hospital:** It was recognized that there should be at least one psychiatrist attached to every district hospital as an integral part of the district health services. The district hospital should have 30–50 psychiatric beds. The psychiatrist in a district hospital was envisaged to devote only a part of his time to clinical care and a greater part in training and supervision of non-specialist health workers.

d. **Mental hospitals and teaching psychiatric units:** Major activities of these higher centers of psychiatric care include:
- Help in care of 'difficult' cases
- Teaching
- Specialized facilities like occupational therapy units, psychotherapy, counseling and behavioral therapy

2. Rehabilitation

The components of this sub-program include treatment of epileptics and psychotics at the community level and development of rehabilitation centers at both the district level and higher referral centers.

3. Prevention

The prevention component is to be community-based with initial focus on prevention and control of alcohol-related problems. Later on, problems like addictions, juvenile delinquency and acute adjustment problems like suicidal attempts are to be addressed.

District Mental Health Program

The District Mental Health Program (DMHP) was launched under National Mental Health Program in the year 1996 (in 9th Five Year Plan). The DMHP was based on 'Bellary Model'.

Aim

To extend mental health services to persons suffering from mental disorders in the district through the existing health care personnel and institutions.

Objectives

- To provide sustainable basic mental health services to the community and to integrate these services with other health services
- Early detection and treatment of patients within the community itself
- To ensure that patients and their relatives do not have to travel long distances to visit the hospital
- To take the pressure off from mental hospitals
- To reduce the stigma of mental illness through public awareness
- To treat and rehabilitate mental patients discharged from the mental hospital within the community

Components

- Training programs for all workers in the mental health team at the identified Nodal Institute in the State, imparting short-term training to general physicians for diagnosis and treatment of common mental illnesses with limited number of drugs under the guidance of specialist. Training of health workers in identifying mentally ill persons.
- Public education in mental health to increase awareness and reduce stigma.
- Outpatient and indoor services for early detection and treatment.
- Providing valuable data and experience at the level of community to the State and Centre for future planning, improvement in service and research.

❖ Team of workers at the district under the program consists of—A Psychiatrist, a Clinical Psychologist, a Psychiatric Social worker, a Psychiatry/Community Nurse, a Program Manager, a Program/Case Registry Assistant and a Record Keeper.

Activities of DMHP

❖ Integration of mental health care into the existing general health services by training of PHC personnel (doctors, nurses, health workers and pharmacists) to offer basic mental care. To implement this activity mental health professional from nearby medical college will conduct/organize training programs for primary healthcare personnel to provide essential mental healthcare in the district.

❖ Early identification and treatment for mental illnesses in the community through active case identification by health workers, conducting periodic mental health camps in each taluk of the district.

❖ Referring all persons with mental health problems to their respective primary health unit or to the taluk hospital after initial evaluation and initiation of treatment in the camps.

❖ Intensive education to the community about availability of treatment for mental disorders, universal nature of mental illness, and regarding the need for regular follow-up in the primary health center. These efforts will bring in large number of persons with mental disorders into care and consequent reduction in stigma and discrimination.

❖ Facilitate adequate psychosocial care of the recovered mentally ill person in the community by making appropriate linkages with NGOs in the local area.

❖ Promotive and preventive activities for positive mental health. For example, school mental health services, life skill education, college counseling services, work place stress management and suicide prevention services.

❖ Linking psychosocial care and public education with social welfare departments (public private partnership).

❖ The DMHP in urban location will address the mental health needs through the existing public healthcare infrastructure such as municipality hospitals/corporation hospitals/other specialty hospitals, mental hospitals and medical college hospitals.

❖ Under DMHP, a small amount of ₹ 50,000/- will be available for research purpose. Non-governmental agencies in the district, medical college department of psychiatry can be encouraged to take-up research work **(Figure 2.5)**.

Nurse's Role

The National Mental Health Program for India (1982) recommended the formation of a District Mental Health Team (DMHT) in order to decentralize mental health care at the district level with two qualified psychiatric nurses and one psychiatrist. The role of the psychiatric nurse in the district mental health program is to provide care to the in-patients. The care includes meeting their basic needs, conducting occupational therapy, recreational therapy and individual and group therapy along with mental health education to families and the public in general. In addition to the above, qualified psychiatric nurses will actively participate in decentralized training to professionals and non-professionals working at taluk and Primary Health Centers (PHCs). They will also supervise the task of multipurpose workers in mental healthcare delivery. They will assist psychiatrists in research activities and in monitoring mental healthcare at district and PHC levels. Their active participation in mental health education to the public will go a long way in creating public awareness in the care of individuals with various mental disorders.

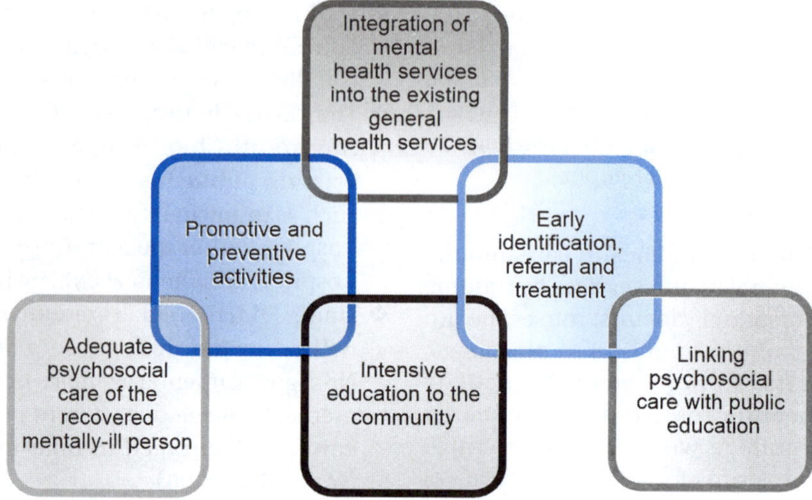

Figure 2.5: Activities of DMHP

- The occurrence of mental illness has been documented since the ancient times.
- Prior to 1860, psychiatric nursing was non-existent as custodial care was emphasized. Over the years, the role of a professional psychiatric nurse has grown in complexity.
- The role of psychiatric nursing began to emerge in the early 1950s. This development was significantly influenced by use of psychotropic drugs.
- In the 1960s, the focus of psychiatric nursing began to shift to primary prevention and implementation of care and consultation in the community. The Community Mental Health Centres Act facilitated the expansion of psychiatric mental health.
- Over the years, the role of a professional psychiatric nurse has grown in complexity. In contemporary psychiatric nursing practice, the role includes parameters of clinical competence, patient advocacy, fiscal responsibility, professional collaboration, social accountability, legal and ethical obligations. Digital revolution expanded the scope of psychiatric nurses to provide digital services to mentally ill patients as well.
- The essential components of psychiatric nursing practice include promotion of mental health, prevention of mental health problems, care and treatment of persons with psychiatric disorders and rehabilitation of mentally ill individuals.
- Areas of concern for a psychiatric nurse include a wide range of actual or potential mental health problems.
- Psychiatric nurses provide patient centered comprehensive psychiatric care in a variety of settings across the entire continuum of care. The continuum of care levels span from illness to wellness states.
- There are two levels of psychiatric mental health nurses: The generalist (registered psychiatric nurse) and the specialist (CNS). The scope and roles of both the generalist and the specialist are guided by nurse practice acts and standards of care.
- Being an integral part of the healthcare delivery system, the psychiatric mental health nurse is responsible for promotion, maintenance and restoration of mental health.

❖ The Government of India launched the National Mental Health Program (NMHP) in 1982. The aims are prevention and treatment of mental disorders, use of mental health technology to improve general health and application of mental health principles in national development to improve quality of life.

❖ The District Mental Health Program was launched under NMHP in the year 1996 (9th Five-year Plan).

REVIEW QUESTIONS

Long Essays

1. Describe historical development of psychiatric nursing.
2. Explain the scope of psychiatric nursing.
3. Narrate current trends in mental health nursing.
4. Describe contemporary roles of a psychiatric nurse.

Short Essays

1. Explain role of a nurse in district mental health program.
2. Explain focused areas of psychiatric nursing practice.
3. Explain components of National Mental Health Program.

Give the Meaning of the Following

1. Forensic psychiatric nurse
2. Psychiatric consultation-liaison nurse

Fill in the Blanks

1. Electroconvulsive therapy (ECT) was used for the treatment of psychoses in the year __________.
2. Psychoanalytical theory was developed by __________.
3. __________ and __________ theorists contributed immensely to shape the practice of psychiatric nursing.
4. __________ introduced therapeutic community.
5. In the year __________ INC made psychiatric nursing subject a component of the GNM course.

State the following Statements are True or False

1. Psychiatric mental health nursing is a specialized area of nursing practice.
2. Home health care is one of the aspects of community health nursing.
3. A forensic psychiatric nurse works with individuals who have mental illness and are detained in psychiatric hospitals.
4. A forensic psychiatric nurse who practices in medical settings provides consultation to medically ill individuals.
5. Geropsychiatric nurse is specialized in caring for older adults with a diagnosis of emotional and behavioral disorders.

Multiple Choice Questions

1. **The Indian Nursing Council included psychiatric nursing subject as a component of general nursing and midwifery course during __________.**
   a. 1956   b. 1965
   c. 1974   d. 1986

2. **The Indian Society of Psychiatric Nurses was founded during the year:**

a. 1986   b. 1989
c. 1991   d. 1995

3. **Following are the approaches of National Mental Health Program, *except*:**
   a. Integration of mental health care services in existing general health services
   b. Eradication of stigma regarding mental illness
   c. Utilization of existing infrastructure in health services to deliver mental healthcare services
   d. Imparting training to existing health staff in mental health care

4. **Government of India launched the National Mental Health Program in the year:**
   a. 1982   b. 1989
   c. 1995   d. 2000

5. **The main aim of National Mental Health Program is:**
   a. Prevention and treatment of mental illnesses
   b. Curing of mental illnesses
   c. Eradication of stigma

d. Formulation of acts related to mental illness

6. **Who is the first psychiatric nurse?**
   a. Hildegard Peplau
   b. Betty Neuman
   c. Linda Richards
   d. Florence Nightingale

7. **Who introduced therapeutic community?**
   a. Maxwell Jones
   b. Philippe Pinel
   c. Benjamin Rush
   d. Bleuler

8. **Chlorpromazine drug was introduced in:**
   a. 1942   b. 1952
   c. 1962   d. 1972

9. **ECT was first used for the treatment of psychosis in:**
   a. 1938   b. 1949
   c. 1952   d. 1955

10. **The Indian Mental Health Act was passed in the year:**
    a. 1912   b. 1952
    c. 1980   d. 1987

ANSWER KEY

Fill in the Blanks

1. 1938	2. Sigmund Freud	3. Hildegard Peplau and June Mellow	4. Maxwell Jones	5. 1986

State the Following Statements are True or False

1. True	2. True	3. False	4. False	3. True

Multiple Choice Questions

1. d	2. c	3. b	4. a	5. a
6. c	7. a	8. b	9. a	10. d

Mental Health Assessment

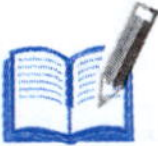

CHAPTER OUTLINE

- Effective Interview Skills
- Psychiatry History Taking
- Mental Status Examination

Mental health assessment involves the collection, organization and analysis of information about the patient's mental health. It is designed to diagnose mental health condition and differentiate between mental and physical health problems. This assessment includes a combination of questions and a physical examination and sometimes use of questionnaires. The nurse obtains assessment data from several sources such as interviewing patient and his family, history taking, physical examination, mental status examination, previous health records and reports, use of psychological tests and laboratory investigations. For obtaining relevant and adequate mental health assessment data the nurse should have effective interviewing skills **(Box 3.1)**.

HISTORY TAKING

History taking and mental status examination are core clinical skills of psychiatry. History

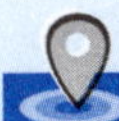

BOX 3.1: Effective interview skills

- Conduct the interview in a quiet place, ensure privacy
- Be relaxed and maintain an unhurried posture
- Maintain eye contact with the patient
- Be interested and attentive to what he says
- Pick up verbal and nonverbal cues of distress
- Allow the patient to talk freely without any interruption
- When the patient deviates from the theme or loses track, guide him back to the main theme politely
- Use open-ended questions
- Use active listening
- Do not offer premature conclusions or assurance on treatment outcome

taking should be collected under following categories **(Figure 3.1)**:

1. Identification and Demographical Details

This includes patient's name, age, sex, religion, address, socioeconomic status, hospital

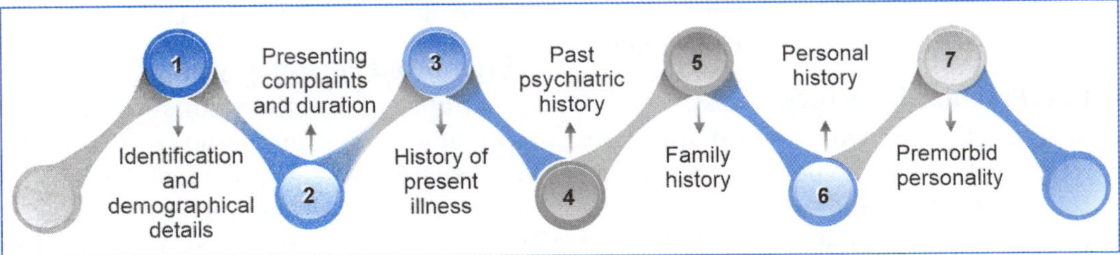

Figure 3.1: Categories of history taking

number, marital status, occupation, details of informant, and information relevant or not, adequate or not.

2. Presenting Complaints and Duration

Here symptoms are listed in a chronological order with their duration. Sometimes the patient may deny the existence of any symptoms and say that he was forcibly brought to the hospital by his relatives. In such cases, information is collected from his relatives. It is preferable to use patient's own words verbatim, without translating or interpreting their meaning. For example, sleeplessness—3 weeks, loss of appetite and hearing voices—2 weeks.

3. History of Present Illness

Under this are recorded the evolution of patient's symptoms from the time they were first noted till the time of consultation. Details of each symptom should be collected. Patient's history may have to be supplemented with data available from other sources.

It is ideal to use patient's own words. Look for and also ask for any precipitating factors. An attempt should also be made to identify any possible secondary gain to the patient because of his symptoms.

The mode of onset of illness may be acute or insidious. Progress may be steady and progressive or diminishing and reappearing periodically or staying the same way throughout. These should also be enquired into. Sometimes the patient is able to point out some antecedent stressful event alluded as precipitants. Temporal relation of the event with illness, severity of the stress, patient's preoccupation with the events and the value attached to the event by him may all give a clue to the presence and nature of the precipitant.

4. Past Psychiatric History

Enquire whether the patient had any psychiatric illness in the past. If so its nature, duration, treatment and outcome should be noted down. If treatment was discontinued in the middle, enquire the reason for this as well as the reason for switching over to other models of therapy.

5. Family History

Enquire about the type and size of family and the general family environment. The presence of psychiatric illness on the paternal or maternal side should be routinely asked. It would be useful to construct a family tree depicting the living members, their age, deceased members and their age at death. Mark whether any of them has or had similar illness and if known, the type of treatment they received and the outcome. Note specifically any history of suicide, mental retardation, epilepsy or any genetically transmittable disorders **(Figure 3.2)**.

6. Personal History

Personal history includes the developmental, educational, occupational as well as the sexual history of the patient. Developmental history includes details of pregnancy and delivery, developmental milestones, health during childhood and adolescence, neurotic symptoms and occurrence of any significant event (for example, separation from parents, bereavements, etc. are recorded). Educational history relates to details regarding the level of performance in school, relationship with peers and teachers, academic achievements and extracurricular activities. While collecting occupational history, enquiry should be made about the types of work, job satisfaction, whether jobs were changed frequently and if so, reasons thereof, work skills and relationship with colleagues. Sexual history includes details about sexual development, practices and attitudes towards sex. In marital history enquiry should be made about married life and details about spouse and children.

7. Premorbid Personality

Personality of a patient consists of those habitual attitudes and patterns of behavior which characterize an individual. Personality sometimes changes after the onset of illness. The nurse has to get a description of the personality before the onset of illness and

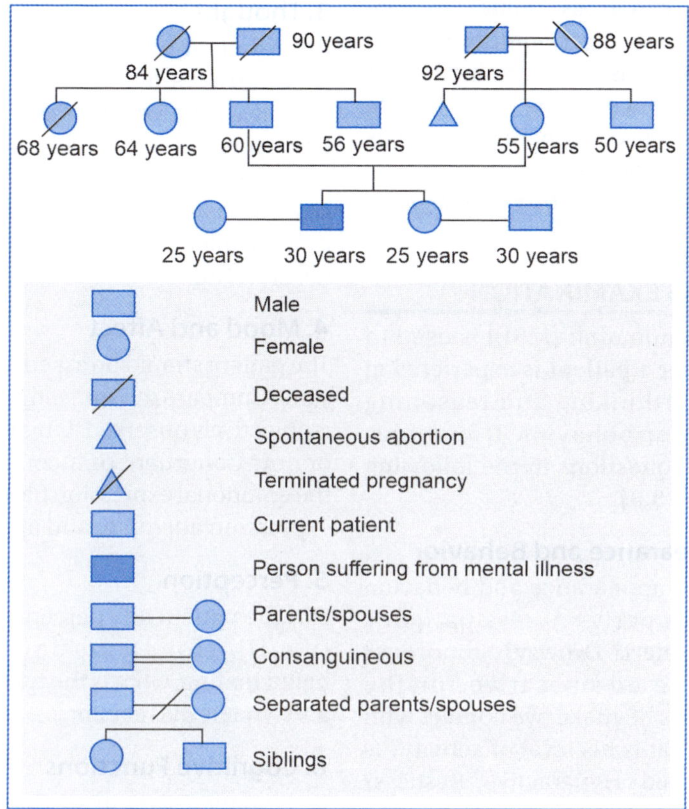

Figure 3.2: Family genogram

aim to build up a picture of the individual, not a type. Enquiry in the following areas has to be made:

❖ **Attitude to others in social, family and sexual relationship**: Ability to trust others, make and sustain relationships, anxious or secure, leader or follower, level of participation, ability to take up responsibility, capacity to make a decision, dominant or submissive, friendly or emotionally cold, etc. Difficulty in role taking—gender, sexual and familial.

❖ **Attitude to self**: Egocentric, selfish, indulgent, dramatizing, critical, depreciatory, over concerned, self-conscious, satisfaction or dissatisfaction with work. Attitude towards health and bodily functions. Attitude to past achievements and failure, and to the future.

❖ **Moral and religious attitudes and standards**: Evidence of rigidity or compliance, permissiveness or over conscientiousness, conformity or rebellion. Enquire specifically about religious beliefs. Excessive religiosity.

❖ **Mood**: Enquire about stability of mood, mood swings, whether anxious, irritable, worrying or tense. Whether lively or gloomy. Ability to express and control feelings of anger, anxiety or depression.

❖ **Leisure activities and hobbies**: Interest in reading, playing, music, movies, etc. Enquire about creative ability. Whether leisure time is spent alone or with friends. Is the circle of friends large or small?

❖ **Fantasy life**: Enquire about content of day dreams and dreams. Amount of time spent in day dreaming.

❖ **Reaction pattern to stress**: Ability to tolerate frustrations, losses, disappointments and circumstances arousing anger, anxiety or depression. Evidence for the excessive use of particular defense mechanisms such as denial, rationalization, projection, etc.
(See Appendix 1 for History Taking Format in Psychiatric Nursing)

MENTAL STATUS EXAMINATION

Mental status examination (MSE) is used to determine whether a patient is experiencing abnormalities in thinking and reasoning ability, feelings or behavior. It includes observations and questions in the following categories **(Figure 3.3)**.

1. General Appearance and Behavior

Describe patient's appearance and behavior. Is he dressed properly? Assess patient's sensorium. Is he alert? Drowsy? Stuporous? Comatose? Is he co-operative for the examination? Does he make eye contact with the examiner? What is his level of activity? Is he excited? Retarded? Hyperactive? Restless? Does he have any mannerisms? Gestures? Tics? Involuntary movements?

2. Speech

The manner of speaking and its defects are recorded under speech, whereas the content and form of speech are recorded under thought disorders. Does he speak spontaneously or only responds to posed questions? Assess the rate, quantity and flow of speech. It is worthwhile to record a sample of speech for later analysis.

3. Thought

Inference about the thought process and its disorders are made from the speech sample or the writing sample of the patient. Disorders of form, progression, content and possession may be present. Does the patient have delusions, obsessive ruminations and thought alienation? How does delusion affect his behavior?

4. Mood and Affect

The patient should be asked about his affective state. Compare the subjective report with what is objectively observed. Is his mood appropriate or not? Congruent or incongruent? Labile? Is the emotional expression blunt? Is the affective expression adequate and appropriate?

5. Perception

Has the patient any perceptual abnormalities like illusions and hallucinations? If hallucinating, what is the type of hallucination and what is his reaction?

6. Cognitive Functions

Is the patient attentive? Can his attention be easily aroused and sustained? How is his level of concentration? To assess cognitive function some simple tests can be administered. The patient is asked to name the days of the week or names of the months forwards and backwards. He may be asked to serially subtract 7 or 3 from 100 and spell out the numbers.

Is the patient oriented to time, place and other persons? Orientation to time involves the ability to tell correctly the time of day, date, week, month, year and other related data. Orientation

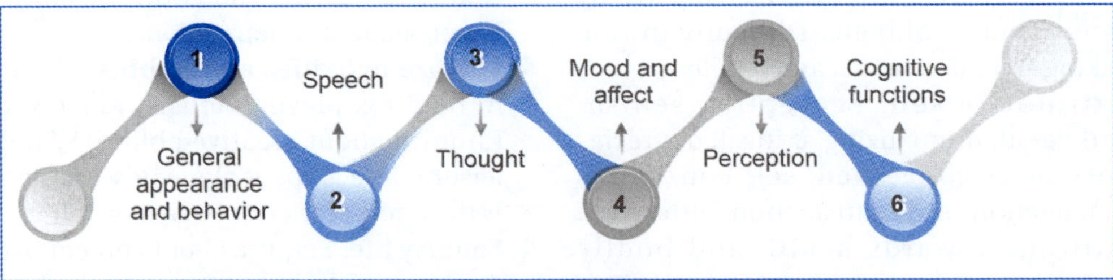

Figure 3.3: Categories of Mental Status Examination (MSE)

to a place includes correct information of his whereabouts, how he came to be there and other details. Correct identification of people around him ensures orientation to other persons.

Patient's intelligence can be inferred from his conversation and behavior, educational level, vocabulary, ability for abstract thinking and reasoning, general information, etc. Specific tests are used when a more accurate measurement of intelligence is needed. Patient's awareness of his disabilities and readiness for treatment are reflected in insight. Judgment may be inferred from his plans for the future.

(See Appendix 2 for MSE Format)

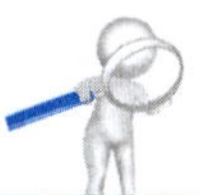

REVIEW QUESTIONS

Short Essays

1. Mental status examination.
2. Describe various methods of assessment in psychiatry.

Short Answers

1. Components of MSE.
2. List effective interview skills.
3. Categories of history taking in psychiatry.

Fill in the Blanks

1. _______ symbol is used to denote female.
2. _______ symbol is used to denote terminated pregnancy.
3. _______ symbol is used to denote consanguineous marriage.
4. _______ is used to determine whether a patient is experiencing abnormalities in thinking, feeling and reasoning ability.
5. Patient's awareness of his disabilities and readiness for treatment are reflected in _______.

State the Following Statements are True or False

1. An enquiry about type, size and general family environment is called family history.
2. Premorbid personality includes personality before the onset of illness.
3. Perceptual abnormalities are delusions.
4. While collecting history focus on both verbal and nonverbal cues.
5. While collecting psychiatric history use open-ended questions.

Multiple Choice Questions

1. **Nurse asks a patient to remember three words: house, garden and rain. About 10 minutes later she asks the patient to repeat those words. Which aspect of memory is the nurse testing?**
   a. Immediate memory
   b. Recent memory
   c. Remote memory
   d. Delayed memory

2. **All of the following are components of MSE, *except*:**
   a. General appearance and behavior
   b. Speech
   c. Mood
   d. Language

ANSWER KEY

Fill in the Blanks

1. ♀	2. 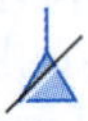	3. 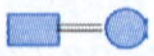	4. Mental status examination	5. Insight

State the Following Statements are True or False

1. True	2. True	3. False	4. True	5. True

Multiple Choice Questions

1. b	2. d			

Therapeutic Communication and Nurse–Patient Relationship

Therapeutic communication is an interpersonal interaction between the nurse and the patient during which the nurse focuses on the patient's specific needs to promote an effective exchange of information. All nurses need skills in therapeutic communication to apply the nursing process effectively and meet standards of care for their patients.

THERAPEUTIC NURSE–PATIENT RELATIONSHIP

The therapeutic nurse–patient relationship is an interaction between the nurse and the patient in which the contributions of both participants help in therapeutic process. It establishes trust and rapport with a specific purpose, facilitates therapeutic communication and engages the client in decision making regarding their plan of care.

In a healthcare system both the nurse and the patient interact with each other with a goal to assist the patient in using personal resources to meet his or her unique needs **(Box 4.1)**.

Characteristics of Therapeutic Nurse–patient Relationship

❖ Therapeutic nurse–patient relationship is the corner stone of psychiatric-mental health nursing, where observation and understanding of behavior and

> **BOX 4.1:** Goals of therapeutic nurse–patient relationship
>
> - Facilitating communication of distressing thoughts and feelings
> - Assisting the patient with problem solving
> - Helping patients examine self-defeating behaviors and test alternatives
> - Promoting self-care and independence

communication are of great importance. It is a mutual learning experience and a corrective emotional experience for the patient.

❖ Nature of the therapeutic relationship is characterized by the mutual growth of individuals who "dare" to become related to discover love, growth and freedom.

❖ Therapeutic relationship is based on the belief that the patient has potential, and as a result of the relationship, "will grow to his fullest potential".

❖ In a therapeutic relationship, the nurse and the patient work together towards the goal or towards assisting the patient in regaining his inner resources to meet life challenges and facilitate growth. The interaction is purposefully established, maintained and carried out with the anticipated outcome of helping the patient to gain new coping and adaptation skills.

Components of Therapeutic Nurse–Patient Relationship

A therapeutic nurse–patient relationship has many components, stages and benefits associated with it. Although each nurse–patient relationship is unique, there are some key components that are essential **(Figure 4.1)**:

Rapport

Rapport is a close and harmonious relationship in which the people understand each other's feelings or ideas and communicate well. It is the crux of a therapeutic relationship. Establishing a rapport is the primary task in relationship development between a nurse and the patient. The nurse establishes rapport through demonstration of understanding, warmth and non-judgmental attitude. When rapport develops, the patient feels comfortable with the nurse finding it easier to self-disclose. The nurse also feels comfortable and recognizes that an interpersonal bond or alliance is developing.

Empathy

Empathy is the ability to feel with the patient while retaining the ability to critically analyze the situation. It is the ability to put oneself in another person's circumstances and feelings. The nurse need not necessarily have to experience it but has to be able to imagine the feelings associated with the experience.

In this process, the nurse receives information from the patient with an open, non-judgmental acceptance, and communicates this understanding of the experience and feelings so that the patient feels understood. This serves as a basis for the relationship.

Sympathy is often confused with empathy. In sympathy, the nurse actually feels what the patient feels but in the process objectivity is lost and the nurse becomes focused on relief of personal distress rather than on assisting the patient to resolve the problem. In empathy, while understanding patient's thoughts and feelings the nurse is able to maintain sufficient objectivity to allow the patient achieve problem resolution with minimal assistance.

Warmth

Warmth is the ability to help the patient feel cared for and comfortable. It shows acceptance of the patient as a unique individual. It involves a non-possessive caring for the patient as a person and a willingness to share his joys and sorrows.

Genuineness

Genuineness involves being one's own self. This implies that the nurse is aware of her thoughts, feelings, values and their relevance in the immediate interaction with a patient. The nurse's response to the patient is sincere and reflects her internal response. It is also important that the nurse's verbal and non-verbal communication corresponds with each other.

Phases and Tasks of Therapeutic Relationship

Hildegard Peplau (1909–1999) known as the mother of psychiatric nursing developed the theory of interpersonal relations. She stressed the need for strong interpersonal relations to overcome many nursing problems, as it is through such relationships that problems are identified and resolutions got. In her theory she identified four distinct stages in the

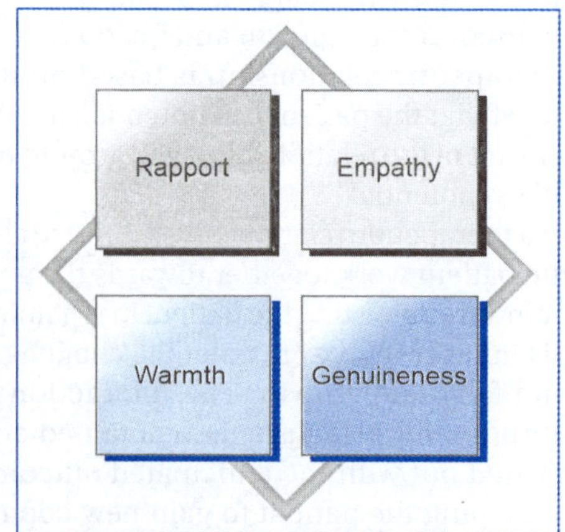

Figure 4.1: Components of therapeutic nurse–patient relationship

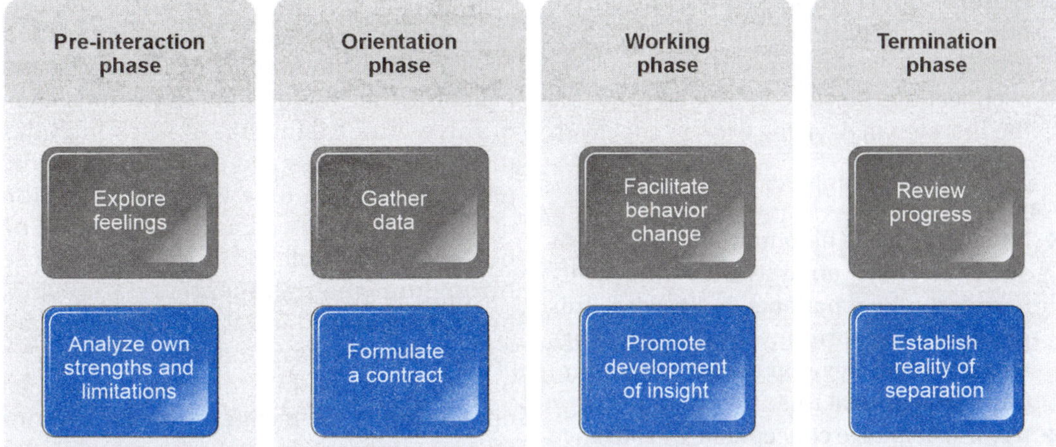

Figure 4.2: Phases of nurse–patient relationship

nurse–patient relationship namely orientation, identification, exploitation and resolution. In this textbook tasks in the relationship have been categorized into four phases **(Figure 4.2)**:

1. Pre-interaction Phase

This phase begins when the nurse is assigned to initiate a therapeutic relationship. It involves preparation for the first encounter with the patient and includes all that the nurse thinks, feels or does immediately prior to the first interaction with the patient. The nurse's initial task is one of self-exploration. The nurse may have misconceptions and prejudices about psychiatric patients and may have feelings and fears common to all novices. Many nurses' express feelings of inadequacy and fear of hurting or exploiting the patient. Another common fear of nurses is related to the stereotyped psychiatric patients' abusive and violent behavior.

The nurse should also explore feelings of inferiority, insecurity, approval-seeking behaviors, etc. This self-analysis is a necessary task because, to be effective she should have a reasonably stable self-concept and an adequate amount of self-esteem.

Nurse's tasks in the pre-interaction phase
❖ Explore own feelings, fantasies and fears
❖ Analyze own professional strengths and limitations

❖ Gather data about patient whenever possible
❖ Plan for first meeting with patient

Problems encountered
❖ **Difficulty in self-analysis and self-acceptance:** Promoting a patient's self-realization and self-acceptance is facilitated by the nurse's acceptance of herself and behaving in ways congruent with her own personality. Also, the nurse should have enough sources of satisfaction and security in her non-professional life to avoid temptations or using her patient for the pursuit of her personal satisfaction or security. If she does not have sufficient personal fulfillment, she should realize it and the source of dissatisfaction clarified so that it does not interfere with the success of the therapeutic relationship.
❖ **Anxiety:** Quite frequently, the nurse may experience anxiety of varying intensity during the pre-interaction phase due to role threat, feeling of incompetence, fear of being hurt or of causing distress, fear of losing control and fear of rejection. The nurse needs to become aware of what is being experienced, identify the threat, and decide what needs to be done about it. This is important so that the patient is not unduly affected by nurse's anxiety.

❖ **Others**: Apart from anxiety, the nurse may also experience boredom, anger, indifference, and depression. The cause of such feelings must be identified, which is the first step in devising ways to cope with them.

Ways to overcome

❖ The nurse needs help from her supervisor and peers in self-analysis and facing reality in order to help patients do likewise. This provides an opportunity to explore feelings and fears and develop useful insight into one's professional role.

❖ It is also helpful to conceptualize in advance what she wishes to accomplish during the relationship. The nurse may in consultation with her supervisor identify by writing goals for the initial interaction and decide upon the methods to be used for achieving them.

❖ The nurse also needs to be consciously aware of the reasons for choosing a particular patient. She may also attempt to assess the patient's anxiety level as well as her own. The nurse who is able to analyze herself and recognize her assets and limitations, is able to use this information in relating to patients in a natural, congruent and relaxed manner.

2. Introductory or Orientation Phase

It is during the introductory phase that the nurse and the patient meet for the first time. One of the nurse's primary concerns is to find out why the patient sought help. This forms the basis of nursing assessment and helps the nurse to focus on the patient's problem and determine the patient's level of motivation.

Nurse's tasks in the orientation phase

❖ Establish rapport, trust and acceptance
❖ Establish communication; assist in the verbal expression of thoughts and feelings
❖ Formulate contract
❖ Gather data including patient's feelings, strengths and weaknesses
❖ Define patient's problems; set priorities for nursing intervention
❖ Set goals mutually

Formulating a contract

Formulating a contract is a mutual process. It begins with the introduction of the nurse and patient, exchanging of names, and explanation of roles. An explanation of roles includes the responsibilities and expectations of the patient and the nurse with a description of what the nurse can and cannot do. The nurse is responsible for providing guidance throughout the therapeutic relationship, protecting confidential information, and maintaining professional boundaries. The patient is responsible for attending agreed upon sessions, interacting during the sessions and participating in the nurse–patient relationship. This is followed by a discussion on the purpose of the relationship in which the nurse emphasizes that the focus of it will be the patient and the patient's life experiences and areas of conflict.

Discuss the contract dates, time and place of meetings, duration of each meeting, when meetings will terminate, who will be involved in the treatment plan. Nurse should maintain confidentiality at all times, evaluate progress with patient, and document sessions. At the outset, both nurse and patient should agree on these responsibilities in an informal or verbal contract. In some instances, a formal or written contract may be appropriate **(Box 4.2)**.

Problems encountered

❖ Major problems encountered during this phase are related to the manner in which the nurse and patient perceive each other. A nurse may react to a patient not in terms of his uniqueness but in terms of the nurse's

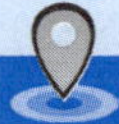

> **BOX 4.2:** Elements of a nurse–patient contract
>
> ❑ Exchanging names of nurse and patient
> ❑ Explanation of roles of nurse and patient
> ❑ Explanation of responsibilities of nurse and patient
> ❑ Discussion of purpose
> ❑ Discussion of date, time and place
> ❑ Description of meeting conditions for termination
> ❑ Confidentiality

stereotyped view of a 'psychiatric patient', or she may because of her theoretical background, read in terms of diagnostic categories. Sometimes the nurse may relate to a patient as if he were a significant individual from the past. The nurse may then displace to the patient the feelings she has for the significant individual. Since interaction is a reciprocal process, the patient also perceives the nurse in his own idiosyncratic manner.

❖ Problems may also arise related to establishing an agreement or pact between the nurse and patient. The patient may feel that since the nurse is here only for a few weeks, much help cannot be expected from her in the short span of time. The same feelings may be experienced by the nurse in that she feels she cannot do much for the patient during his stay in the hospital due to factors like limited time, overwork or the nurse's opinion that the patient is suffering from a 'major psychiatric problem'. Because the establishment of an agreement or pact to work together is a mutual process such misperceptions can greatly hinder it.

Ways to overcome

❖ The nurse must be willing to relate honestly to her perceptions, thoughts and feelings, and share the data collected during the nurse–patient interaction with her supervisors. The supervisor must provide an atmosphere in which the nurse feels free to reveal self without any fear of criticism.

❖ Difficulties may be faced in assisting a nurse who perceives a patient as if he were someone from her past life. She is usually not aware of doing so since most of this behavior is unconsciously determined. An alert supervisor can usually detect that the nurse is distorting the patient by viewing him as someone else. It may be necessary to bring the problem to the nurse's attention so that she can examine her behavior. Gradually, with assistance the nurse is able to audit her own behavior and then change it.

3. Working Phase

Most of the therapeutic work is carried out during the working phase. The nurse and the patient explore relevant stressors and promote the development of insight in the patient. By linking perceptions, thoughts, feelings and actions, the nurse helps the patient to master anxieties, increase independence and coping mechanisms. Actual behavioral change is the focus of attention in this phase of the relationship.

Nurse's tasks in the working phase

❖ Gather further data; explore relevant stressors
❖ Promote patient's development of insight and use of constructive coping mechanisms
❖ Facilitate behavioral change; encourage him to evaluate the results of his behavior
❖ Provide him with opportunities for independent functioning
❖ Evaluate problems and goals and redefine as necessary

Problems encountered

❖ **Testing of the nurse by the patient**: The patient may test the nurse in a number of ways and for a number of reasons. For example, he may wish to check her ability to set limits and abide by them. A patient with problems related to aggression may deliberately attempt to provoke the nurse to determine whether or not she will become punitive.

❖ **Progress of the patient**: Another barrier is the nurse's unrealistic assumption as to the progress the patient should be making. It is common for the patient to show desirable behavioral changes in the beginning and then stagnate by neither progressing nor regressing. A nurse who was initially enthusiastic about patient's improvement may then become discouraged when he does not progress at the anticipated rate.

❖ **Nurse's fear of closeness**: If the nurse fears closeness too much, she may react by being indifferent, rejecting or being cold towards the patient. She may find it difficult to interact with kindness and concern, and with objectivity and professional interest.

❖ **Life stresses of the nurse**: A nurse who has difficulty in coping with her own life problems cannot help a patient in making appropriate behavioral changes.

❖ **Resistance behaviors**: Resistance is the patient's attempt to remain unaware of anxiety-producing aspects within himself which may manifest in various forms. Some of them were identified by Wolfberg:
  - Suppression and repression of relevant information
  - Intensification of symptoms
  - Helpless outlook on the future
  - Breaking appointments, coming late for sessions, being forgetful, silent and sleepy during interactions
  - Acting out or irrational behavior
  - Expressing an excessive liking for the nurse and claiming that nobody can replace her
  - Reporting physical symptoms which may occur only during the time the patient is with the nurse
  - Hostility, dependence, provocative remarks, sexual interest in the nurse

❖ **Transference and counter transference reactions**: These are in fact a form of resistance behavior. Transference is the unconscious transfer of qualities or attributes originally associated with another individual by the patient. Transference occurs because the patient brings frustrations, conflicts and feelings of dependence from a past relationship into the therapeutic relationship. The patient may express feelings of aggression, rejection or hostility that are too intense for the current situation. These responses are often not appropriate for the nurse–patient relationship.

Counter transference is the reverse of transference. The nurse may have unresolved problems from an earlier relationship. She may unconsciously transfer inappropriate attributes experienced in the earlier relationship to the patient. Patient's transference provokes the nurse's counter transference reactions.

Ways to overcome

❖ Conferences with supervisors and group discussions with other members of the staff are some ways in which the nurse can best be assisted to overcome barriers encountered during the working phase. It is during this phase that the supervisor helps the nurse to increase her ability to collect and interpret data, apply concepts and synthesize the data obtained.

❖ There will be times when the nurse believes she is making little or no progress either in helping the patient or in gaining knowledge. It is at such times that emotional support is needed and is the task of the supervisor to encourage the nurse to persevere.

❖ At one time or another, most nurses may exhibit reluctance to write and analyze process records or engage in a discussion with the supervisor about the content of records. This can be due to many reasons such as fatigue, boredom, discouragement or an apparent impasse in interacting with the patient. A discussion on the meaning of such behavior and ways to overcome it is essential.

❖ **Handling resistances**: The nurse may find the experience of transference and counter transference particularly difficult. The relationship can become stalled and non-beneficial if the nurse is not prepared for patient's expression of feelings or is so preoccupied by her own needs and problems that she cannot clearly perceive what is happening.
  - The first thing the nurse must do in handling resistance is to listen. When she recognizes resistance, she then uses clarification and reflection of feelings. While clarification helps to give the nurse a more focused idea of what is happening, reflection of content helps the patient to become aware of what has been going on in his own mind.
  - It is not sufficient to merely identify that resistance is occurring; behavior

must be explored and possible reasons for its occurrence analyzed. Ignoring transference can perpetuate the pattern. Also, being overly critical of the patient, withholding information or being over involved in making decisions for the patient can encourage the dysfunctional behavioral pattern. It is important that the nurse maintains open communication with her supervisor who can then guide her in making adequate progress in handling such resistance reactions.

4. Termination Phase

This is the most difficult and also the most important phase of the therapeutic nurse–patient relationship. The goal of this phase is to bring a therapeutic end to the relationship. At this point the patient is expected to be successful in all the activities discussed and now has the capacity to make individual decisions. Here it is important to ensure that the patient does not develop any dependency on the nurse.

Criteria for determining patient's readiness for termination

- Patient experiences relief from presenting problems
- Patient's social function has improved and isolation reduced
- Patient's ego functions are strengthened and he has attained a sense of identity
- Patient employs more effective and productive defense mechanisms
- Patient has achieved the planned treatment goals

Nurse's tasks in termination phase

- Establish reality of separation
- Mutually explore feelings of rejection, loss, sadness, anger and related behavior
- Review progress of therapy and attainment of goals
- Formulate plans for meeting future therapy needs

Problems encountered

It is the task of the nurse to prepare the patient for termination of the relationship. However, patients differ in their reactions to the nurse's attempts to prepare them for termination. An ill person who has experienced trust, support and the warmth of caring may be reluctant to discontinue the nurse–patient contact.

Some behaviors exhibited in this regard can be:

- Patients may perceive termination as desertion and thereby demonstrate angry behavior.
- Some patients attempt to punish the nurse for this desertion by not talking during the last few interactions or by ignoring termination completely; they may act as if nothing has changed and the interactions will go on as before.
- Other patients react to the threatened loss by becoming depressed or assuming an attitude of not caring.
- Fault-finding is another behavior; the patient may state that the therapy is not beneficial or not working; he may refuse to follow through on something that has been agreed upon before.
- Resistance often comes in the form of "flight to health", which is exhibited by a patient who suddenly declares that there is no need for therapy; he claims to be all right and wants to discontinue the therapeutic relationship; this may be a form of denial or fear of the anticipated grief over separation.
- "Flight to illness" occurs when a patient exhibits sudden return of symptoms; this is an unconscious effort to show that termination is inappropriate and that the nurse is still needed; the patient may disclose new information about him or more problems or even threaten to commit suicide in an attempt to delay parting.
- Barriers to goal accomplishment during this phase also seem to be related to the nurse's inability or unwillingness to make specific plans and implement them. While the plans for termination are essential, the nurse needs to conceptualize these plans in advance. A nurse who does not discuss frankly the reasons for termination or elicit from the patient his thoughts and feelings about the impending termination cannot help to prepare him psychologically.

Similarly, a nurse who cannot explore her own thoughts and feelings about separation from the patient is also unable to accomplish the goals related to termination.

Ways to overcome

- ❖ The nurse should be aware of patient's feelings and be able to deal with them appropriately. The nurse can assist the patient by openly eliciting his thoughts and feelings about termination. For some patients, termination is a critical experience because many of their past relationships were terminated in a negative way that left them with unresolved feelings of abandonment, rejection, hurt and anger. Learning to bear the sorrow of loss while incorporating positive aspects of the relationship into one's life is the goal of termination in therapeutic nurse–patient relationship.
- ❖ During this phase, the supervisor may notice that the nurse is showing less interest in the patient than shown earlier and may be disengaging self from the patient several days before the final interaction. This may be a psychological defense mechanism by which she tries to decrease or delay the anxiety she is experiencing as a result of the impending termination of relationship. The task of the supervisor is to discuss frankly with the nurse the meaning of such behavior. The supervisor then initiates action to assist the nurse to persevere and intensify her efforts to prepare both self and patient for his eventual release from the hospital.

Importance of Therapeutic Nurse–Patient Relationship

It can help nurses to accomplish many goals of nursing care such as:

- ❖ Establish a therapeutic nurse–patient relationship
- ❖ Identify the most important patient needs
- ❖ Assess patient's perception of the problem
- ❖ Facilitate patient's expression of emotions
- ❖ Implement interventions designed to address patient needs

To have an effective therapeutic communication, the nurse must consider privacy, have respect for boundaries, use of touch, and active listening and observation.

COMMUNICATION SKILLS

Communication is the fundamental aspect of human interaction that permits individuals to establish, maintain and improve relations with others. It is a broad soft skills category. The word communication originates from 'communis' a Greek word meaning 'to make common'. Communication is a process by which people exchange ideas, facts, feelings or impressions in a way that each gains a 'common understanding' of the meaning, intent and use of a message.

In general, communication refers to the giving and receiving of information, ideas, facts, opinions, beliefs, feelings and attitudes through verbal or non-verbal means between people. It includes listening and understanding with respect as well as expressing views and ideas and passing information to others in a clear manner. It is the means by which people influence the behavior of another. Thus, good communication skills constitute the ability to not only speak confidently but also listen, empathize and present well whenever necessary.

Elements of Communication

Communication is the vehicle used to establish a therapeutic relationship involving three elements: the sender, the message and the receiver. The sender prepares or creates a message when a need occurs and sends the message to a receiver or listener, who then decodes it. The receiver may then return a message or give feedback to the sender or initiator of the message **(Figure 4.3)**.

Types of Communication

Communication takes place on two levels: verbal and non-verbal

1. Verbal communication occurs through words, spoken or written.

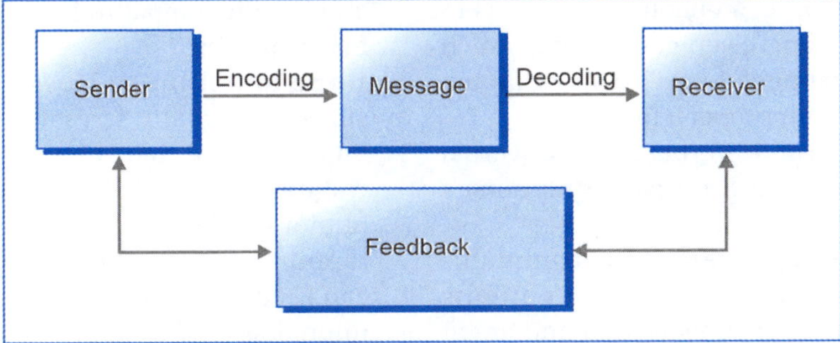

Figure 4.3: Communication process

2. Non-verbal communication occurs through gestures or behaviors that do not involve spoken or written words. Various types of non-verbal communication include vocal cues, gestures, physical appearance, space, posture, touch and facial expression. Non-verbal communication may more accurately reveal patient feelings than verbal communication.

Components of Communication

Better communication between the nurse and the patient builds confidence and improves compliance with treatment. While subject knowledge and practical skills are science of nursing practice, communication skills are the art of nursing practice. The key components for establishing communication with patients are presented in **Box 4.3**.

Therapeutic Communication Techniques

Therapeutic communication techniques are specific methods used to provide patients with support and information while focusing on their concerns. Skilled use of these techniques helps the nurse to understand and empathize with patient's experience and assist them in setting goals and select strategies for their plan of care based on their needs, values, skills and abilities. When using therapeutic communication, nurses often use open-ended statements and questions, repeat information, or use silence to prompt patients to work through problems on their own. The important therapeutic communication techniques are described in **Figure 4.4**.

1. **Active listening:** It is an active process of receiving information. It refers to showing interest in what the patients have to say, acknowledging them, and engaging with them throughout the conversation. For example, responses on the part of the nurse such as maintaining eye-to-eye contact, nodding, gesturing and other forms of receptive non-verbal communication convey to the patient that he is being listened to and understood. Verbal cues

BOX 4.3: Key components for establishing communication with patient

- ❑ Open the discussion
- ❑ Gather information
- ❑ Understand patient's perspective
- ❑ Comprehend information and explain it
- ❑ Share information
- ❑ Reach an agreement on problems and plans
- ❑ Be able to listen

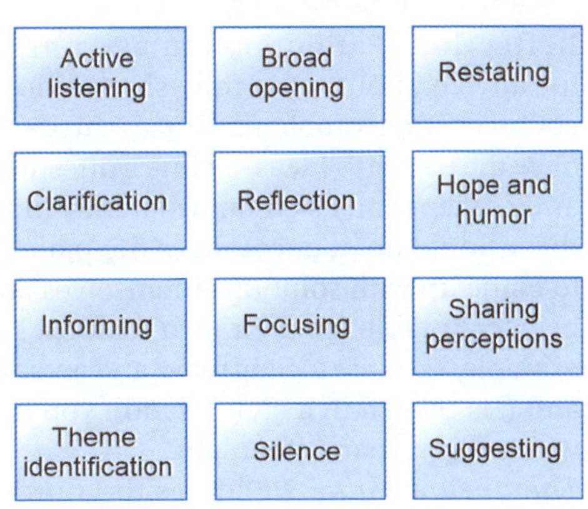

Figure 4.4: Therapeutic communication techniques

such as "I see" can encourage patients to continue talking. Even general leads such as "What happened next?" can guide the conversation or propel it forward.

Therapeutic value: Verbal and non-verbal cues communicate to the patient the nurse's interest and acceptance.

2. **Broad opening:** Therapeutic communication is most effective when patients direct the flow of conversation and are at a liberty to select topics for discussion. For example, "What would you like to talk about?" or "What are you thinking about?" can be a good way to allow the patient an opportunity to discuss what's on their mind.

Therapeutic value: Indicates acceptance by the nurse and the value of patient's initiative.

3. **Restating:** Repeating the main thought expressed by the patient.

Therapeutic value: Indicates that the nurse is listening and validates, reinforces or calls attention to something important that has been said.

4. **Clarification:** Similar to active listening, it is an attempt to put vague ideas or unclear thoughts of the patient into words so as to enhance nurse's understanding or asking the patient to explain what he means. For example, "I am not sure what you mean. Could you tell me about that again?"

Therapeutic value: It helps the nurse to understand the actual feelings, ideas and perceptions of the patient and provides an explicit correlation between them and the patient's actions.

5. **Reflection:** Patients often ask nurses for advice about what they should do to counter certain problems. Nurses can direct back the patient's ideas, feelings, questions and content and ask them what they think they should do. It encourages the patients to come up with solutions themselves and be accountable for their own actions. For example, "You are feeling tense and anxious and it is related to a conversation you had with your husband last night."

Therapeutic value: Validates the nurse's understanding of what the patient is saying and signifies empathy, interest and respect for the patient.

6. **Hope and humor:** Hospital visits and stays are usually stressful for patients. Sharing hope that the current situation will improve and lightening of mood with humor can both help the nurses establish rapport quickly. Though this technique can keep the patients in a positive state of mind, it is vitally important to know when and how to use humor with patients. For example, "That gives a whole new meaning to the word nervous" or "I understand how difficult this must be. We'll try to get to the bottom of this and do everything we can to have you up and running again soon."

Therapeutic value: Can promote insight by making repressed material conscious, resolving paradoxes, tempering aggression and revealing new options, and is a socially acceptable form of sublimation.

7. **Informing:** The skill of information giving. For example, "I think you need to know more about your medications."

Therapeutic value: Helpful in health teaching or patient education about relevant aspects of patient's well-being and self-care.

8. **Focusing:** When something important is being mentioned by a patient during conversation, the nurse can focus on the main thought thereby prompting the patient to take it further. As impartial observers, nurses can more easily pick out on the topics on which to focus. For example, "I think that we should talk more about your relationship with your father."

Therapeutic value: Allows the patient to discuss central issues and keep the communication process goal-directed.

9. **Sharing perceptions:** Asking the patient to verify the nurses understanding of what the patient is thinking or feeling. For example, "You are smiling, but I sense that you are really very angry with me."

Therapeutic value: Conveys nurse's understanding to the patient, has the potential for clearing up confusing communication.

10. **Theme identification:** It involves identification of underlying issues or problems experienced by the patient that emerge repeatedly during the course of nurse–patient relationship. For example, "I noticed that you said, you have been hurt or rejected by the man. Do you think this is an underlying issue?"
    Therapeutic value: It allows the nurse to promote patient's exploration and understanding of important problems.

11. **Silence:** Lack of verbal communication for a therapeutic reason. For example, sitting with a patient and non-verbally communicating interest and involvement.
    Therapeutic value: At times, it's useful to not speak at all. Deliberate silence can give both nurses and patients an opportunity to think through and gain insight. It slows the pace of the interaction and encourages the patient to initiate conversation while enjoying nurse's support, understanding and acceptance.

12. **Suggesting:** Presentation of alternative ideas for the patient's consideration relative to problem solving. For example, "Have you thought about responding to your boss in a different way when he raises that issue with you? You could ask him if a specific problem has occurred."
    Therapeutic value: Increases the patient's perceived notions or choices.

Ineffective/Non-therapeutic Communication/Barriers to Establish Therapeutic Communication

Non-therapeutic responses block the patient's communication of their feelings and ideas. These are depicted in **Figure 4.5**.

1. **Giving personal opinion:** It means giving one's own opinion, evaluating by using words such as 'this is right', 'you shouldn't do that way', etc. Personal opinion of the nurse reduces the decision-making ability of the patient. To improve decision making ability use words such as 'let's talk about more options to solve this issue' etc.

2. **False reassurance**: It means trying to be kind and offering false hope to the patient. False reassurance is not based on facts or reality. Example, saying 'Do not worry, everything will be alright'. These statements tend to discourage the patient from expressing his feelings. A better therapeutic response would be, 'We have to wait for the lab result to know the status'. A better response might be to explain when the lab result will be expected, the next line of treatment and clarify patient doubts.

3. **Changing subject**: It means asking new questions not related to the discussion. Example, saying let us not talk about this issue, this is the time for your personal prayer. This kind of response demonstrates lack of empathy and blocks further communication. The therapeutic response would be 'we will talk about this issue after your prayer'.

4. **Giving contradictory responses**: It simply means giving conflicting messages. It also refers to incongruence in verbal and non-verbal messages. Example, while the patient is communicating with the nurse she asks him to describe the complaints in detail, however she repeatedly keeps looking at her watch during the explanation process conveying a contradictory message. The patient is confused with the incongruence

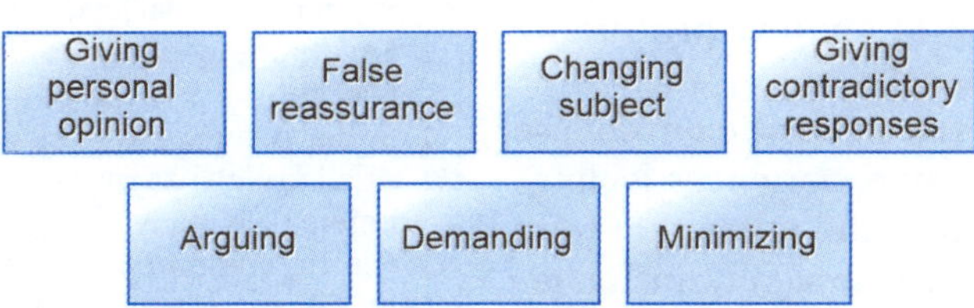

Figure 4.5: Non-therapeutic communication

in verbal and non-verbal message and fails to understand which message to accept. The therapeutic response would be to display congruence in the verbal and non-verbal message.

5. **Arguing:** Invalidating the patient's perception. Example, 'How can you say that you did not sleep well last night, I heard you were snoring'. It implies that the nurse does not believe the patient. This can lead to the patient getting angry. The skillful nurse should avoid such arguments and provide information in a way that avoids arguments. Example, let me know for how many hours you slept last night?

6. **Demanding:** Asking why questions, inappropriate questions, personal questions, probing sensitive areas. These questions make the patient feel uncomfortable. Example, 'Why did you divorce Mrs A?'. The more therapeutic response would be, 'Can you describe your relationship with Mrs A?'

7. **Minimizing:** It means not listening, not maintaining eye contact, answering before the patient finishes his question, using clinches, not responding to patient communication, etc. More therapeutic response would be nodding the head, maintaining eye-to-eye contact while communicating with the patient, etc.

THERAPEUTIC IMPASSES AND ITS MANAGEMENT

Therapeutic impasses are blocks in the progress of nurse–patient relationship. Impasses provoke intense feelings in both the nurse and the patient which may range from anxiety and apprehension to frustration, love or intense anger **(Figure 4.6)**.

1. **Resistance:** It is the patient's attempt to remain unaware of anxiety producing aspects within the self.

2. **Transference:** It is an unconscious response in which the patient experiences feelings and attitudes toward the nurse that were originally associated with significant figures in the patient's early life. For example, a

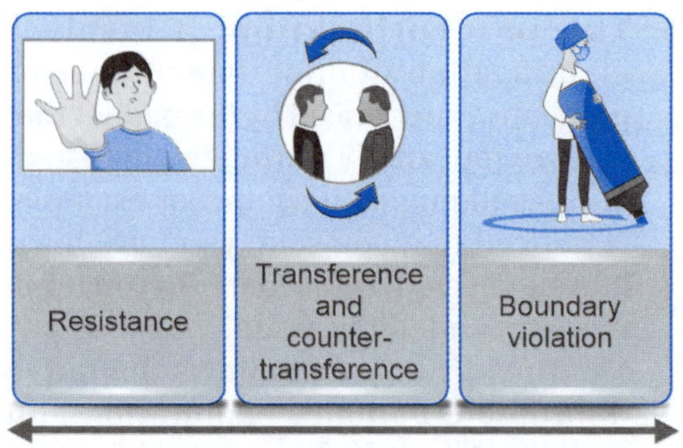

Figure 4.6: Therapeutic impasses

patient perceives the nurse as acting the way that his mother did, regardless of how the nurse is truly acting. Transference can be positive if patients view the nurse as helpful and caring. Negative transference is more difficult because of unpleasant emotions that interfere with treatment such as anger and fear.

3. **Counter transference:** It refers to a specific emotional response of the nurse towards the patient that is inappropriate to the content and context of the therapeutic relationship or inappropriate in its emotional intensity. Counter transference reactions are usually of three types: Reactions of intense love or caring, reactions of intense hostility or hatred and reactions of intense anxiety often in response to a patient's resistance **(Box 4.4)**.

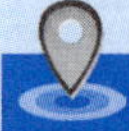

BOX 4.4: Forms of counter transference displayed by nurses

- Difficulty in empathizing with patient in certain problem areas
- Recurrent anxiety, unease, or guilt related to patient
- Personal or social relationship with patient
- Encouraging patient's dependency, praise or affection
- Sexual or aggressive fantasies towards patient
- Arguing with patient or tendency to "push" patient before he is ready
- Feeling angry or impatient because of patient's unwillingness to change

4. **Boundary violation**: Occurs when a nurse goes beyond the boundaries of therapeutic relationship and establishes a social, economic or personal relationship with a patient **(Box 4.5)**.

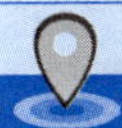

> **BOX 4.5:** Possible boundary violations
>
> ❑ Accepting free gifts from the patient
> ❑ Having personal or social relationship with patient
> ❑ Attending social functions of patient
> ❑ Regularly revealing personal information to the patient
> ❑ Routinely hugging or having physical contact with the patient
> ❑ Doing business with or purchasing services from the patient

Interventions to Overcome Therapeutic Impasses

❖ The nurse must have knowledge of the impasses and recognize behaviors that indicate their existence.

❖ She must reflect on feelings and explore reasons behind such behavior.

❖ Co-workers are more likely than others to recognize the phenomenon initially and give feedback to the nurse about it.

❖ Nurses must examine their strengths, weaknesses, prejudices, and values before they can interact more appropriately with patients.

❖ Transference reactions of patients must also be examined, gently but directly.

❖ Nurses must be open and clear about their genuine reactions when patients misperceive behavior.

❖ Nurses should also state actions that they can and cannot take to meet patient's needs.

❖ Limit setting is useful when patients act inappropriately towards the nurse.

❖ Nurses must maintain open communication with their supervisor, who can then guide them in making adequate progress in handling such resistance reactions.

❖ Therapeutic communication is an interpersonal interaction between the nurse and the patient during which the nurse focuses on the patient's specific needs to promote an effective exchange of information.

❖ Interpersonal relationship is an interaction between two or more people who communicate or exchange their opinions and values.

❖ In healthcare system the nurse establishes interpersonal relationships with a goal to assist the patient in utilizing his own resources for healing.

❖ The therapeutic nurse–patient relationship is an interaction between the nurse and the patient in which the contributions of both participants help in therapeutic process. It establishes trust and rapport with a specific purpose, facilitates therapeutic communication and engages the client in decision making regarding their plan of care.

❖ The key components that are essential in therapeutic nurse–patient relationship are rapport, empathy, warmth and genuineness.

❖ Hildegard Peplau in her theory identified four distinct stages in the nurse–patient relationship namely orientation, identification, exploitation and resolution.

❖ Pre-interaction involves preparation for the first encounter with the patient and includes all that the nurse thinks, feels or does immediately prior to the first interaction with the patient.

❖ During the introductory phase that the nurse and the patient meet for the first time. One of the nurse's primary concerns is to find out why the patient sought help.

❖ During working phase, the nurse and the patient explore relevant stressors and promote the development of insight in the patient.

❖ The goal of termination phase is to bring a therapeutic end to the relationship.

❖ Therapeutic impasses are blocks in the progress of nurse–patient relationship. These are resistance, transference, counter transference and boundary violation.

❖ Therapeutic communication techniques are specific methods used to provide patients with support and information while focusing on their concerns.

❖ Therapeutic communication techniques include active listening, broad opening, restating, clarification, reflection, hope and humor, informing, focusing, sharing perception, theme identification, silence and suggesting.

❖ Ineffective or non-therapeutic techniques include failure to listen, conflicting verbal or non-verbal messages, judgmental attitudes, false reassurance, giving of advice, inability to receive information.

❖ Process recording is the recording of conversation during interaction or interview between the nurse and the patient in psychiatric set up with nurse's inference.

REVIEW QUESTIONS

Long Essays

1. Explain in detail therapeutic communication techniques.
2. Define therapeutic nurse–patient relationship. Explain the various phases and tasks of therapeutic relationship.
3. Explain in detail therapeutic impasses and its intervention.

Short Essays

1. Characteristics of therapeutic communication.
2. Components of therapeutic relationship.
3. Explain nurse's activities during working phase.
4. Describe characteristics of therapeutic nurse–patient relationship.
5. Explain problems encountered during orientation phase.

Short Answers

1. Goals of therapeutic relationship

2. List the activities of a nurse during pre-interaction phase
3. List the elements of nurse–patient contract
4. What is the criteria for determining patient's readiness for termination?

Differentiate between

1. Rapport and resistance
2. Empathy and sympathy
3. Transference and counter transference

Give the Meaning of the Following

1. Nurse–patient relationship
2. Counter transference
3. Empathy
4. Warmth
5. Genuineness

Fill in the Blanks

1. ___________ is known as the mother of psychiatric nursing who developed the theory of interpersonal relations.

2. In __________ phase of nurse–patient relationship, the nurse formulates contract with the patient.

3. In __________ phase of nurse–patient relationship, the nurse facilitates behavioral change and promotes patient's development of insight.

4. __________ is the patient's attempt to remain unaware of anxiety producing aspects within himself.

5. __________ is the ability to feel with the patient while retaining the ability to critically analyze the situation.

State the Following Statements are True or False

1. Patient experiences relief from presenting problems is one of the criteria for determining termination of relationship.

2. Establishment of reality of separation occurs in orientation phase of nurse-patient relationship.

3. Nurse reviews patient's progress during pre-interaction phase of the nurse-patient relationship.

4. Repeating the main thoughts expressed by the patient are called restating.

5. Giving personal opinion is one of the therapeutic communication techniques.

Multiple Choice Questions

1. **Nurse's ability to be open, honest and real in interactions with clients is described as:**
   a. Genuineness
   b. Empathy
   c. Objectivity
   d. Harmony

2. **A nurse is communicating with a newly admitted patient. Which communication technique can interfere with the establishment of a therapeutic relationship?**
   a. Clarification

   b. Summarizing
   c. Giving opinion
   d. Providing information

3. **Which of the following is a goal of therapeutic communication?**
   a. Identifying important needs of patient
   b. Facilitating patient's expression of emotions
   c. Implementing the interventions
   d. All of the above

4. **What is the meaning of restating?**
   a. Repeating the main thoughts expressed by the patient
   b. Directing back the patient's ideas
   c. Asking the patient to verify nurse's understanding
   d. All of the following

5. **Which of the following is a barrier to therapeutic communication?**
   a. Focusing
   b. Giving advice
   c. Restating
   d. Listening

6. **Which of the following is an ineffective/non-therapeutic communication?**
   a. Judgmental attitude
   b. Silence
   c. Focusing
   d. Informing

7. **A relationship occurring between two individuals having emotional commitment to each other is:**
   a. Social relationship
   b. Intimate relationship
   c. Therapeutic relationship
   d. Distant relationship

8. **Empathy means:**
   a. An ability to feel with the patient
   b. An ability to put oneself in patient situation
   c. An ability to imagine the feelings associated with the experience
   d. All of the above

9. **For a nurse to be able to develop effective communication skills, she should:**
   a. Be able to communicate effectively with all patients
   b. Identify her own beliefs, thoughts and motivations
   c. Understand causes of mental disorders
   d. Have knowledge of various treatment modalities

10. **Following is a task of the orientation phase in nurse–patient relationship.**
    a. Encouraging verbalization of feelings
    b. Exploring alternate behavior
    c. Implementing various interventions
    d. Evaluating plan of action

11. **In which of the following phases of therapeutic nurse–patient relationship are patient problems noted and coping skills identified?**
    a. Pre-introductory phase
    b. Introductory phase
    c. Working phase
    d. Termination phase

12. **Unconscious transfer of qualities originally associated with another individual by the patient is called:**
    a. Transference
    b. Counter transference
    c. Rapport
    d. Empathy

13. **Unconscious transfer of inappropriate attributes originally associated with another individual by the nurse is called:**
    a. Transference
    b. Counter transference
    c. Rapport
    d. Empathy

14. **During an interview ________ are used.**
    a. Closed ended questions
    b. Open ended questions
    c. Derogatory questions
    d. Critical questions

15. **Process recording is:**
    a. A written documentation of patient education
    b. A written documentation of patient care
    c. A written documentation of verbal interaction with the patient
    d. A written documentation of abnormal patient behavior

ANSWER KEY

Fill in the Blanks

1. Hildegard Peplau	2. Orientation phase or Introductory phase	3. Working	4. Resistance	5. Empathy

State the Following Statements are True or False

1. True	2. False	3. False	4. True	5. False

Multiple Choice Questions

1. a	2. c	3. d	4. a	5. b
6. a	7. b	8. d	9. b	10. a
11. b	12. a	13. b	14. b	15. c

Mental Disorders and Nursing Interventions

Mental disorders constitute a wide spectrum ranging from sub-clinical states to very severe forms of disorders. Mental health problems are classified as major mental disorders and minor mental disorders. Major mental disorders are easy to recognize and commonly seen in mental hospitals, whereas minor mental disorders are commonly seen in community.

PSYCHOPATHOLOGY OF MENTAL DISORDERS

- ❖ Psychopathology is the scientific study of mental disorders including efforts to understand their genetic, biological, psychological and social causes; effective classification schemes; course across all stages of development; manifestations and treatment.
- ❖ Psychopathology is the scientific study of mental disorders including their theoretical underpinnings, ethology, progression, symptomatology, diagnosis and treatment.
- ❖ Psychopathology is that branch of psychiatry which deals with the study of manifestations of behavior and experiences indicative of mental illness.
- ❖ The scientific discipline of psychopathology was founded by Karl Jaspers in 1913 with an objective to study 'mental phenomena'. Psychopathology involves various specialties with an aim to describe symptoms and syndromes of mental illness for the diagnosis of individual patient. While neuroscientists focus on brain changes related to mental illness, psychiatrists are interested in descriptive psychopathology.
- ❖ Before diagnosing a psychological disorder, clinicians must study the abnormalities within psychological disorders. These are deviance, distress, dysfunction and danger. These themes are known as four Ds. Below is the description of four Ds while defining an abnormality:
  - ○ *Deviance*: The individual actions are deviant or abnormal when his or her behavior is deemed unacceptable by the culture he or she belongs to.
  - ○ *Distress:* The individual feels deeply troubled and affected by his illness.
  - ○ *Dysfunction:* It is a maladaptive behavior that impairs the individual's ability to perform normal daily functions.

○ *Danger:* It involves dangerous or violent behavior directed at the individual or others in the environment.

SIGNS AND SYMPTOMS OF MENTAL ILLNESS (DISORDERS OF THOUGHT, MOTOR ACTIVITY, PERCEPTION, MOOD SPEECH, MEMORY, CONCENTRATION AND JUDGEMENT)

Every mental disorder has specific set of symptoms that can vary from person to person and also based on severity. The common signs and symptoms of mental illnesses are described in **Box 5.1**:

1. Alterations of Personality and Behavior

Personality refers to the sum total of an individual's thinking, feeling and behavior which is more or less stable and enduring. Any alteration in personality may be the initial or only symptom which a patient exhibits as suggestive of illness. A confirmed atheist observing religious rituals and turning into a God-fearing individual overnight or a habitually social and outgoing person isolating himself from others are examples.

2. Alterations of Biological Functions

❖ **Sleep**: Disturbances of sleep are very common complaints in psychiatry. Sleep is disturbed in several ways in its pattern,

---

> **BOX 5.1:** Signs and symptoms of mental illness

- ❑ Alterations of Personality and Behavior
- ❑ Alterations of Biological Functions
- ❑ Disorders of Consciousness
- ❑ Disorders of Attention and Concentration
- ❑ Disorders of Orientation
- ❑ Volitional Disturbances
- ❑ Disorders of Motor Activity
- ❑ Disorders of Perception
- ❑ Disorders of Mood
- ❑ Disorders of Memory
- ❑ Disorders of Thought
- ❑ Disorders of Intelligence
- ❑ Disorders of Insight and Judgment

---

quality and duration. In some pathological conditions like mania, insomnia may occur. Delay in falling asleep (initial insomnia) occurs in anxiety. Depression is characterized by early waking up (late insomnia) and the sleep is usually non-refreshing. The sleep-wake pattern is reversed in certain organic conditions like delirium and dementia. The patient sleeps in daytime and remains awake during the night (reversal of rhythm).

Various types of impairment occur in schizophrenia. Sleeping for excessively long periods at night is called hypersomnia. Somnolence is abnormal drowsiness in the daytime. Hypersomnia and somnolence may occur to compensate insufficient night-time sleep and pathologically in many central nervous system (CNS) diseases.

❖ **Appetite**: Appetite reduces in anxiety states and depression and increases in conditions like mania and thyrotoxicosis. Overeating may sometimes be a feature of anxiety. In schizophrenia, appetite is increased or decreased or perverted (pica). Pica refers to eating inedible items like soil, paper, hair, etc. It is also seen in conditions like mental retardation, brain damage and autism.

❖ **Sexual desire**: Sexual desire is altered in many psychiatric conditions. It increases in conditions like mania and certain cerebral lesions, and reduces in conditions like anxiety, depression and drug abuse. Loss of libido, erectile dysfunctions, ejaculatory disturbances and pain are the presenting symptoms in psychosexual disorders.

3. Disorders of Consciousness

Consciousness is awareness of self and environment. Unconsciousness is lack of awareness of self and environment, and lack of subjective experience. Alterations of sensorium are usually indicative of organic pathology. Levels of consciousness range from full alertness to coma with intervening stages of clouding, drowsiness and stupor. Etiology is multiple and non-specific like intoxication, infections, trauma, metabolic disorders and others.

❖ **Clouding of consciousness**: There is diminution of alertness. It occurs in several organic conditions as well as in functional psychosis where it is a part of an overall cognitive deficit.

❖ **Drowsiness**: Though the patient appears awake he may slip into sleep unless constantly stimulated. Patient's thinking is muddled, speech slurred and activities sluggish though all reflexes are preserved.

❖ **Coma**: In coma, the patient is unconscious and in a state of non-responsiveness to external stimuli. In deep coma the patient is no longer in a state of arousal even with painful stimuli and his reflexes are lost.

❖ **Qualitative changes in consciousness**: Some quantitatively different alterations of consciousness are confusion, delirium, somnolence, twilight states, automatisms, fugue and dissociation and stupor. Confusion refers to the inability to think clearly. The person is disoriented to time, place and person and wears a perplexed look. It occurs both in organic and functional disorders. Delirium is a state of impaired consciousness with global disturbances of cognitive functions. Somnolence is excessive daytime sleepiness. Twilight states are transient states of altered sensorium during which patient's perceptions are faint and indistinct. Activities carried out during this period may be simple or complex. The patient is not aware of these activities later on. Automatisms are repetitive stereotypic behavior of which the patient is not aware of and over which he has no control. These occur in a confusional setting and are a result of brain dysfunction. Both twilight states and automatisms occur as epilepsy related events.

❖ **Fugue and dissociation**: Dissociation is a reversible and temporary alteration in the integrative functions of consciousness and identity during which the patient has no memory of his previous identity or events of that period. Fugue is similar to dissociation. The patient has a mistaken identity and tends to wander away from normal surroundings. Both dissociation and fugue resemble states of alteration of consciousness but have no true organic dysfunction.

❖ **Stupor**: Stupor in psychiatry refers to a state where the patient though conscious, is unresponsive to his environment. He is mute and immobile though his eyes are open. Retrospectively, he may be able to give an account of the happenings around while he was in stupor indicating that there was no loss of consciousness. Stupor occurs in catatonia and depression.

4. Disorders of Attention and Concentration

While attention is the focus of consciousness on a particular object or idea, concentration refers to persistence of attention to the same stimulus or "focused attention". Distraction is the inability to shut of irrelevant stimuli so that any stimulus in the environment takes away his attention. Disorders of attention are present in the form of narrowing of attention and its span, undue distractibility and lack of concentration. Narrowing of attention occurs when a person is able to focus his attention only on small part of his awareness field. Attention is impaired in anxiety, mania, depression, schizophrenia and organic states. Fatigue and substance abuse disrupt attention and concentration.

5. Disorders of Orientation

Orientation is the proper and continuous awareness of time, place and person in relation to self and surroundings. In several organic conditions this may fluctuate from time to time or diurnally. Disorientation to time occurs first in a progressive illness followed by disorientation to place and person in that order. Disorientation to one's own identity (i.e., failing to recognize one's own name and identity) indicates an advanced stage of deterioration.

6. Volitional Disturbances

Volition is the willful initiation and control of one's behavior. Volitional disturbances are seen in organic and functional disorders. Lesions of midbrain, the area of brain where centers of biological drives are located (sleep, appetite, thirst, etc.) cause volitional disturbances by reducing drives. Will and motivation are affected in functional psychosis as in schizophrenia, presenting as lack of initiative and other negative symptoms. In its extreme form, volitional disturbances may present themselves as immobility, mutism and stupor.

7. Disorders of Motor Activity

a. Disturbances in the Level of Activity

❖ **Increased activity level (hyperactivity):** Hyperactivity may or may not be goal-directed. In mania and hypomania though it appears as goal-directed and purposeful, the goal is often not reached due to distraction. Impulsivity implies lack of forethought or deliberation of the consequences of action and is often carried out forcefully. Restlessness is the inability to remain still and being uneasily active. Agitation is restlessness with anxiety or depression, generally seen in several psychiatric conditions, organic and functional such as dementia, epilepsy, depression and schizophrenia. Excitement is an emotionally roused state with added hyperactivity shown as accelerated speech, motor activity and hypervigilance.

❖ **Decreased activity level (retardation):** The level of activity is reduced in depression and in some types of schizophrenia. There is slowness in initiation and in carrying out an activity. In its extreme form it is present as stupor which is a state of akinesia (lack of movement), mutism and non-responsiveness to environment. Stupor is common in depression, schizophrenia and also certain organic conditions.

b. Qualitative Disturbances in Movement

❖ Tics are sudden involuntary twitching of small groups of muscles. They are brief, repetitive and stereotypic and may be single or multiple. Typically, they involve the face like blinking or distortion of expression. But other variations include sniffing, lip smacking, throat clearing, tongue darting or shoulder shrugging. Tics involving the diaphragm are present as grunting or coughing. In one variety they are multiple, associated with vocalization (usually obscene words or curses—coprolalia) and are known as Gilles de Tourette's Syndrome (GTS).

❖ Mannerisms are odd stilted and idio syncratic movements or activities characteristic of the particular individual. They may or may not be goal-directed, and are intentional and purposeful. Bizarre mannerisms are characteristic of schizophrenia?

❖ Tremors are rhythmic oscillatory movements due to alternative contraction of agonist and antagonist muscles. Simple tremors involve only a single group of muscles but in compound tremors several groups of muscles are involved. They may be slow in frequency or rapid, coarse or fine in amplitude. They may be present at rest or may be related to posture, movement or specific tasks.

❖ Stereotype is a repetitive and non-purposeful movement which is carried out uniformly in the absence of any external stimulus. Perseveration is continuation of a goal-directed activity even beyond the fulfillment of purpose where the patient is unable to stop the action. It is a common feature of frontal lobe dysfunction and a symptom commonly associated with neurological disorders such as autism spectrum disorder, obsessive-compulsive disorder, and traumatic brain injury.

❖ Negativism is resistance to all passive movements or commands of the examiner. Automatic obedience is a pathological compliance to the examiner's commands, like automation.

c. Disturbances of Posture and Expression

Disturbance in posturing is a voluntary assumption of inappropriate and bizarre positions of the body. Waxy flexibility is the maintenance of a particular posture imposed on the patient by the examiner even though it is bizarre and uncomfortable. Some patients lie with their head raised a few inches above the bed and maintain this posture for very long periods ("psychological pillow").

Expressive movements are exaggerated, diminished or distorted. In mania, the patient is extremely cheerful or irritated at any trifling provocation and uses wide expansive gestures. Face is expressionless in some types of schizophrenia. Grimacing and facing contortions are distortions of expression.

d. Disturbances of Motor Speech

Echolalia is repetition of words or sentences uttered by another person. Palilalia is a variant of echolalia where only the last word or syllable is repeated.

8. Disorders of Perception

Perception is the meaningful organization of sensory data and their interpretation in the light of one's past experience. Anomalies of perception are of four types: sensory distortions, sensory deceptions (false perceptions), perceptual disturbances of time and space, perceptual disturbances of body image.

a. Sensory Distortions

These occur in all sensory modalities and involve changes in intensity and quality. In hyperesthesia sensations become more intense and vivid with sounds appearing louder, colors looking brighter and pain becoming unbearable. It occurs under intense emotions, acute psychoses and prior to epileptic seizures. However, in hypoesthesia they are all diminished. It occurs in depression and delirium where more intense stimuli are needed to arouse the patient.

b. Sensory Deceptions

They occur in all sensory modalities and can mainly be classified into two types: illusions and hallucinations.

❖ Illusions are misperceptions of external stimuli. In the fading light a rope is misperceived as a snake. Illusions may occur in normal life when the sensory data are inadequate or when one is fearful and apprehensive.

❖ Hallucinations are false perceptions which occur in the absence of corresponding sensory stimuli and mostly during intoxication, delirium, sensory deprivations, epilepsy and in psychotic conditions like schizophrenia and depression. Hallucinations may be described in terms of their sensory modality as visual, auditory, olfactory, gustatory and tactile.

○ *Visual hallucinations:* False perception involving sight consisting of both formed images (for example, people) and unformed images (for example, flashes of light); most common in medically determined disorders.

○ *Auditory hallucinations:* It is a false perception of sound which is by far the most common and may be experienced as noise, music or voices. Voices may seem to address the patient directly (second-person hallucinations) or talk to one another referring to the patient as 'he' or 'she' (third-person hallucinations). Third-person hallucinations may be experienced as voices commenting on the patient's intentions or actions. Such commentary voices are strongly suggestive of schizophrenia.

○ *Olfactory hallucination:* False perception of smell; most common in medical disorders.

○ *Gustatory hallucination:* False perception of taste that is often strange or unpleasant (often a metallic taste). It is a relatively common symptom in people with epilepsy and medical disorders.

○ *Tactile (haptic) hallucination:* False perception of touch or surface sensation as from an amputated limb (phantom limb); crawling sensation on or under the skin (formication).

c. Perceptual Disturbances of Time and Space

Disturbances of time perception take several forms. The passage of time is perceived as too slow in depression and anxiety and too fast in mania and drug abuse. Depressed patients often report that time is standing still. Anxious patients often fear that they would not be able to complete a task in stipulated time (pressure of time). Disturbances of space perception are experienced as seeing objects being nearer and larger (macropsia) and smaller and far away (micropsia). This occurs in schizophrenia, delirium and as premonitory symptoms of epilepsy.

d. Perceptual Disturbances of Body Image

In organic lesions, there are disturbances of bodily experience like right-left disorientation, anosognosias (ignoring the presence of an illness like paralysis) and autotopagnosia (inability to recognize one's own body parts). The body appears mishapen and grotesque, body parts appear reduplicated. Parts of body like the nose appear to have assumed change in size or are misplaced. The body may appear to be floating in space. Such changes occur in drug intoxications and under the influence of hallucinogenic drugs. Phantom limb and autoscopy are other examples of bodily disturbances.

9. Disorders of Mood

Affect is a feeling tone and refers to the emotional state of an individual. Affect sustained for a long time is called mood. These two terms are akin to the terms 'weather' and 'season'. Disorders of mood are present in several ways such as their abnormal presence, abnormality in depth and duration, inappropriateness, and their abnormal swings.

a. Abnormal Presence

Fear, anxiety, depression, elation and anger are examples.

b. Abnormality in Depth and Duration

Emotions vary in their depth. They may be excessive and out of proportion to the event or markedly reduced (blunted or flattened) and lost (apathetic). Blunting refers to lack of emotional sensitivity, whereas flattening is a limitation of the usual range of emotions. Blunting and apathy are common in schizophrenia, whereas the others are characteristic of affective disorders. Anhedonia is the total inability to enjoy or experience pleasure. It is seen in depression and schizophrenia.

c. Inappropriateness

A mood is said to be appropriate and congruent when it is proper to the occasion, thinking and action and inappropriate when it is not proper to the occasion (feeling happy when a tragedy strikes) and incongruent (laughing when a sad event is narrated). Incongruent affect is very common in schizophrenia.

d. Abnormal Swings

A mood is said to be labile when the emotional changes are very rapid i.e., from sorrow to joy. Emotional incontinence refers to spilling of emotions and the patient's inability to control them. Lability and incontinence are particularly common in organic conditions and in cerebral arteriosclerosis. Ambivalence refers to coexistence of contradictory feelings and attitudes towards the same object simultaneously. It is observed in schizophrenia.

10. Disorders of Memory

Disorders of memory are present as: amnesias, hypermnesias and paramnesias.

a. Amnesias

Amnesia is the partial or total failure to recall past happenings and is due to disturbances of memory. Defective registration occurs when the level of consciousness is diminished, person is inattentive, drowsy or under the effect of drugs like alcohol. It also occurs in various lesions of the brain due to trauma, infection, etc.

b. Hypermnesias

Hypermnesia is not truly abnormal. It is an extreme degree of retention and recall of events. Every minor detail is recalled accurately. This is seen in mania, delusional disorders and obsessive-compulsive disorders.

c. Paramnesias

Paramnesias are distorted or falsified recall of events in relation to details or their temporal relationships.

❖ Confabulation is the unintentional filling of gaps of memory with material which is untrue and fanciful. Such recall changes from moment to moment and occurs in clear consciousness where organically determined amnesias coexist.

- ❖ Déjà vu is an error of recognition where an event or situation though occurring for the first time strikes a familiar chord as if it had happened earlier. In contrast, jamais vu is a feeling of strangeness to familiar situations or events. Both déjà vu and jamais vu are not primarily disorders of memory but disturbances of the associated familiarity feeling.
- ❖ Ganser syndrome otherwise known as the 'syndrome of approximate answers', is an example of psychologic paramnesia characterized by:
  - ○ Approximate answers (For example, Q. "How many legs do cows have?" Ans. "Three")
  - ○ Somatic conversion features
  - ○ Pseudohallucinations
  - ○ Clouding of consciousness

11. Disorders of Thought

Thought disorders are of four types: disorders of form, progression, content and possession.

a. Disorders of Form

Disordered form of thought is present as various logical and syntactical errors of conceptualization. Some of the common errors are as follows:

- ❖ **Incoherence**: The sequential connection between one idea and the next is lost so that the talk seems to be muddled up and incoherent. In extreme cases, the speech is full of jargon and meaningless. For example, the term word "animal" is followed by, "I think it is delightful for the cylindrical dog and my scooter to go flying."
- ❖ **Illogical thinking**: Here the thought is totally illogical. For example, "Suresh has a beard. I have a beard, so I am Suresh."
- ❖ **Over inclusion**: Themes irrelevant to the context and only distantly related to the main theme are included in thinking.
- ❖ **Neologism**: Neologism refers to coining new words which almost always have a private meaning known to the patient alone.

For example, "The Malitors are coming to get me." These new words are indicative of disconnected thought process.

b. Disorders of Progression

They are disorders of productivity, tempo and direction.

- ❖ **Disorders of productivity (volume)**: The rate at which thoughts are produced is altered in different clinical settings. It may be rapid (logorrhea) giving rise to crowding of thoughts and pressure of speech. On the other hand, there may be low productivity and poverty of ideas.
- ❖ **Disorders of tempo (speed)**: The tempo is accelerated and the flow of words rapid in several conditions like mania. In a flight of ideas, the patient flies from one topic to another so rapidly that it is often incomprehensible even to the extent of being incoherent. In thought block, there is a sudden break in the flow of thought or speech and the patient feels that his mind has gone blank.
- ❖ **Disorders of direction**: Direction of thoughts is lost in 'derailment' and the thought goes away from the intended theme. In circumstantiality the thought reaches its ultimate goal in a long and round about manner taking too many digression and irrelevant elaborations on its way. The goal is not reached in tangentiality where the thought is sidetracked more and more away from the natural end. Tangentiality is a form of derailment.

c. Disorder of Content

Disturbances of thought content are seen as various abnormal beliefs and convictions, obsessions, phobias and strange experiences.

- ❖ Overvalued ideas are abnormal beliefs, unique to the individual which dominates his life. They differ from delusions in being less intense and less 'unbelievable.'
- ❖ Fantasies are vivid imaginations with a wishful content perceived as unreal by the individual. In 'autism,' they predominate the psychic life of the individual.

❖ Ideas of reference are false interpretations with a self-referential quality. All happenings around are interpreted as having special reference to the individual. A man spitting on the ground is taken by the patient as spitting at him.

❖ Delusions are defined as fixed false beliefs which are not shared by others, are out of keeping with one's educational, social and cultural background and are unshakable in the face of evidence to the contrary. Delusions are classified in several ways. Primary (autochthonous) delusions spring up suddenly with no preceding mental events. For example, the patient has a sudden revelation that his neighbor has plans to kill him. Secondary delusions can be understood in the light of happenings which preceded the delusion. Delusions are called systematized when they are well organized and several interrelated beliefs are 'logically' woven into them. Unsystematized delusions are fragmented and poorly organized. Partial delusions are less 'sticky' and less strong than the complete ones. Simple delusions retain only a few delusional elements unlike the complex ones **(Table 5.1)**.

Themes of delusions

The themes of delusions are influenced by the patient's educational and cultural background as well as to a great degree by the type of illness.

TABLE 5.1: Types of delusions

Parameter	Types
Depending on origin	Primary and secondary
Depending on organization	Systematized and non-systematized
Depending on the reality value	Partial and complete
Depending on complexity	Simple and complex
Depending on the theme	Grandiose, persecutory, etc.

Various types of delusions are:
❖ Persecutory delusions
❖ Delusions of references
❖ Delusions of jealousy
❖ Delusions of love
❖ Hypochondriacal delusions
❖ Nihilistic delusions
❖ Somatic delusions
❖ Obsessions and compulsions
❖ Phobias
❖ Strange experiences

d. Disorders of Possession

Normal thinking has a quality of possession i.e., the individual is aware that the thoughts are his own and that he has control over them. He knows that his thoughts cannot be revealed to another person without his will. This is lost in some thought disorders and the patient believes that other persons can play upon his thinking.

In thought insertion the patient thinks that others' thoughts are inserted in his mind. In thoughts withdrawal his own thoughts are taken away from him. In thought diffusion the patient thinks that thoughts escape from his mind and become accessible to others. In its severe form the patient might say that his thoughts are read aloud in public. This is called thought broadcasting. Disorders of thinking are elicited through patient's speech or writing samples.

12. Disorders of Intelligence

Mental retardation is a subnormal level of intellectual functioning. It is of several grades: mild, moderate, severe and profound, depending on the IQ level. Intellectual deterioration occurs in dementias and other organic conditions and in schizophrenia.

13. Disorders of Insight and Judgment

Judgment is impaired in many organic conditions and psychoses. It is usually intact in neuroses. Insight is the patient's awareness of his disability and the need for help. There are several grades of insight. When there is total lack of insight the patient denies any illness and the need for treatment. Preservation of insight implies awareness of his own symptoms and their causal relationship to his psychic life.

It implies a readiness to effect a change by altering his behavior and to follow medical advice.

ETIOLOGY: BIOPSYCHOSOCIAL FACTORS

Many factors are responsible for the causation of mental illness. These factors may predispose an individual to mental illness, precipitate or perpetuate the mental illness.

Predisposing Factors

These are risk factors that determine an individual's susceptibility to mental illness. For example, previous mental disorder, heredity, negative self-concept, unemployment are some of the predisposing factors for schizophrenic patients. They interact with precipitating factors resulting in mental illness. Some of the predisposing factors are:

- Genetic makeup
- Physical damage to the central nervous system
- Adverse psychosocial influence

Precipitating Factors

These are events that occur shortly before the onset of a disorder and appear to have induced it. For example, abuse of substances, repeated unpleasant experiences, financial problems are some of the precipitating factors for schizophrenic patients. The precipitating factors are:

- Physical stress
- Psychosocial stress

Perpetuating Factors

These are factors or conditions in the patient, family, community or larger systems that are responsible for aggravating or prolonging the diseases already existing in an individual rather than subsiding it. Psychosocial stress is an example.

Etiological Factors of Mental Illness

Mental illnesses are caused by a combination of biological, physiological, environmental, psychological and social factors (**Figure 5.1**).

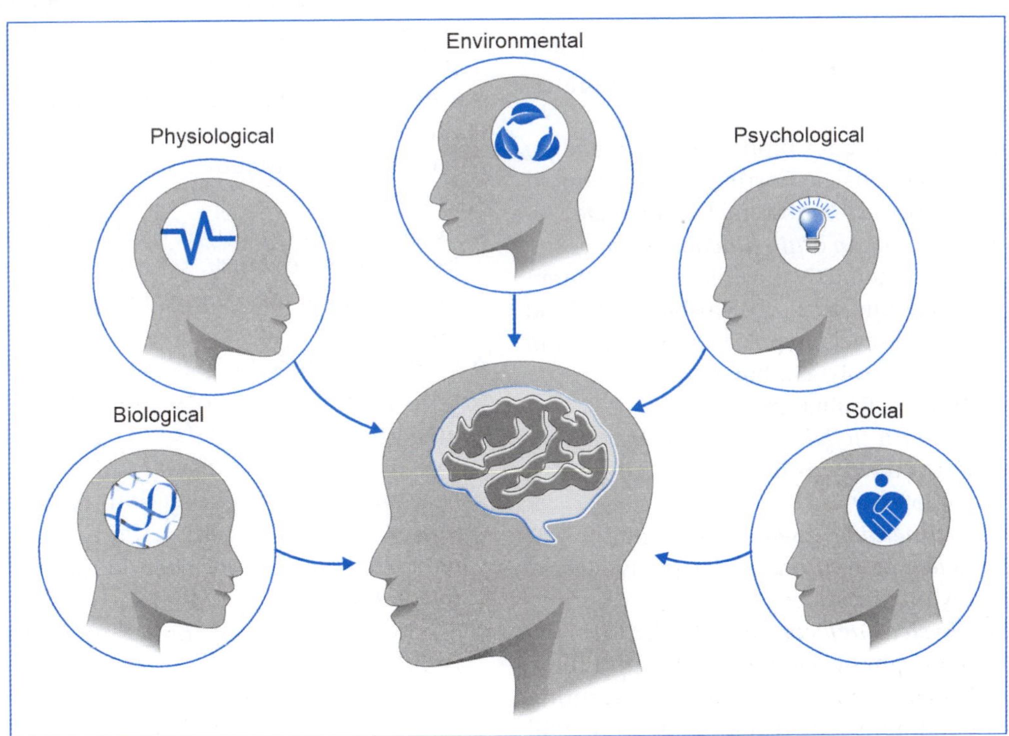

Figure 5.1: Etiological factors of mental illness

Biological Factors

Biological factors involved in causation of mental illnesses are as follows:

- ❖ **Heredity**: What one inherits is not the illness or its symptoms but a predisposition to the illness which is determined by genes that we inherit directly. Studies have shown that three-fourths of mental defectives and one-third of psychotic individuals owe their condition mainly to unfavorable heredity.
- ❖ **Biochemical factors**: Biochemical abnormalities in the brain are considered to be the main cause for psychiatric disorders. Disturbance in neurotransmitters in the brain is found to play an important role in the etiology of psychiatric disorders.
- ❖ **Brain damage**: Any damage to the structure and functioning of the brain can give rise to mental illness. Damage to the structure of the brain may be due to one of the following causes:
  - ○ *Infection*: Example, Neurosyphilis, encephalitis, HIV infection, etc.
  - ○ *Injury*: Loss of brain tissue due to head injury
  - ○ *Intoxication*: Damage to brain tissue due to toxins such as alcohol, barbiturates, lead, etc.
  - ○ *Vascular:* Poor blood supply, bleeding (intracranial hemorrhage, subarachnoid hemorrhage, subdural hemorrhage)
  - ○ *Alteration in brain function:* Changes in blood chemistry that interfere with brain functioning such as disturbance in blood glucose levels, hypoxia, anoxia, and fluid and electrolyte imbalance
  - ○ *Tumors:* Brain tumors
  - ○ *Vitamin deficiency and malnutrition:* Particularly deficiency of vitamin B complex
  - ○ *Degenerative diseases:* Dementia
  - ○ *Endocrine disturbances:* Hypothyroidism, thyrotoxicosis, etc.
  - ○ *Physical defects and physical illness:* Acute physical illness as well as chronic illnesses with all their handicapping conditions may result in loss of mental capacities.

Physiological Changes

It has been observed that mental disorders are more likely to occur at certain critical periods of life, namely—puberty, menstruation, pregnancy, delivery, puerperium and climacteric. These periods are marked not only by physiological (endocrine) changes but also by psychological issues that diminish the adaptive capacity of the individual. Thus, the individual becomes more susceptible to mental illness during this period.

Environmental Factors

Environmental factors associated with mental illness are pregnancy risk factors such as infections, malnutrition, exposure to heavy metals; perinatal risk factors such as birth complications; childhood environment factors such as poverty, maltreatment, bullying and drug use in adolescence.

Psychological Factors

- ❖ It is observed that some specific personality types are more prone to develop certain psychological disorders. For example, those who are unsocial and reserved (schizoid) are vulnerable to schizophrenia when they face adverse situations and psychosocial stresses.
- ❖ Strained interpersonal relationships at home, place of work, school or college, bereavement, loss of prestige, loss of job, etc.
- ❖ Childhood insecurities due to parents with pathological personalities, faulty attitude of parents (over-strictness, over leniency), abnormal parent–child relationship (over-protection, rejection, unhealthy comparisons), deprivation of child's essential psychological and social needs, etc.
- ❖ Social and recreational deprivations resulting in boredom, isolation and alienation.
- ❖ Marriage problems like forced bachelor hood, disharmony due to physical,

emotional, social, educational or financial incompatibility, childlessness, too many children, etc.
- ❖ Sexual difficulties arising out of improper sex education, unhealthy attitudes towards sexual functions, guilt feelings about masturbation, pre and extramarital sex relations, worries about sexual perversions.
- ❖ Stress, frustration and seasonal variations are sometimes noted in the occurrence of mental diseases.

Social Factors
- ❖ Poverty, unemployment, injustice, insecurity, migration, urbanization
- ❖ Gambling, alcoholism, prostitution, broken homes, divorce, very big family, religion, traditions, political upheavals and other social crises.

CLASSIFICATION OF MENTAL DISORDERS

Classification is a process by which complex phenomena are organized into categories, classes or ranks so as to bring together such aspects that most resemble each other and separate those that differ. It is important because it allows scientists to identify and group patterns of abnormal behavior.

Purposes of Classification

At present there are two major classifications in psychiatry namely ICD-11 (2022) and DSM-5-TR (2022). In both forms of classification mental disorders are grouped by their symptoms in categories that compose the classification. Classifications currently used in psychiatry serve following purposes:
- ❖ To make generally acceptable diagnosis
- ❖ To provide standardized vocabulary that permits effective communication between psychiatrists, other doctors and professionals
- ❖ To make generalizations in treatment response, course and prognosis of individual patients
- ❖ To make framework for research in psychiatry
- ❖ To facilitate statistical records for public health institutions

1. ICD-11

The International Classification of Diseases (ICD) provides a common language that allows health professionals to share standardized information across the world. ICD-11 came into in effect in January 2022 for the national and international recording and reporting of causes of illness, death and more.

Special Features of ICD-11
- ❖ The 11th revision contains around 17,000 unique codes.
- ❖ Smart coding algorithm
- ❖ Digital reference guide and multilingual browser and coding tool
- ❖ 35 countries are using ICD-11
- ❖ Used for certification and reporting of cause of death; morbidity coding; assessing and monitoring the safety, efficacy and quality of care; rare disease coding; grade and stage coding for cancers, clinical description and diagnostic requirements for mental health; digital documentation of COVID-19 vaccination status and test results and many more.

ICD-11 Categories

Chapter 06 (6A00-6E8Z) of ICD-11 describes mental, behavioral or neurodevelopmental disorders. According to ICD-11 mental behavioral and neurodevelopmental disorders are syndromes characterized by clinically significant disturbance in an individual's cognition, emotional regulation or behavior that reflects a dysfunction in the psychological, biological or developmental processes that underline mental and behavioral functioning. These disturbances are usually associated with distress or impairment in personal, family, social, educational, occupational or other important areas of functioning. Major categories of ICD-11 are presented in **Box 5.2.**

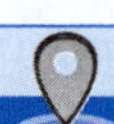

BOX 5.2: Major categories of ICD-11

1. Neurodevelopmental disorders
2. Schizophrenia or other primary psychotic disorders
3. Catatonia
4. Mood disorders
5. Anxiety or fear related disorders
6. Obsessive compulsive disorders
7. Disorders specifically associated with stress
8. Dissociative disorders
9. Feeding or eating disorders
10. Elimination disorders
11. Disorders of bodily distress or bodily experience
12. Disorders due to substance use or addictive behaviors
13. Impulse control disorders
14. Disruptive behavior or dissocial disorders
15. Personality disorders
16. Paraphilic disorders
17. Factitious disorders
18. Neurocognitive disorders
19. Mental or behavioral disorders associated with pregnancy, child birth or the puerperium
20. Psychological or behavioral factors affecting disorders classified elsewhere
21. Secondary mental or behavioral syndromes associated with disorders or diseases classified elsewhere

ICD-10 (International Statistical Classification of Disease and Related Health Problems)—1992

This is WHO's classification for all diseases and related health problems. The chapter 'F' classifies psychiatric disorders as mental and behavioral disorders and codes them on an alphanumeric system from F00 to F99. Main categories in ICD10 are:

F00–F09	Organic, including symptomatic, mental disorders
F10–F19	Mental and behavior disorders due to psychoactive substance use
F20–F29	Schizophrenia, schizotypal and delusional disorders
F30–F39	Mood (affective) disorders
F40–F48	Neurotic, stress-related and somato form disorders
F50–F59	Behavioral syndromes associated with physiological disturbances and physical factors
F60–F69	Disorders of adult personality and behavior
F70–F79	Mental retardation
F80–F89	Disorders of psychological development
F90–F98	Behavioral and emotional disorders with onset usually occurring in childhood and adolescence
F99	Unspecified mental disorder

2. DSM-5

The Diagnostic and Statistical Manual of Mental Disorders (DSM) is the handbook widely used by clinicians and psychiatrists in the United States to diagnose psychiatric illnesses. It is published by the American Psychiatric Association (APA). Published in 2013, DSM-5 refers to the fifth edition of handbook overriding the DSM-IV-TR. In the United States, the DSM serves as a universal authority for psychiatric diagnosis. DSM-5-TR (text revision) is the latest version released in March 2022.

DSM uses multiaxial or multidimensional approach for diagnosing mental disorders. It helps clinicians to make comprehensive evaluations of a patient's level of functioning because mental illnesses often impact many different life areas. The five axes of DSM are:

1. **AXIS I:** Clinical psychiatric diagnosis
2. **AXIS II:** Personality disorder and mental retardation
3. **AXIS III:** General medical conditions
4. **AXIS IV:** Psychosocial and environmental problems
5. **AXIS V:** Global assessment of functioning

DSM-5 uses unified system of clinical assessment that is aligned with international classification systems. It combines the first three axes into one that contains all mental and other medical diagnoses. Doing so removes artificial distinctions among conditions benefitting both clinical practice and research

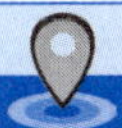

BOX 5.3: The DSM-5 diagnostic chapters

1. Neurodevelopmental disorders
2. Schizophrenia spectrum and other psychotic disorders
3. Bipolar and related disorders
4. Depressive disorders
5. Anxiety disorders
6. Obsessive-compulsive and related disorders
7. Trauma and stressor related disorders
8. Dissociative disorders
9. Somatic symptom and related disorders
10. Feeding and eating disorders
11. Elimination disorders
12. Sleep–wake disorders
13. Sexual dysfunctions
14. Gender dysphoria
15. Disruptive, impulse control, and conduct disorders
16. Substance related and addictive disorders
17. Neurocognitive disorders
18. Personality disorders
19. Paraphilic disorders
20. Other mental disorders and additional conditions

use. The diagnostic chapters of DSM-5 are presented in **Box 5.3**.

PREVALENCE OF PSYCHIATRIC DISORDERS

Prevalence is defined as total number of persons in the population who have a psychiatric disorder at a point or period of time. It includes both new and old cases. The World Health Organization reports that psychiatric disorders are the leading cause of disability globally. To estimate prevalence of psychiatric disorders several epidemiological studies are conducted in India since 1960s.

In India, National Mental Health Survey (NMHS) was conducted in 2016 to assess the prevalence of psychiatric disorders. This NMHS is a multisite nationwide household survey conducted across India using a uniform methodology. As per NMHS the prevalence of mental disorders is as follows:

❖ The overall weighted prevalence for any mental morbidity was 13.7% lifetime and 10.6% current.

❖ The age group between 40–49 years were predominantly affected with psychotic disorders, bipolar affective disorders, depressive disorders and neurotic and stress related disorders.

❖ The prevalence of substance use disorders was 29.4%, it was highest in the 50–59 year age group, the gender prevalence of psychotic disorders was near similar.

❖ Male predominance was observed in alcohol use disorders and for BPAD. A female predominance was observed for depressive disorders, neurotic and stress related disorders.

❖ Residents from urban metro had a greater prevalence across the different disorders.

❖ Persons from lower income were observed to have a greater prevalence of one or more mental disorders.

❖ The suicide risk among individuals in the past one month was observed to be 0.7 (moderate risk) to 0.9% (high risk). It was highest in the 40–49 year age group, greater amongst females and those from urban metros.

❖ Intellectual disability (ID) screener positivity rates were 0.6% and epilepsy screener positivity rate was 0.3%; it was greater amongst the younger age group, among males and those from urban metro areas.

❖ The prevalence of morbidity amongst adolescents was 7.3% with a similar distribution between males and females.

❖ Treatment gap for mental disorders ranged between 70 to 92% for different disorders.

❖ At least half of those with a mental disorder reported disability in all three domains of work, social and family life and was relatively less among alcohol use disorder. Greater disability was reported among persons with epilepsy, depression and bipolar affective disorders.

[*Source*: National Mental Health Survey of India, 2015-2016 Prevalence, Patterns and Outcomes, Supported by Ministry of Health and Family Welfare, Government of India, and Implemented by National Institute of Mental Health and Neurosciences (NIMHANS) Bengaluru: In Collaboration with Partner Institutions; 2015-2016].

PERSONALITY DISORDER

The term personality refers to enduring qualities of an individual that are shown in his ways of behaving in a wide variety of circumstances. Personality disorders result when personality traits become abnormal, i.e., become inflexible and maladaptive and cause significant social or occupational impairment or significant subjective distress. In ICD-11, they are listed under the section on Personality disorders and related traits (6D10).

Meaning

- Personality disorder reflects adaptive failure involving impaired sense of self-identity or failure to develop effective interpersonal functioning.
- An abnormal personality is one in which there are, "deeply ingrained maladaptive patterns of behavior recognizable by the time of adolescence or earlier and continuing through most of adult life. Because of this, the patient suffers or others have to suffer, and there is an adverse effect on the individual or on society."
- Personality disorders are a group of mental health conditions that are characterized by inflexible and atypical patterns of thinking, feeling and behaving.

Incidence

Prevalence of personality disorders in the general population is 5–10%. Occurrence of mixed personality disorders is more common than a single personality disorder in an individual.

Etiology

The exact cause of personality disorders is unknown; most likely they represent a combination of genetic, biological, social, psychological, developmental and environmental factors.

Genetic Factors

Genetic factors influence the biological basis of brain function as well as basic personality structure. Genetic predisposition can be responsible for a psychopathic personality.

Biological Factors

Some researchers suspect that poor regulation of the brain circuits that control emotion increases the risk for a personality disorder when combined with such factors as abuse, neglect or separation. For a biologically predisposed person, the major developmental challenges of adolescence and early adulthood (such as separation from the parents, identity and independence) may trigger a personality disorder.

Psychodynamic Theories

These theories propose that personality disorders stem from deficiencies in ego and superego development. These deficiencies may relate to mother-child relationships marked by unresponsiveness, over protectiveness or early separation.

Other Factors

- Maternal deprivation especially in *antisocial* personality
- **Borderline** personalities are more likely to report physical and sexual abuse in childhood.
- **Histrionic** personality is said to occur as a result of failure to resolve oedipal complex and excessive use of repression as a mechanism of defense.
- **Dependent** personality may be due to fixation in the oral stage of development.
- **Paranoid** personality is due to absence of trust which results from lack of parental affection in childhood and persistent rejection by parents leading to low self-esteem.

Clinical Features of Abnormal Personalities

According to DSM-5 the four core features of all personality disorders are:

1. **Distorted thinking patterns:** They may be unaware of how their behaviors cause problems for themselves and others.
2. **Problematic emotional responses:** They have issues in understanding realistic and acceptable ways to treat others and behave around them.

3. **Over or under regulated impulse control:** They are unable to control their impulses.
4. **Interpersonal difficulties:** Their behavior is inconsistent, frustrating and confusing to loved ones and others.

Paranoid Personality Disorder (Mistrust and Suspicion)

This disorder is marked by a distrust of other people and a constant unwarranted suspicion that others have sinister motives. Persons with paranoid personality disorder search for hidden meanings and hostile intentions in everything others say and do. The signs and symptoms are **(Box 5.4)**:

❖ Suspicious
❖ Mistrustful
❖ Sensitive
❖ Argumentative
❖ Stubborn
❖ Self-important
❖ Hypersensitive
❖ Jealous and irritable

Schizoid Personality Disorder (Disinterest in Others)

Schizoid personality disorder is characterized by detachment and social withdrawal. People with this disorder are commonly described as loners, with solitary interests and occupations and no close friends; typically, they maintain a social distance even from family members and seem unconcerned about other's praise

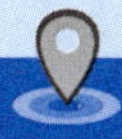 **BOX 5.5:** Case vignette—Schizoid personality disorder

Ms Leena, a 20-year-old college student stays in the hostel. She does not interact with others and races back to the hostel soon after the classes. Her classmates describe Ms Leena as absent-minded. She does not have friends, no interest in events happening in the campus, does not like to go home even during holidays.

or criticism. The signs and symptoms are **(Box 5.5)**:

❖ Emotionally cold
❖ Aloof
❖ Detached
❖ Humorless
❖ Introspective
❖ No desire for or enjoyment of close relationship
❖ Inability to experience pleasure

Schizotypal Disorder (Eccentric Ideas and Behavior)

This disorder is marked by odd thinking and behavior, a pervasive pattern of social and interpersonal deficits and acute discomfort with others. The signs and symptoms are:

❖ Inappropriate affect
❖ Odd beliefs or magical thinking
❖ Social withdrawal
❖ Odd, eccentric or peculiar behavior
❖ Lack of close relationships
❖ Social isolation
❖ Not fitting easily with others

Antisocial (Dissocial) Personality Disorder (Sociopath, Psychopath)

Antisocial personality disorder is characterized by chronic antisocial behavior that violates others' rights or social norms which predisposes the affected person to criminal behavior. The person is unable to maintain consistent, responsible functioning at work, school or as a parent. The signs and symptoms are:

❖ Failure to sustain relationships
❖ Disregard for feelings of others
❖ Impulsive actions
❖ Low tolerance to frustration

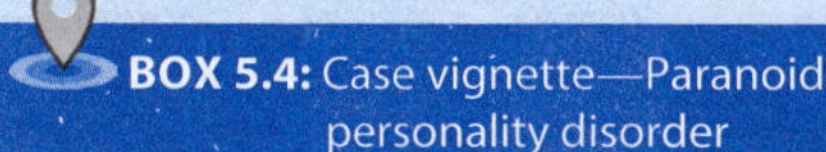 **BOX 5.4:** Case vignette—Paranoid personality disorder

Jimmy has paranoid personality disorder. He performed exceptionally well at school and also achieved high grades. Most of the time he was rude, making fun of those who could not score good marks, he even corrected his teachers, laughed and mocked at them and thought he was better than everyone else. At school he was considered to be arrogant. He was always suspicious about others stealing his ideas and thereby could not form trust with anyone. Later he was employed at a company where he showed hostility towards his co-workers and suspected that they are stealing his ideas. He got fired from his job. Jimmy got married to a co-worker, later got divorced due to his suspicious behavior.

- Tendency to cause violence
- Lack of guilt
- Failure to learn from experience
- Reckless disregard for own or others safety
- Impulsivity and failure to plan ahead
- Manipulative behavior for self-gratification
- Inability to maintain close personal or sexual relationship

Histrionic Personality Disorder (Attention Seeking and Excessive Emotionality)

Patients with this disorder characteristically have a pervasive pattern of excessive emotionality and attention seeking behavior and are drawn to momentary excitements and fleeting adventures. This disorder is more common in females. People with this disorder need to be the center of attention at all times. The signs and symptoms are:

- Dramatic emotionality (emotional blackmail, angry scenes, demonstrative suicide attempts, etc.)
- Craving for novelty and excitement
- Shallow and labile affectivity
- Attention-seeking behavior
- Over concern with physical attractiveness
- Exaggerated, vague speech
- Self-dramatization
- Impulsivity
- Suggestibility
- Ego-centricity, self-indulgence and lack of consideration for others

Narcissistic Personality Disorder (Self-grandiosity and Lack of Empathy)

Patient with narcissistic personality disorder is self-centered, self-absorbed and lacking in empathy for others. He typically takes advantage of people to achieve his own ends, and uses them without regard to their feelings. The signs and symptoms are:

- Inflated sense of self-importance
- Attention-seeking, dramatic behavior
- Unable to face criticism
- Lack of empathy
- Exploitative behavior
- Arrogance
- Preoccupation with fantasies of success, power, beauty, brilliance or ideal love

Borderline Personality Disorder (Inner Emptiness and Emotional Dysregulation)

Borderline personality disorder is marked by a pattern of instability in interpersonal relationships, mood, behavior and self-image. The four main categories of signs and symptoms are **(Box 5.6)**:

- Unstable relationships
- Unstable self-image
- Unstable emotions
- Impulsivity

Other symptoms include:

- Lack of control on anger
- Recurrent suicidal threats or behavior
- Uncertainty about personal identity
- Chronic feelings of emptiness
- Efforts to avoid abandonment
- Transient stress-related paranoid or dissociative symptoms
- Acting out of feelings instead of expressing them appropriately or verbally

Anxious (Avoidant) Personality Disorder (Avoidance of Interpersonal Contact)

Anxious personality disorder is marked by feelings of inadequacy, extreme social anxiety, social withdrawal and hypersensitivity to others' opinions. People with this disorder

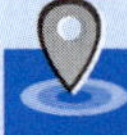

BOX 5.6: Case vignette—Borderline personality disorder

Mrs Meena, 24-year-old women is taking supportive therapy in the outpatient clinic for her borderline personality disorder. She presents with a history of self-injurious behavior, cutting her fore arms and legs. She made two suicidal attempts by consuming overdose of prescribed medications during her teenage period. She says that suicide attempts provide her relief. She has limited and unstable relationship with others. There is a history of changing her hobbies, style of clothing and sometimes even the job as well. At times she is over caring towards her partner, impulsively buys lavish gifts, prepares tasty dishes, and expresses caring words. At other times she ignores or yells and throws things at him. Soon after such an incident she reports guilt for her behavior. She also reports frequent engagement in unsafe behaviors with unknown people. She has several tattoos on her arm, back and neck.

have low self-esteem and poor self-confidence; they dwell on the negative and have difficulty viewing situations and interactions objectively. The signs and symptoms are **(Box 5.7)**:

❖ Persistent feeling of tension and apprehension
❖ Inferiority complex
❖ Fear of criticism, disapproval or rejection
❖ Unwillingness to become involved with people
❖ Excessive preoccupation with being criticized or rejected in social situations

Many people with avoidant personality disorder have other psychiatric disorders like social phobia, anxiety disorder, obsessive compulsive disorder, depressive disorders, somatoform disorders, dissociative disorder and schizophrenia.

Dependent Personality (Submissiveness)

This disorder is characterized by an extreme need to be taken care of, which leads to submissive, clinging behavior and fear of separation or rejection. People with this disorder let others make important decisions for them and have a strong need for constant reassurance and support. The signs and symptoms are:

❖ Subordination of one's own needs
❖ Unwillingness to make even reasonable demands on other people
❖ Inability to take decision

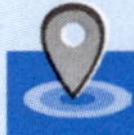

BOX 5.7: Case vignette—Avoidant personality disorder

Mr Manoj a 22-year-old male, studying engineering course hailing from middle socioeconomic status came to psychiatric OPD along with his parents with the following complaints: avoiding close relatives, crowded places, scared to talk to neighbors and ladies, avoiding almost all activities outside home. He had several fears and phobias, frequent anger outbursts and inability to study. Insidiously symptoms started over a period of 3 years and gradually worsened. For the past 2 years, he is not attending classes, spending most of the time sleeping and watching television. He was more or less home bound.

❖ Feeling uncomfortable or helpless when alone
❖ Low self-esteem and lack of self-confidence
❖ Hypersensitivity to criticism

Obsessive-Compulsive (Anankastic) Personality Disorder (Perfectionism, Rigidity and Obstinacy)

This disorder is marked by a pervasive desire for perfection and order at the expense of openness, flexibility and efficiency. The individual places a great deal of pressure on himself and others not to make mistakes. There is a constant sense of righteous indignation and feeling of anger and contempt for anyone who disagrees with him, believes his way of doing something is the only right way, may force himself and others to follow right moral principles and to conform to extremely high standards of performance and insist on literal compliance with authority and rules. The signs and symptoms are:

❖ Feeling of excessive doubt and caution
❖ Preoccupation with details, rules, lists, order or schedule
❖ Perfectionism
❖ Rigidity and stubbornness
❖ High standards

Treatment Modalities

Personality disorder is often difficult to treat. Drug treatment has a very limited role and may be used if associated mental illness like depression or psychosis is present. Individual and group psychotherapy, therapeutic community and behavioral therapy may be beneficial. Manipulation of social environment can be tried.

❖ Group therapy helps patients improve interaction skills in addition to gaining an understanding of how they are perceived by others. Patients can learn how to ventilate anxiety and trust others in a safe environment. Problem-solving methods can be practiced within the group to resolve community issues.
❖ Individual therapy helps patients gain insight into their thinking and behavior.

Ways can be explored for them to modify their behavior to a more functional level.

- Occupational therapy allows patients to increase their level of functioning so that they become more independent. Task completion skills can also be evaluated and enhanced by these activities.
- Recreation therapy can assist patients to ventilate feelings and increase socialization skills.
- Interaction and guidance by the therapist can provide patients with constructive ways to deal with anger and other self-destructive behaviors.
- Medications if needed.

Nursing Interventions for Patients with Personality Disorders

Providing care for people with personality disorders is very challenging for nurses. The nurse must identify personal feelings about the patient's behaviors and maintain a continuous awareness to provide appropriate interventions. Nursing actions may include the following:

- Show acceptance of the person at all times by separating the person from his behaviors
- Provide a safe environment, especially important for patients who exhibit self-mutilating behavior
- Set and maintain limits with consequences
- Explain all unit rules and enforce them fairly and consistently
- Require the patient to take responsibility for his or her own behavior
- Identify inappropriate behavior and discuss possible alternative behavior with the patient
- Do not make exceptions or show favoritism
- Encourage the patient to openly express feelings and thoughts
- Identify triggers of acting-out behaviors
- Maintain alertness to manipulative behaviors of patients
- Communicate problems with manipulative patients to other team members

- Provide positive feedback to patients who are making efforts to change behavior
- Approach patients from the front and speak clearly. This is especially true for the patient with paranoia
- Monitor medication
- Encourage the patient to participate in unit activities
- Assess for suicidal ideation
- Develop a no-harm contract with the patient with self-destructive tendencies
- Assist and educate the patient in the problem-solving process
- Demonstrate a matter-of-fact attitude when patients act-out or exaggerate events
- Encourage the patient to keep a private journal of thoughts and feelings
- Discuss with the patient how his or her behavior affects others and assist to explore alternative actions
- Observe and intervene before escalation of behavior occurs
- Use time-out for curbing acting-out behavior if patient is resistant to redirection

ORGANIC MENTAL DISORDERS

Organic mental disorders are behavioral or psychological disorders associated with transient or permanent brain dysfunction. In ICD-11 these are classified under neurocognitive disorders. These disorders represent a decline from a previously attained level of functioning. Neurocognitive disorders are characterized by primary clinical deficits in neurocognitive functioning that are acquired rather than developmental.

Delirium
(Acute Organic Brain Syndrome)

According to ICD-11, delirium is an acute organic mental disorder characterized by disturbance of attention, orientation and awareness that develops within a short period of time typically presenting as significant confusion or global neurocognitive impairment with transient symptoms that may fluctuate depending on the etiology.

Incidence

Delirium is an acute medical emergency with psychiatric manifestations. Highest prevalence is observed in intensive care units (ICUs) and palliative care settings. About 10–25% of medical-surgical inpatients, and about 20–40% of geriatric patients meet the criteria for delirium during hospitalization. This percentage is higher in postoperative patients, ICU patients and palliative care patients.

Etiology

There are two groups of risk factors related to delirium: predisposing and precipitating factors.

❖ The predisposing factors are old age, dementia, functional disability, male gender, poor visibility and hearing.

❖ The precipitating factors include surgery, anesthesia, hypoxia, untreated pain, infections, acute illness and acute exacerbation of chronic illness.

Delirium can result from an imbalance in neurotransmitters especially acetylcholine.

Some of the common causes of delirium are presented in **Figure 5.2**.

❖ **Drug interactions or sensitivity**: Any new medications, increased dosage, drug interaction, alcohol, when long-term sedation or pain drugs are stopped, etc.

❖ **Dehydration**: Electrolyte disturbances

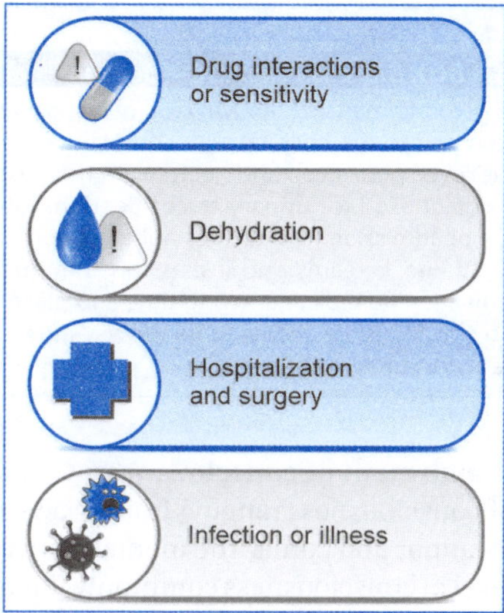

Figure 5.2: Causes of delirium

❖ **Hospitalization and surgery**: Major surgery, anesthesia, untreated pain

❖ **Illness/infections**: Urinary or respiratory tract infections, myocardial and lung diseases, brain infections, hemorrhage, stroke or tumor

Clinical Features

Delirium is a sudden and severe change in brain function that causes a person to appear confused or disoriented, difficulty in thinking, remembering recent events with a fluctuating course (**Figure 5.3 and Box 5.8**).

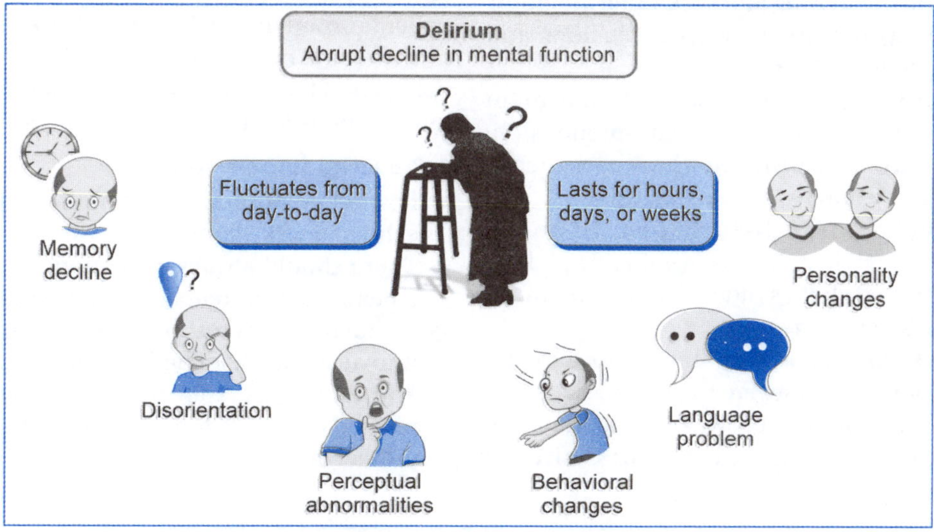

Figure 5.3: Clinical features of delirium

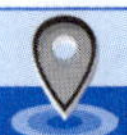

> **BOX 5.8:** Case vignette—Delirium
>
> A 78-year-old man with known case of hypertension is admitted to the hospital with complaints of low-grade fever, poor sleep and nocturia. In the hospital he is diagnosed for urinary tract infection. After 4 hours of admission he becomes agitated, confused, pulls IV line, screams and insists to go home. On examination he is disoriented to time and place and unable to focus. He seems to be drowsy in the day time and irritable in the night.

* **Impairment of consciousness**: Clouding of consciousness ranging from drowsiness to stupor and coma. The mental status and level of consciousness commonly fluctuate throughout the day. Symptom patterns of delirium tend to fall into one of the two categories:
  1. *Hyperactive delirium*: Also called 'excited delirium' it involves higher activity levels and includes agitation, aggression, combativeness and mood swings.
  2. *Hypoactive delirium*: It is harder to diagnose as it involves lower activity levels and is usually mistaken for fatigue or depression. Symptoms include apathy and lack of interest in what's happening around, sluggishness and slowed movements.
* **Impairment of attention**: Difficulty in shifting, focusing and sustaining attention
* **Perceptual disturbances**: Illusions and hallucinations, most often visual
* **Disturbance of cognition**: Impairment of abstract thinking and comprehension, impairment of immediate and recent memory, increased reaction time
* **Psychomotor disturbance**: Hypo- or hyperactivity, aimless groping or picking at the bed clothes (flocculation), enhanced startle reaction
* **Disturbance of the sleep-wake cycle**: Insomnia or in severe cases total sleep loss or reversal of sleep-wake cycle, daytime drowsiness, nocturnal worsening of symptoms, disturbing dreams or nightmares which may continue as hallucinations after awakening
* **Emotional disturbances**: Depression, anxiety, fear, irritability, euphoria, apathy
* **Other symptoms**: Difficulty maintaining focus, change the subject frequently, disoriented to place and time. Tremors is common in withdrawal states.

Course and Prognosis

The onset is usually abrupt. Duration of the episode is usually brief, lasting for about a week.

Investigations

Blood tests, urine tests, chest X-ray, CT scan, lumber puncture, EEG testing, etc.

Treatment

* Identification of cause and its immediate correction. For example, 50 mg of 50% dextrose IV for hypoglycemia, O_2 for hypoxia, 100 mg of B_1 IV for thiamine deficiency, IV fluids for fluid and electrolyte imbalance.
* Symptomatic measures: Benzodiazepines (10 mg diazepam or 2 mg lorazepam IV) or antipsychotics (5 mg haloperidol or 50 mg chlorpromazine IM) may be given.

Nursing Interventions

Nurses play a crucial role in identifying patients experiencing delirium. Nurses are the one who first notice any changes in cognitive behavior of the patient. The common nursing interventions for a delirium patient are:

1. Providing Safe Environment

* Restrict environmental stimuli, keep unit calm and well-illuminated.
* There should always be somebody at the patient's bedside reassuring and supporting.
* As the patient is responding to a terrifying unrealistic world of hallucinatory illusions and delusions, special precautions are needed to protect him from himself and to protect others.

2. Alleviating Patient's Fear and Anxiety

- ❖ Remove any object in the room that seems to be a source of misinterpreted perception
- ❖ To the best extent possible have the same person all the time by the patient's bedside
- ❖ Keep the room well lighted especially at night

3. Meeting the Physical Needs of the Patient

- ❖ Appropriate care should be provided after physical assessment
- ❖ Use appropriate nursing measures to reduce high fever, if present
- ❖ Maintain intake and output chart
- ❖ Mouth and skin should be taken care of
- ❖ Monitor vital signs
- ❖ Observe the patient for any extreme drowsiness and sleep as this may be an indication that the patient is slipping into a coma

4. Facilitate Orientation

- ❖ Repeatedly explain to the patient where he is and what date, day and time it is
- ❖ Introduce people with name even if the patient misidentifies the people
- ❖ Have a calendar in the room and tell him what day it is
- ❖ When the acute stage is over take the patient out and introduce him to others

Dementia
(Chronic Organic Brain Syndrome)

Dementia is an acquired global impairment of intellect, memory and personality but without impairment of consciousness. It is a general term used to describe brain disorders that primarily affect person's memory and behavior.

According to ICD-11, dementia is characterized by the presence of marked impairment in two or more cognitive domains relative to that expected given the individual's age and premorbid level of cognitive functioning which represents a decline from the individual's previous level of functioning.

Dementia can be defined as a clinical syndrome characterized by a cluster of symptoms and signs manifested by difficulties in memory, disturbances in language and other cognitive functions, changes in behaviors, and impairments in activities of daily living.

Incidence

Dementia occurs more commonly in the elderly than in the middle-aged. It increases with age from 0.1% in those below 60 years of age to 15–20% in those aged 80 years and above.

Causes

Various neurodegenerative disorders and factors contribute to the development of dementia through a progressive and irreversible loss of neurons and brain function.

- ❖ **Alzheimer's disease**: This is the most common of all dementing illnesses which accounts for 60–70% of all cases of dementia. It is characterized by amyloid plaques and beta tangles.
- ❖ **Frontotemporal dementia**: Characterized by deterioration of frontal and temporal lobes of the brain, it is associated with abnormal amount of the protein tau.
- ❖ **Lewy body dementia**: It is caused by Lewy body protein deposits on nerve cells. It prevents transmission of nerve cell chemical signals in the brain resulting in lost messages, delayed reactions and memory loss.
- ❖ **Parkinson's disease**: Individuals with advanced Parkinson's disease may develop dementia. Symptoms of this particular type of dementia includes problems with reasoning and judgment, irritability, depression and paranoia.
- ❖ **Vascular/multi-infarct dementia**: A form of dementia caused by conditions that damage blood vessels in the brain or interrupt the flow of blood and oxygen to the brain. Example: strokes, brain injury, etc.
- ❖ **Other diseases**: Dementia due to Huntington's disease, HIV, Creutzfeldt-Jakob disease, Korsakoff syndrome.

Other Factors

- ❖ **Environmental factors**: Infections such as meningitis and syphilis, metals and toxins (excessive amounts of metal ions like zinc and copper in the brain).

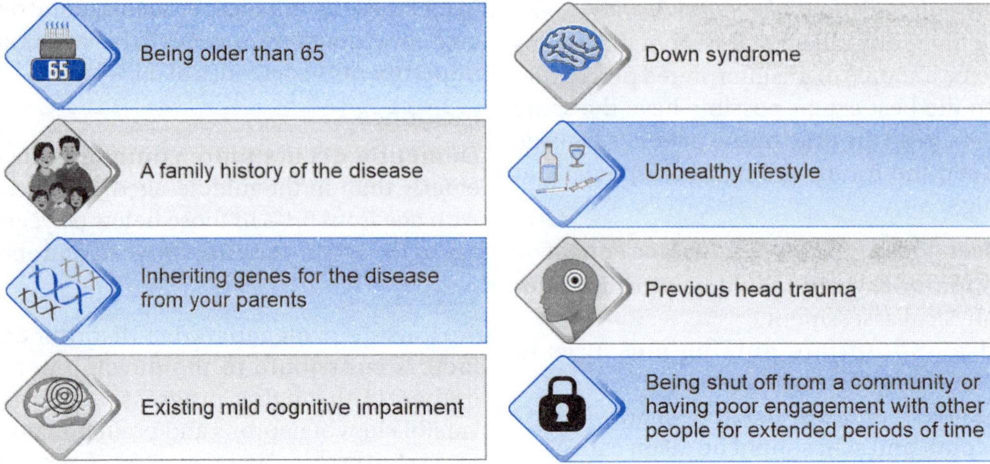

Figure 5.4: Risk factors for dementia

❖ Other possible factors being researched are:

○ *Deficiencies of vitamins B_6, B_{12} and folate*: Possible risk factor due to increased levels of homocysteine (amino acid that may interfere with nerve cell repair).

○ *Early depression*: Common genetic factors seen in those with early depression and Alzheimer's disease.

○ *Serious head injury*: Possible link between injury in early adulthood and later development of Alzheimer's disease. The various risk factors for dementia are presented in **Figure 5.4**.

Pathophysiology

❖ Alzheimer's disease attacks nerves and brain cells as well as neurotransmitters. It causes degeneration of brain neurons especially in the cerebral cortex. Destruction of these parts produces amyloid beta peptide. It is proposed to be an early toxic event in the pathogenesis of Alzheimer's disease.

❖ Accumulation of beta amyloid, an insoluble protein forms sticky patches (neurotic plaques and tangles) around the brain's cells. The presence of neurofibrillary tangles (twisted nerve cell fibers that are the damaged remains of microtubules) and plaques, containing beta-amyloid cells start to destroy more and more connections between the brain cells.

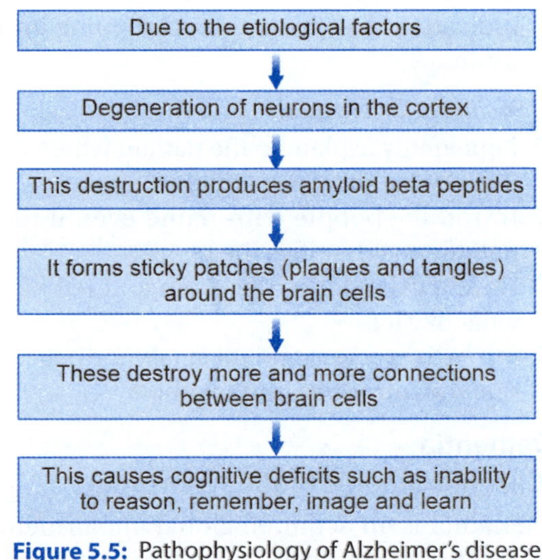

Figure 5.5: Pathophysiology of Alzheimer's disease

❖ This significant loss of brain cells (neurons) and volume in brain regions devoted to memory and higher mental functioning causes inability to reason, remember, imagine and learn **(Figure 5.5)**.

Stages of Dementia

In most cases though dementia is progressive it differs from individual to individual. Common stages of dementia are presented in **Figure 5.6**. **Stage I: Mild cognitive impairment—no mental impairment**

❖ Forgetfulness

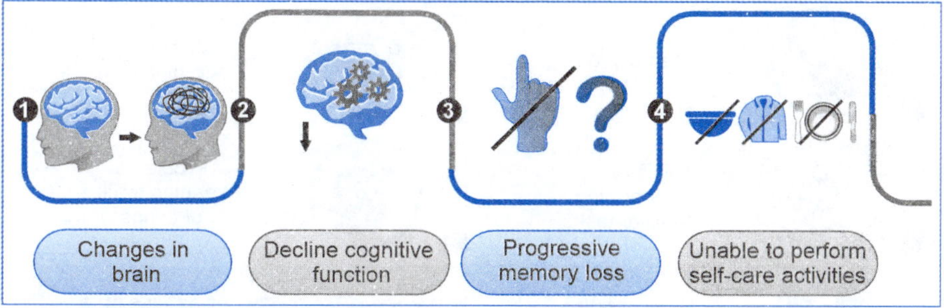

Figure 5.6: Stages of dementia

❖ Trouble recalling words and short-term memory

Stage II: Mild dementia—able to function independently

❖ Short-term memory lapses
❖ Forgetfulness
❖ Personality changes including anger or depression
❖ Difficulty with complex tasks
❖ Difficulty expressing emotions or ideas

Stage III: Moderate dementia—may need assistance for daily activities

❖ Progressive memory loss
❖ Increasing confusion and frustration
❖ Needing help for bathing and dressing
❖ Has difficulty in following simple instructions
❖ Irritable, anxious
❖ Wandering
❖ Neglects personal hygiene
❖ Social isolation
❖ Declining interest in environment
❖ Significant personality changes

Stage IV: Severe dementia—worsening of physical and mental symptoms

❖ Require full-time assistance
❖ Inability to maintain bodily functions including walking, bladder control and swallowing
❖ Marked loss of weight because of inadequate intake of food
❖ Unable to communicate
❖ Does not recognize family
❖ Loses the ability to stand and walk
❖ Increased risk of infections

Warning Signs of Alzheimer's Dementia

Memory loss itself does not mean that person is suffering with dementia. There is a difference between occasional forgetfulness and routine forgetfulness. The warning signs of Alzheimer's dementia are very vague and may not be immediately obvious (**Figure 5.7**). Family members should be aware of early warning signs which may suggest that one of the older members may be on the verge of developing Alzheimer's disease. Early diagnosis and intervention can be beneficial to both the patient and the family. As the disease progresses, the family remains the main pillar of support for the patient.

Clinical Features for Alzheimer's Type

Signs and symptoms of dementia result when once healthy neurons in the brain stop working, lose connections with other brain cells and die. As the age progresses everyone loses some neurons but people with dementia experience greater loss of neurons (**Box 5.9**).

❖ **Personality changes**: Lack of interest in day-to-day activities, taking longer to complete normal daily tasks, easy mental fatigability, self-centered, withdrawn, decreased self-care.
❖ **Memory impairment**: Recent memory is prominently affected.
❖ **Thought impairment**: Difficulty in understanding and expressing thoughts such as difficulty in speaking, reading and writing, using unusual words to refer to familiar objects, experiencing delusions.

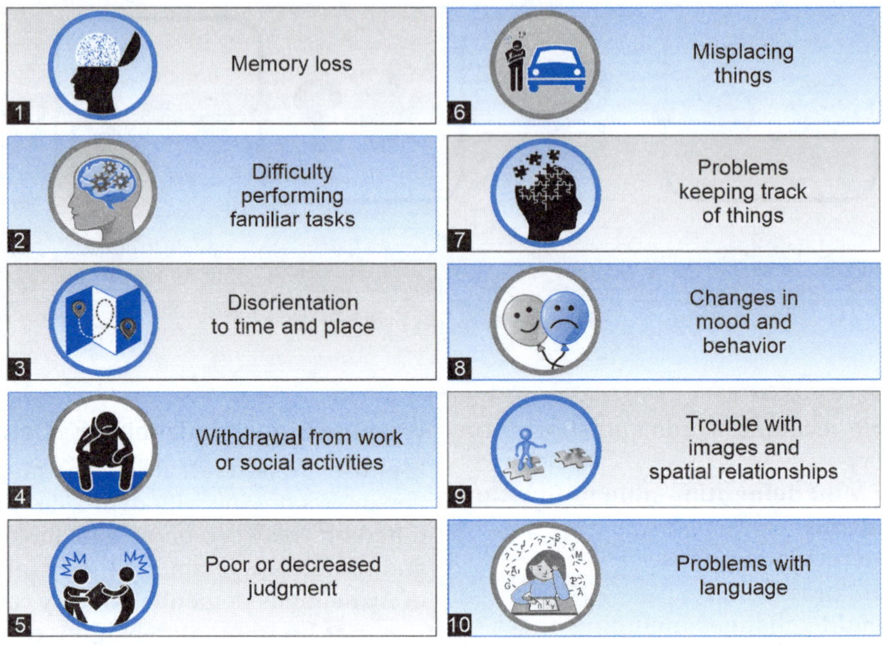

Figure 5.7: Warning signs of dementia

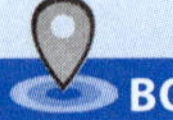

A 76-year-old man is referred to geriatric clinic with following complaints. His family members stated that there has been a gradual decline in memory over the past two years. Forgetfulness of the patient had progressed from subtle changes like forgetting where he kept his money or spectacles to his daily chores such as eating and bathing. History of slurred speech, slowness in performing daily activities, confusion, lack of concentration, decreased attention span, repeatedly asking same questions, unable to remember previous day issues and being withdrawn from family members. On examination he is conscious, alert, co-operative, and responsive to commands. MMSE score is 16/30. Cranial nerves, motor and sensory evaluation was within normal limits. No other pathologies were found on general examination.

❖ **Cognitive impairment**: Trouble handling money and paying bills, disorientation, confusion, poor judgment, difficulty in abstraction, decreased attention span.

❖ **Affective impairment**: Labile mood, irritableness, depression, not caring about other people's feelings.

❖ **Perceptual impairment**: Hallucinations

❖ **Behavioral impairment**: Stereotyped behavior, alteration in sexual drives and activities, wandering and getting lost in a familiar neighborhood, repeating questions, acting impulsively, losing balance and problems with movement.

❖ **Neurological impairment**: Aphasia, apraxia, agnosia, seizures, headache.

❖ **Catastrophic reaction**: Agitation, attempt to compensate for defects and avoid demonstrating failures in intellectual performances by indulging in activities such as changing the subject, cracking jokes or otherwise diverting the interviewer.

❖ **Sundowner syndrome**: It is characterized by drowsiness, confusion, ataxia; accidental falls may occur at night when external stimuli such as light and interpersonal orienting cues are diminished.

Course and Prognosis

Insidious onset but slow progressive deterioration occurs. Life expectancy of the people with this disease is reduced. The mean life expectancy following diagnosis is approximately 7 years. Men have a less favorable survival prognosis than women. Pneumonia and dehydration are the most frequent immediate causes of death.

Diagnosis

Following tests are used for diagnosis:

❖ **Cognitive and neurological tests**: These are used to evaluate thinking and physical functioning such as assessments of memory, problem solving, language skills and math skills as well as balance, sensory response and reflexes.

❖ **Functional dementia scale**: To assess severity of dementia.

❖ **Brain scan**: These tests identify strokes, tumors, brain structures and functions. These include CT scan, X-rays, magnetic resonance imaging (MRI), positron emission tomography (PET).

❖ **Cerebrospinal fluid analysis**: To measure the levels of proteins or other substances in CSF.

❖ **Psychiatric evaluation**: To evaluate behavioral and mood changes, recommended to determine depression and other symptoms.

❖ **Blood tests**: To measure the levels of beta-amyloid, a protein that is accumulated abnormally in people with Alzheimer's.

Treatment Modalities

❖ **Medications used in the treatment of Alzheimer's disease and other dementias are**:
  - *Cholinesterase inhibitors:* Inhibit the enzyme acetylcholinesterase in the CNS, increasing the level of acetylcholine. The drug may temporarily improve cognitive function and delay the worsening of symptoms in patients with Alzheimer's disease. Example, Donepezil and galantamine.
  - *N-Methyl d-aspartate receptor anta gonist:* It is NMDA receptor antagonist, used to delay the cognitive and behavioral symptoms. Example, Memantine
  - *Aducanumab-avwa (Aduhelm) and Lecanemab-irmab (Leqembi):* These two drugs are approved by the FDA to treat Alzheimer's disease. These are monoclonal antibodies that lessen the buildup of amyloid plaques in the brain.
  - Antipsychotic medications such as risperidone and haloperidol may be used to reduce verbal and physical aggressiveness, and alleviate hallucinations and delusions.
  - Benzodiazepines for insomnia and anxiety
  - Antidepressants for depression
  - Anticonvulsants to control seizures
  - Medicines to control blood pressure and cholesterol can prevent additional damage to the brain due to vascular dementia

❖ **Psychosocial interventions**:
  - Brief psychotherapy techniques such as reality orientation and memory retraining to aid patients during certain stages.
  - Other therapies helpful to retain certain skills include behavior therapy to maintain skills and to teach new skills, reminiscence therapy, validation therapy, supportive psychotherapy, cognitive oriented approach.

Nursing Management

Nursing care for patients of Alzheimer's disease is most important whether at home or in an acute hospital environment or a day-care center or in a long-term stay institution. Caregivers must be trained to promote patient's remaining intellectual abilities; help them maintain their independence in attending to their usual functions and avoid injuries; and provide for a good quality of life **(Figure 5.8)**.

Nursing Assessment

Assessment data for the patient with dementia should include a past health and medication history **(Box 5.10)**.

Nursing Interventions

1. **Maintain daily routine:** Maintaining a daily routine includes drawing up a fixed time table for the patient for waking up in the morning, toilet, exercise and meals. This gives the patient a sense of security.

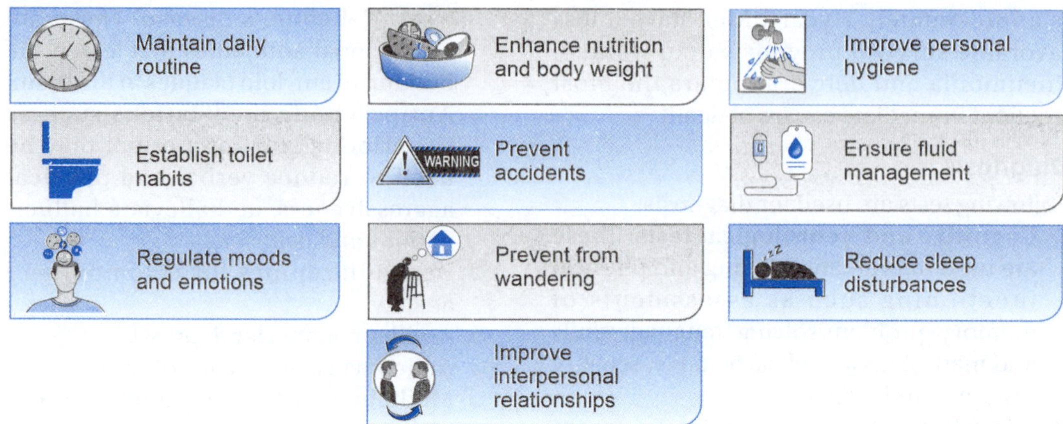

Figure 5.8: Nursing interventions for dementia patient

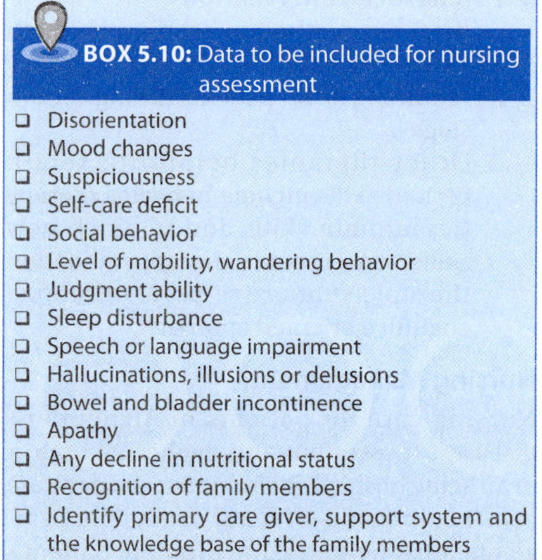

BOX 5.10: Data to be included for nursing assessment

- Disorientation
- Mood changes
- Suspiciousness
- Self-care deficit
- Social behavior
- Level of mobility, wandering behavior
- Judgment ability
- Sleep disturbance
- Speech or language impairment
- Hallucinations, illusions or delusions
- Bowel and bladder incontinence
- Apathy
- Any decline in nutritional status
- Recognition of family members
- Identify primary care giver, support system and the knowledge base of the family members

Patients often deteriorate after dark, a phenomenon known as 'sun downing'. Additional care must be taken during the evening and at night. Orient the patient to reality in order to reduce confusion; clocks with large faces aid in orientation to time. Use calendar with large writing and a separate page for each day. Provide newspapers which stimulate interest in current events. Orientation of place, person and time should be given before approaching the patient.

2. **Enhance nutrition and body weight:** Patient should be provided a well-balanced diet rich in protein and high in fiber with adequate amount of calories. Allow plenty of time for meals. Tell the patient which meal it is and what is there to eat; food served should neither be too hot nor too cold. Many patients have sugar craving. Care should be taken that such patients do not gain weight. The diet should take into account other medical illnesses which require diet modification such as diabetes or high blood pressure. Semi-solid diet is the safest while liquids are the most dangerous as these can be easily aspirated into the lungs.

3. **Improve personal hygiene:** Particular care should be taken about patient's personal hygiene which includes brushing of teeth, bathing, keeping the skin clean and dry particularly in areas prone to perspiration such as the armpits and groin. Caustic substances such as spirit or antiseptic solutions should not be used routinely on the skin. Remember to check finger and toe nails regularly and cut them if the person cannot do it by himself.

People with dementia may have a problem with the lock on the bathroom door; if this happens it is advisable to remove the lock.

Compliment the patient when he/she looks good.

4. **Establish toilet habits to reduce incontinence:** Toilet habits should be established as soon as possible and maintained as a rigid routine. This includes conditioned behavior such as going for bowel movement immediately after a cup of tea. The patient should be taken to urinate at fixed intervals depending on the season and amount of fluid intake. Prostate trouble common in elderly men leads to discomfort as it causes urgency and frequency of urination particularly in winters. A doctor should check this.

Incontinence is very distressing to the patient and family. Once incontinence sets in, the undergarments, pants of the patient and the house in general start reeking of foul smell. Toilet habits established in healthy years must be maintained as long as possible by gently persuading the patient to go to the toilet and use it. When the first sign of incontinence appears doctor should check for an underlying cause if any, such as urinary infection or urinary tract damage.

Constipation is a frequent cause of discomfort to the patient. The quantity of feces passed each morning should be checked to ensure that the patient is not constipated.

Constipation can be avoided by adding fiber supplements and roughage to the diet on a daily basis.

5. **Prevention of accidents:** Great care should be taken to avoid accidents caused by tripping over furniture, falling down the stairs or slipping in the bathroom. The reasons for falling include loose and poorly fitting footwear and wrinkled carpets. Ideally, patients should be made to wear soft slip-on shoes with straps which fit securely. Any floor covering must be firmly secured.

In modern cities most people including the older ones are dependent on their personal cars for transportation. Once early signs of the disease appear, patients should be gently persuaded to stop driving as this can pose a hazard to them and others.

Make sure that lights are bright enough. Keep matches, bleach, and paints out of reach. Do not allow the patient to take medication alone.

6. **Ensure fluid management:** Patients require as much fluid as normal people and this depends on the season. Ideally, sufficient fluid should be given during the day and only the minimum essential amount of fluid (some water with dinner) after 6 PM. The last cup of tea should be given around 5 PM. After that no beverages, including tea, coffee, cocoa or any other caffeine containing drinks should be given as all these promote urination. Proper fluid management will reduce bed-wetting and also reduce the number of times the patient will need to get up during the night.

7. **Regulate moods and emotions:** Some patients of Alzheimer's disease have abrupt change in their moods and emotions. These changes can be unpredictable. Mood changes are best controlled by keeping a calm environment with fixed daily routine. The patients should not be questioned repeatedly or given too many choices such as what they want to eat or what they want to wear. Mood changes are also amenable to distraction particularly if topics related to the past are discussed or favorite pieces of music played. For example, if music that reminds the patients of their childhood is played, the pleasant associations put them in a nostalgic mood. If patient behavior and emotions are distressing to the family members, the doctor may prescribe some medications to calm the patient.

8. **Prevent from wandering:** Patients of Alzheimer's disease often lose their geographic orientation and get lost even in familiar surroundings. They may be

found wandering aimlessly either in the neighborhood or far away. It is advisable to have some identification bracelet or card always in their possession. The doors of the house should be securely locked so that the patients cannot leave unnoticed. The patient should always be accompanied while going for walks or for simple chores outside the house.

9. **Reduce sleep disturbances:** Sleep disturbances are extremely distressing to the family. If the patient is restless at night or wanders and talks at night, the entire family is disturbed. Sleep patterns must be maintained. Napping during the day should be avoided. Sleeping pills are best avoided as their effect is temporary and frequently unpredictable in patients of Alzheimer's disease. Causes of discomfort at night such as pain, uncomfortable temperature or prostate trouble should be checked.

10. **Improve Interpersonal relationship:** Verbal communication should be clear and unhurried. Questions that require 'yes' or 'no' answers are best. Reinforce socially acceptable skills. Give necessary information repeatedly. Focus on things the person does well rather than on mistakes or failures. Try to make sure that each day has something of interest for the patient—it might be going for a walk, listening to music; talk about the day's activities. Try to involve him with old friends for a chat, reminiscing about the past.

Follow-Up, Homecare and Rehabilitation

Programs and services for patients with dementia and their families have increased with the growing awareness of Alzheimer's disease. Home care is available through home health agencies, public health agencies and visiting nurses. These services offer assistance with bathing, medication management and transportation as well as with other support. Residential facilities are available for patients who do not have home caregivers or whose needs have progressed beyond the care that could be provided at home. These patients usually require assistance with activities of daily living such as eating and taking medications.

Role of the Caregiver

Caregivers need to know about dementia and the required patient care, as well as how the patient care should change as the disease progresses. Many caregivers have other demands on their time such as their own families, careers, and personal lives. Caregivers must deal with their feelings of loss and grief as the health of their loved ones continually declines.

Caring for patients with dementia can be emotionally and physically exhausting and stressful. Caregivers may need to drastically change their own lives such as quitting a job to provide care. Role strain is identified when the demands of providing care threaten to overwhelm a caregiver.

Supporting the caregivers is an important component of providing care at home to patients with dementia. Caregivers need outlets for dealing with their own feelings. Support groups can help them to express frustration, sadness, anger, guilt or ambivalence. All these feelings are common. Nurses should offer hope to the family and avoid false reassurance when possible. Teach the family/caregiver strategies that promote patient's existing memory. For example, reminiscence activities, environmental cues, familiar songs, pictures, pets, etc.

Rehabilitative Services

Alzheimer's associations around the world provide practical and emotional help and information to families, healthcare professionals and the community. Alzheimer's and Related Disorders Society of India (ARDSI) started in 1992, a national organization dedicated to dementia care, support and research. World Alzheimer's Day is celebrated on September 21st every year.

SCHIZOPHRENIC DISORDER

The word 'Schizophrenia' was coined by the Swiss psychiatrist Eugen Bleuler in 1908. It is derived from the Greek words skhizo (split) and phren (mind).

Schizophrenia is a long-term mental health condition characterized by disturbances in thought (delusions), perception (hallucinations) and behavior (disorganized behavior) by a loss of emotional responsiveness and extreme apathy and noticeable deterioration in the level of functioning in everyday life.

Schizophrenia is a chronic, severe mental disorder that affects the way a person thinks, acts, expresses emotions, perceives reality and relates to others.

Schizophrenia is characterized by disturbances in multiple modalities including thinking, perception, cognition, volition, affect and behavior.

Prevalence and incidence

Prevalence includes both old and new cases while incidence refers to new cases arising from healthy individuals.

- According to Global burden of disease 2019, Schizophrenia affects approximately 24 million people or 1 in 300 people (0.36%) worldwide. This rate is 1 in 222 people (0.45%) among adults.
- According to the global burden of disease study 1990–2017, in 2017 there were 197.3 million people with mental disorders in India, comprising 14.3% of the total population of the country. Mental disorders contributed 4.7% (3.7–5.6) of the total disability-adjusted life-years (DALYs). The crude prevalence rate of schizophrenia was 0·3%.
- Schizophrenia affects approximately 1% of adults.
- Men are slightly more likely to be diagnosed and have an earlier onset than women.
- Onset is most often during late adolescence. The peak ages of onset are 15–25 years for men and 25 to 35 years for women. About two-thirds of cases are in the age group of 15–30 years.
- It is prevalent in all cultures across the world. About 15% of new admissions in mental hospitals are schizophrenic patients. It has been estimated that patients diagnosed as having schizophrenia occupy 50% of all mental hospital beds.

Etiology

The exact cause of schizophrenia is unknown. Several studies suggest that multiple factors are responsible for causation of schizophrenia **(Figure 5.9)**.

Biological Theories

Biological explanations include biochemical, neurostructural, genetic and perinatal risk factors.

Biochemical Theories

- Many studies hypothesize the functional increase of dopamine at the postsynaptic receptor.
- Other neurotransmitters probably involved are serotonin and alpha-adrenergic hyperactivity or glutaminergic and GABA hypoactivity.

Neurostructural Theories

- Research has found abnormal brain structure in people with schizophrenia.
- Computed tomography and magnetic resonance imaging (MRI) studies of brain structure show enlarged ventricles and mild cortical atrophy in some patients of schizophrenia.
- Positron emission tomography scan shows hypofrontality and decreased glucose utilization in the dominant temporal lobe.

Genetic Theories

- Schizophrenia can run in families.
- The disease is more common among people born of consanguineous marriages.

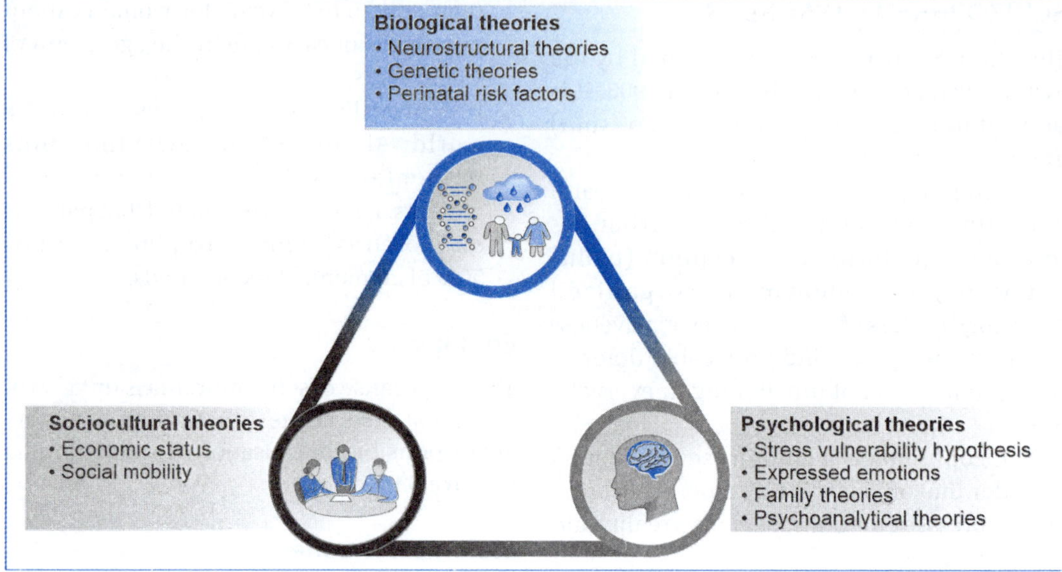

Figure 5.9: Etiology of schizophrenia

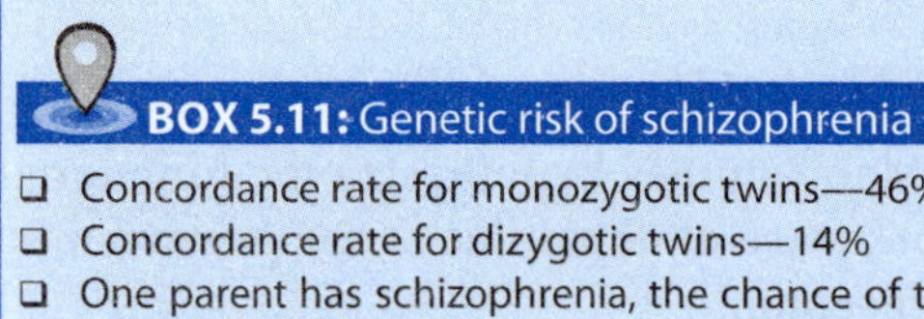

BOX 5.11: Genetic risk of schizophrenia

- Concordance rate for monozygotic twins—46%
- Concordance rate for dizygotic twins—14%
- One parent has schizophrenia, the chance of the child developing schizophrenia—10–12%
- Both the parents have schizophrenia, the chance of the child developing schizophrenia—40%
- First degree relatives have schizophrenia, the chance of developing schizophrenia—8–10%
- Second degree relatives have schizophrenia, the chance of developing schizophrenia—3%
- Third degree relatives have schizophrenia, the chance of developing schizophrenia—2%
- General population—0.5–1% (no affected relative)

❖ Studies show that relatives of schizophrenics have a much higher probability of developing the disease than the general population **(Box 5.11)**.

Perinatal Risk Factors

Following factors are associated with an increased risk of developing schizophrenia in people whose genes make them more likely to get the disorder.

❖ Gestational diabetes
❖ Pre-eclampsia

❖ Abnormal fetal development and low birth weight
❖ Birth complications
❖ Maternal malnutrition and vitamin deficiency
❖ Winter births and urban residence
❖ Viral infections, exposure to toxins like marijuana

Psychological Theories

Psychological explanation includes stress vulnerability hypothesis, expressed emotions, family theories, and psychoanalytical theories.

Stress Vulnerability Hypothesis

❖ According to this theory increased number of stressful life events before the onset or relapse probably has a triggering effect on the onset of schizophrenia among genetically vulnerable individuals.
❖ Stressful life events can precipitate the disease in predisposed individuals.
❖ Higher the genetic vulnerability in a person, lessor the environmental stress needed to precipitate a relapse.

Expressed Emotions

Increased expressed emotions such as hostility, critical comments, emotional over-involvement of significant others in the family can lead to an early relapse.

Family Theories

❖ Several early theories have been advocated in the past but are currently of doubtful value. Some of these theories were unfortunately responsible for arousing a sense of unnecessary guilt in parents for causation of schizophrenia in their children.

❖ These include schizophrenic mother (cold, over protective and domineering), lack of real parents, dependency on mother, anxious mother, parental marital schism or skew (hostility between parents), double blind theory (parents convey two or more conflicting and incompatible messages at the same time).

Psychoanalytical Theories

❖ According to Freud there is regression to the oral stage of psychosexual development with the use of defense mechanisms of denial, projection and reaction formation.

❖ The individuals have poor ego boundaries, ambivalent relationships and arrested psychosexual development.

Sociocultural Theories

Sociocultural explanation includes economic and social mobility.

Economic Status

Some studies show that schizophrenia was found to be more common in people with very lower socioeconomic status.

Social Mobility

Higher rates of schizophrenia have been found among some migrants.

Clinical Manifestations

According to ICD-11, schizophrenia and other primary psychotic disorders are characterized by significant impairment in reality testing and alterations in behavior. They manifest in:

❖ Positive symptoms such as persistent delusions, persistent hallucinations, disorganized thinking, grossly disorganized behavior and experiences of passivity and control.

❖ Negative symptoms such as blunted or flat affect and avolition and psychomotor disturbances.

❖ Symptoms occurring with sufficient frequency and intensity to deviate from expected cultural or subcultural norms.

❖ Symptoms not arising as a feature of another mental and behavioral disorder. Schizophrenia symptoms are classified into positive, negative and cognitive symptoms **(Figure 5.10).**

❖ **Positive symptoms** are those which cause an excess or distortion of normal function including:
  ○ *Delusions:* Delusions can be paranoid (beliefs of persecution), somatic (false beliefs about physical illness), grandiose (belief of self-importance and having special powers or abilities; belief that one is especially very powerful, rich, born with a special mission in life); delusion of reference (being referred to by others); delusion of control (being controlled by an external force).
  ○ *Hallucinations:* Most commonly auditory or visual characterized by experiences when there are no external stimuli.
  ○ *Disorganized speech and behavior:* Aggression, agitation, odd behavior.
  ○ *Thought disorders:* Thoughts can be blocked or withdrawn from the mind by others.
  ○ *Ideas of reference:* Occurs when a person believes that certain external phenomena such as TV, radio or newspaper articles are reporting about them or talking directly to them (ideas of reference can also be considered delusions if there are beliefs that external happenings relate directly to the individual).

❖ **Negative symptoms** are those that lead to a decrease or loss of normal function including:
  ○ Lack of emotions or restricted range and intensity of emotions (affective flattening)
  ○ Poor or non-existent social functioning
  ○ Lack of motivation, lack of initiative, less energy, withdrawal from family, friends

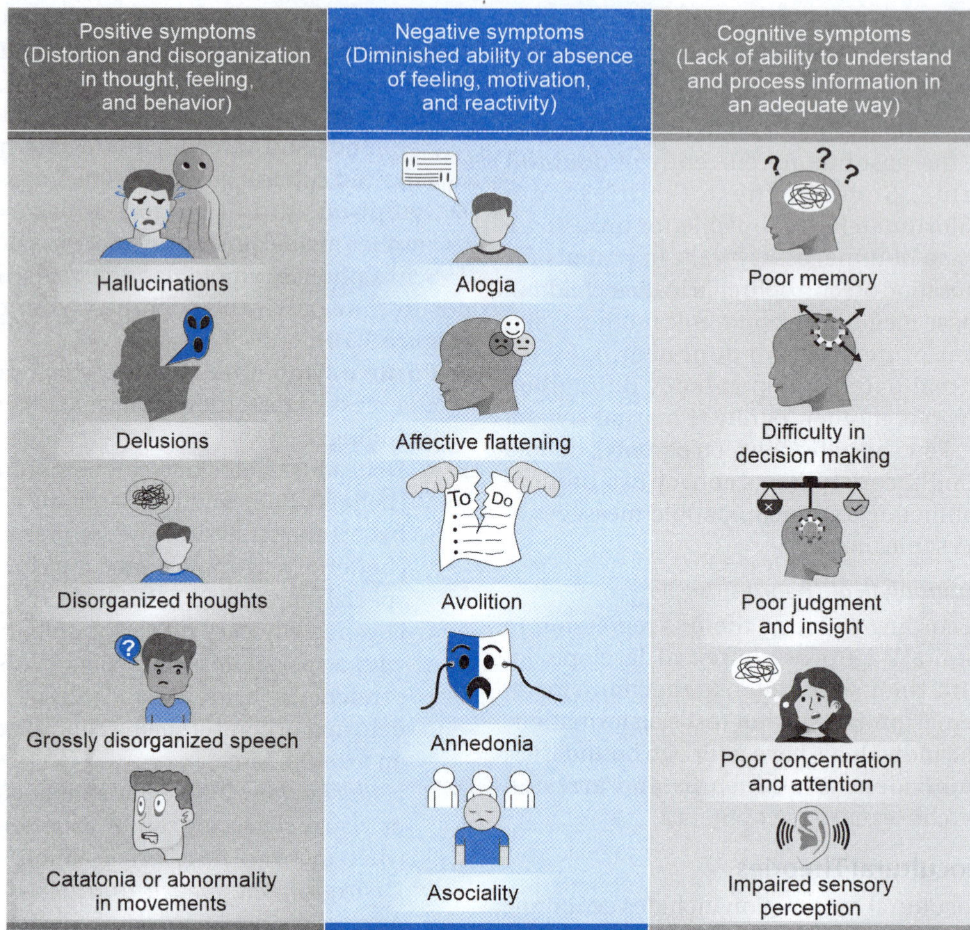

Figure 5.10: Positive, negative and cognitive symptoms of schizophrenia

and social activities, slow movements (avolition)

- Loss of pleasure or interest in life (anhedonia)
- Reduced speech (alogia)
- Ambivalence and poor self-care
- It is common for people with schizophrenia to lack insight to such an extent that they do not believe they are ill.

❖ **Cognitive symptoms** are nonspecific and hence must be severe enough for another individual to notice them. These include:

- Problems in attention, concentration and memory
- Having trouble processing information to make decisions

❖ Having trouble using information immediately after learning it

> 📍 **BOX 5.12:** Bleuler's four A's
>
> ❑ *Associative looseness*: Inability to think logically, stringing together of unrelated topics
> ❑ *Affective disturbance*: Inability to show appropriate emotional responses (inappropriate), blunted or flattened affect
> ❑ *Ambivalence*: Contradictory or opposing emotions, attitudes, ideas or desires for the same person, thing or situation simultaneously
> ❑ *Autistic thinking*: Thought process in which the individual is unable to relate to others or to the environment. Preoccupation with the self, with little concern for external reality

Eugene Bleuler (1857–1939) defined the main symptoms of the disease as Bleuler's 4A's: associations, affect, ambivalence and autism **(Box 5.12).**

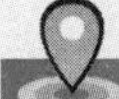

BOX 5.13: Schneider's first-rank symptoms of schizophrenia (SFRS)

- Hearing one's thoughts spoken aloud (audible thoughts or thought echo)
- Hallucinatory voices in the form of statement and reply (patient hears voices discussing him in the third person)
- Hallucinatory voices in the form of a running commentary (voices commenting on one's action)
- Thought withdrawal (thoughts cease and subject experiences them as removed by an external force)
- Thought insertion (subject experiences thoughts imposed by some external force on his passive mind)
- Thought broadcasting (subject experiences that his thoughts are escaping the confines of his self and are being experienced by others around)
- Delusional perception (normal perception has a private and illogical meaning)
- Somatic passivity (bodily sensations especially sensory symptoms are experienced as imposed on body by some external force)
- Made volition or acts (one's own acts are experienced as being under the control of some external force, the subject being like a robot)
- Made impulses (the subject experiences impulses as being imposed by some external force)
- Made feelings or affect (the subject experiences feelings as being imposed by some external force)

Kurt Schneider proposed the first rank symptoms of schizophrenia in 1959. The presence of even one of these symptoms is considered to be strongly suggestive of schizophrenia **(Box 5.13)**.

Predominant clinical features in acute schizophrenia are delusions, hallucinations and interference with thinking. Features of this kind are often called positive symptoms or psychotic features. While most of the patients recover from acute illness, some progress to the chronic phase during which time the main features are negative symptoms. Once the chronic syndrome is established few patients recover completely **(Box 5.14)**.

Course and Prognosis

The classic course is one of exacerbations and remissions. In general, schizophrenia has been described as the most crippling

BOX 5.14: Case vignette—Schizophrenia

Mr Ravi, a 24-year-old male, studying BA final year, resides in village, came to psychiatric OPD with the following complaints. Talking and behaving strangely since 2 months, restless and hostile towards family members, abuses and assaults family members whenever he gets irritated, talking to self and muttering to self, unduly suspicious towards family members, decreased sleep, appetite, poor self-care and not attending college since 2 months. On enquiry he believes that people stare at him and watch his actions. He believes that few of his relatives are trying to harm and kill him. He also informed that he is hearing voices when no one is around, hears the conversations of people who are against him. He hears his own thoughts as if somebody is shouting from somewhere. At other times he can hear a running commentary of his own actions. Because of these experiences, he is scared to move around.

and devastating of all psychiatric illnesses. Prognostic factors of schizophrenia are presented in **Table 5.2.**

TABLE 5.2: Prognostic factors in schizophrenias

Good prognostic factors	Poor prognostic factors
Abrupt or acute onset	Insidious onset
Later onset	Younger onset
Presence of precipitating factor	Absence of precipitating factor
Good premorbid personality	Poor premorbid personality
Paranoid and catatonic subtypes	Simple, undifferentiated subtypes
Short duration: <6 months	Long duration: >2 years
Predominance of positive symptoms	Predominance of negative symptoms
Family history of mood disorders	Family history of schizophrenia
Good social support	Poor social support
Female sex	Male sex
Married	Single, divorced or widowed
Out patient treatment	Institutionalization

Investigations

- ❖ No diagnostic test definitively confirms schizophrenia. Tests may be ordered to rule out disorders that cause psychosis including vitamin deficiencies, uremia, thyrotoxicosis and electrolyte imbalances.
- ❖ CT scan and MRI show enlarged ventricles, enlargement of the sulci on the cerebral surface and atrophy of the cerebellum.

Treatment Modalities

Schizophrenia requires long-term treatment. Medications and psychosocial therapy can control the symptoms effectively. In some cases, hospitalization may be required.

Pharmacotherapy

An acute episode of schizophrenia typically responds to treatment with antipsychotic agents which are most effective in its treatment. Conventional antipsychotics are now used less frequently because of their partial efficacy and adverse effects. Some non-compliant patients may receive fluphenazine or haloperidol depot formulations. These are long-acting IM doses that release the drug gradually over several weeks **(Box 5.15)**.

Atypical antipsychotics control wider range of signs and symptoms than conventional agents do and cause few or no adverse motor affects **(Box 5.16)**.

Other drugs which are used in the treatment of schizophrenia are antidepressants, mood stabilizers, benzodiazepines, etc. (*Refer Appendix 25 for detailed description of these drugs*).

Electroconvulsive Therapy (ECT)

Indications for ECT in schizophrenia include:
- ❖ Drug resistant patients

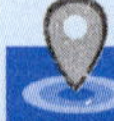

BOX 5.15: Conventional antipsychotics

- ❑ **Chlorpromazine:** 300–1500 mg/day PO; 50–100 mg/day IM
- ❑ **Fluphenazine decanoate:** 25–50 mg IM every 1–3 weeks
- ❑ **Haloperidol:** 5–100 mg/day PO; 5–20 mg/day IM
- ❑ **Trifluoperazine:** 15–60 mg/day PO; 1–5 mg/day IM

BOX 5.16: Commonly used atypical antipsychotics

- ❑ **Clozapine:** 25–450 mg/day PO
- ❑ **Risperidone:** 2–10 mg/day PO
- ❑ **Olanzapine:** 10–20 mg/day PO
- ❑ **Quetiapine:** 150–750 mg/day PO
- ❑ **Ziprasidone:** 20–80 mg/day PO
- ❑ **Aripiprazole:** 10–15 mg/day PO
- ❑ **Paliperidone:** 1.5–12 mg/day PO
- ❑ **Amisulpride:** 400–800 mg/day PO

- ❖ Schizophrenia patients with catatonia, aggression or suicidal behavior
- ❖ ECT combined with pharmacotherapy is a viable option for selected patients

Psychosocial Therapies

Commonly used psychosocial therapies are as follows:

- ❖ **Group therapy:** Social interaction, sense of cohesiveness, identification, and reality testing achieved within the group setting have proven to be highly therapeutic for these individuals.
- ❖ **Behavior therapy:** Behavior therapy is useful in reducing the frequency of bizarre, disturbing and deviant behavior, and increasing appropriate behaviors.
- ❖ **Social skills training:** Social skills training addresses behaviors such as poor eye contact, odd facial expressions and lack of spontaneity in social situations through the use of videotapes, role playing and homework assignments.
- ❖ **Cognitive therapy:** Used to improve cognitive distortions like reducing distractibility and correcting judgment.
- ❖ **Family therapy:** Family therapy typically consists of a brief family education about schizophrenia. It has been found that relapse rates of schizophrenia are higher in families with high expressed emotions (EE) where significant others make critical comments, express hostility or show emotional over-involvement. The significant others are therefore taught to lower expectations and family tensions apart from being given social skills training

to enhance communication and problem solving.

- ❖ **Psychosocial rehabilitation**: This includes activity therapy to develop the work habit, training in a new vocation or retraining in a previous skill, vocational guidance and independent job placement.

Nursing Management

Nursing management for schizophrenia includes assessing symptoms, establishing rapport, enhancing communication, improving general and social functioning level, promoting medication compliance and educating family members.

Nursing Assessment

Data may be obtained from patient, family members, other people familiar with the patient and also from old records. Nursing assessment includes information regarding any previous incidence of mental illness or psychotic episodes.

- ❖ Observe behavior pattern, posturing, psychomotor disturbance, appearance, hygiene.
- ❖ Identify the type of disturbance the patient is experiencing.
- ❖ Ask the patient about feelings while thought alterations are evident.
- ❖ Note the effect and emotional tone of the patient and whether they are appropriate in relation to the thought or present situation.
- ❖ Assess for theme and content of delusional thinking. If the delusion is persecution oriented, assess the nature of threat and risk for violence.
- ❖ Assess speech patterns associated with delusions.
- ❖ Assess for ability to perform self-care activity, i.e., sleep pattern and interaction with other patients.
- ❖ Determine any suicidal intent or recent attempts that may have been made **(Table 5.3)**.

Nursing diagnosis I
Disturbed thought process related to inability to trust, panic anxiety, possible hereditary or

TABLE 5.3: Objective signs and subjective symptoms of schizophrenia

Objective signs	Subjective symptoms
• Withdrawal behavior • Hostility • Inadequate or inappropriate communication/speech • Inadequate food and fluid intake • Psychomotor agitation • Catatonic rigidity • Stereotype behavior • Apathy • Ambivalence • Mutism • Inability to trust others	• Hallucination • Illusions • Paranoid thinking • Anhedonia • Confusion • Ideas of reference • Thought blocking • Retarded thinking • Insomnia

biochemical factors evidenced by delusional thinking, extreme suspiciousness of others.

Objectives: The patient will
- ❖ Eliminate pattern of delusional thinking
- ❖ Demonstrate trust in others
- ❖ Demonstrate decreased anxiety level
- ❖ Demonstrate improved reality orientation

Interventions: See **Table 5.4**.

Barriers to successful intervention
- ❖ Becoming anxious
- ❖ Focusing on delusions
- ❖ Attempting to prove the patient wrong
- ❖ Setting unrealistic goals

Nursing diagnosis II
Ineffective health maintenance related to inability to trust, extreme suspiciousness evidenced by inadequate food and fluid intake, difficulty in falling asleep.

Objectives: The patient will
- ❖ Maintain adequate nutrition, hydration and elimination
- ❖ Maintain adequate sleep and rest
- ❖ Take medication as administered

Interventions: See **Table 5.5**.

TABLE 5.4: Nursing interventions for delusional behavior

Nursing interventions	Rationale
Assess the content of delusion without appearing to probe	Provides baseline data to plan accurate care
Initially clarify meanings, for example, "Who do you think is trying to hurt you?"	Provides baseline data to plan accurate care
Assess the intensity, frequency and duration of delusion	Provides baseline data to plan accurate care
Assess the context and environmental triggers for the delusional experience	Helps to reduce environmental triggering factors
Approach the patient with calmness, empathy and gentle eye contact	Non-verbal nursing approaches foster the development of trust between nurse and the patient
When patients are suspicious they may be afraid of everyone, everything and every interaction around them. The nurse must communicate clearly and directly with simple statements	This communication improves patient's understanding
Misinterpretations of patients are clarified, arguments are avoided	Arguing with a patient about delusion is ineffective, inappropriate and may strengthen patient's beliefs
Distract the patient from delusions that tend to exacerbate aggressive or potentially violent episodes. Promote activities that require attention to physical skills and will help the patient use time constructively	Engaging the patient in constructive activities increases the reality base and decreases the risk for violent episodes that are provoked by delusions
Careful monitoring is required if the delusions lead patients to harm themselves or others	Early intervention may prevent aggressive response to delusions
Discourage long discussions about their irrational thinking. Instead talk about real events and real people	Discussions that focus on false ideas are purposeless and useless and may even aggravate the condition
Following interventions will help highly suspicious patients: • Use the same staff as far as possible • Be honest and keep all the promises • Avoid physical contact in the form of touching the patient • Avoid laughing, whispering or talking quietly where the patient can see but cannot hear what is being said • Avoid competent activities • Use assertive, matter-of-fact yet friendly approach	Promotes trust, prevents the patient from feeling threatened
Encourage the patient to express feelings as much as possible	Provides relief from stress
Patient's participation is encouraged in providing care but not forced	This increases feelings of self-worth and facilitates trust
Educate the patient and family or significant others about patient's symptoms, importance of medication compliance, and follow up visits	This will facilitate learning and increase knowledge base, ensure the patient's continued treatment and prevent relapse after discharge from the hospital

TABLE 5.5: Nursing interventions to improve health

Nursing interventions	Rationale
Assess for malnutrition and dehydration	If patient's delusions are related to food they may refuse to eat because the patient believes that the food is poisoned
Monitor food and fluid intake	Patient's physiological problems are first priority. The patient may be unaware of or may ignore his or her needs for food and fluids
Creative approaches may need to be followed with patients who are not eating, e.g., allowing them to take packed foods, fruits, eggs, etc.	To ensure patient's nutritional needs are met
Provide less stimulating environment (dim light, comfortable bed, less noise, etc.) to suspicious patients as they find it difficult to fall asleep due to nightmares or severe anxiety	Patient may feel more comfortable in less stimulating environment
Administer sedatives if needed	To facilitate normal sleep
Prevent day time naps by involving the patients actively in physical exercises or day treatment programs. Example, referral to rehabilitation programs, job training programs, sheltered workshops, etc.	To facilitate normal sleep pattern
If the patient is suspicious or is reluctant to take medications, allow the patient to open the sealed medication packet	Patient has an opportunity to see medications sealed in packages which may reduce suspicion
If toileting needs are not being met, establish a structured schedule for the patient	A structured schedule will help the patient establish a pattern so that he can develop a habit of toileting independently
Monitor patient's elimination patterns. If constipation occurs use medications to establish regularity	Constipation occurs frequently with use of major tranquilizers, decreased food and fluid intake and reduced level of activity

Nursing diagnosis III

Self-care deficit related to withdrawal, regression, panic anxiety, cognitive impairment, inability to trust evidenced by difficulty in carrying out tasks associated with hygiene, dressing, grooming, eating, sleeping and toileting.

Objectives: The patient will

❖ Demonstrate increased interest in self-care
❖ Complete daily activities with minimum assistance
❖ Demonstrate adequate personal hygiene skills

Interventions: See **Table 5.6.**

TABLE 5.6: Nursing interventions to improve self-care activities

Nursing interventions	Rationale
Assess patient's ability to meet self-care activities	Provides baseline data
Provide assistance with self-care needs as required. Some patients who are severely withdrawn may require total care	Patient's safety and comfort are nursing priorities. Good physical grooming can enhance confidence in social situation
Develop a structured schedule for patient's routine for hygiene, toileting, and meals	A structured schedule will help the patient establish a pattern so that he can develop a habit

Contd...

Contd...

Nursing interventions	Rationale
Encourage the patient to perform as many activities as possible independently	Independent accomplishment enhances self-esteem and promotes repetition of desirable behavior
Praise the patient for completing activities of daily living and initiating self-care activities	Positive reinforcement enhances self-esteem and promotes repetition of desirable behavior
Encourage wearing appropriate clothes for the setting	Appropriate clothing enhances confidence in social situations
Role model appropriate behavior and explain tasks in short simple steps	Short simple steps and role modeling are easier for the patient to perform activities
Allow the patient enough time to complete any task	It may take the patient longer to dress or comb his or her hair because of lack of concentration and short attention span
Withdraw assistance gradually and supervise the patient's grooming or other self-care skills	It will improve patient's independence

Nursing diagnosis IV

Potential for violence, self-directed or at others, related to command hallucinations evidenced by physical violence, destruction of objects in the environment or self-destructive behavior.

Objectives: The patient will

❖ Not injure others or destroy property or self
❖ Verbalize feelings of anger or frustration
❖ Express lesser feeling of agitation, fear or anxiety

Interventions: See **Table 5.7.**

TABLE 5.7: Nursing interventions for violent behavior

Nursing interventions	Rationale
Maintain low level of stimulation (low lighting, low noise, few people, etc.) in patient's environment	Anxiety levels rise in a stimulating environment and may trigger aggression
Observe patient's behavior frequently	Close observation is necessary so that interventions can be provided to ensure patient's or other's safety
Remove all dangerous objects from patient's environment	To prevent the patient from using them to harm self or others in an agitated state
Provide a structured environment with scheduled routine activities of daily living	Lack of structure and unexplained changes usually increase agitation and anxiety. Structure enhances patient's security
Be alert for signs of increasing fear, anxiety or agitation so that we may intervene as early as possible and prevent harm to the patient or others	Earlier the intervention, easier it is to calm the patient and prevent harm
Do not use physical restraints or techniques without sufficient reason	Patient has the right to fewest restrictions possible within the limits of safety
Talk to the patient in a low calm voice	Using a low voice may help to calm the patient
Have sufficient staff available to indicate a show of strength to the patient if necessary	This provides the patient an evidence of control over the situation and physical security for the staff
Administer tranquilizers as prescribed.	If the patient is not calmed by 'talking down', use medications as prescribed

Contd...

Contd...

Nursing interventions	Rationale
Apply mechanical restraints safely for very short duration. Check extremities for color, temperature, and pulse distal to the restraints every 15 minutes	Mechanical restraints applied too tightly can impair circulation of blood
If necessary loosen the restraints one at a time to exercise limbs or change patient's position	The patient may continue to be agitated while in restraints. Loosening one restraint and reapplying it before loosening another can minimize chances of injury to self or others
Perform passive range of motion on restrained limbs and reposition the patient at least every 2 hourly	These actions minimize the deleterious effects of immobility
As agitation subsides encourage the patient to express his feelings	Expression of feelings reduce anxiety
Help the patient identify and practice ways to relieve anxiety such as deep breathing, meditation, listening to music, etc.	These activities reduce anxiety
Redirect violent behavior with physical outlets such as exercises	Physical exercise is a safe and effective way of relieving pent-up tension

Nursing diagnosis V

Risk for self-inflicted or life-threatening injury related to command hallucinations evidenced by suicidal ideas, plans or attempts.

Objective: Patient will not harm self.

Interventions: See **Table 5.8.**

TABLE 5.8: Nursing interventions to prevent self-harm

Nursing interventions	Rationale
Assess the nature and severity of hallucinations by asking the patient to describe	Provides information on risk for self directed behavior
Create a safe environment for the patient, remove all potentially harmful objects from patient's vicinity (sharp objects, straps, belts, glass items, alcohol, etc.)	Improves patient safety
Ask the patient directly, "Have you thought about harming yourself in any way? If so, what do you plan to do? Do you have the means to carry out this plan?"	The risk of suicide is greatly increased if the patient has developed a plan and if means exist for the patient to execute it
Keep the patient near nurses station	To improve patient safety
Do not allow the patient to put the bolt on his side of the door of bathroom or toilet	To improve patient safety

Nursing diagnosis VI

Disturbed sensory-perception (auditory/ visual) related to panic anxiety, possible hereditary or biochemical factors evidenced by inappropriate responses, disordered thought sequencing, poor concentration, disorientation, withdrawn behavior.

Objectives: The patient will
❖ Demonstrate decreased hallucinations
❖ Interact with others
❖ Verbalize plans to deal with hallucinations, if they recur

Interventions: See **Table 5.9.**

TABLE 5.9: Nursing interventions for hallucinatory behavior

Nursing interventions	Rationale
Nurse should be tolerant, show acceptance and use active listening skills	To establish trusting, interpersonal relationship
Assess for type of hallucinations and characteristics of hallucinations	To determine whether hallucinations are command hallucinations that direct the patient to hurt him or others
Ask what voices are saying and whose voice it is. Avoid further discussion on hallucination to prevent reinforcing inappropriate behavior	To determine whether hallucinations are command hallucinations that direct the patient to hurt him or others
Observe the patient for hallucinating behavior like talking to self, laughing to self, stopping in mid sentence	Listening and observing are the key to successful intervention
Determine precipitating factors that may exacerbate patient's hallucinatory experience	Identifying stressors may help to prevent the severity of hallucinating experience
Interrupt hallucination by calling the patient by name or other distraction or move the patient to another area. Be alert to cues that patient is hallucinating	Reduced stimuli provides fewer opportunities for misperception
Help the patient understand the connection between anxiety and hallucinations	If a patient can learn to interrupt escalating anxiety, hallucinations may be prevented
Help the patient learn that he can dismiss hallucinations by humming or whistling or saying 'go away' or 'be quiet'	Helps in dealing with hallucinations
Provide a busy schedule of activity to prevent being all alone. Engage in conversation or a concrete activity of interest to the patient	When engaged in real activities and interactions it becomes much difficult for him to respond to hallucinations
Show acceptance of patient's behavior and of the patient as a person	Patient may need help to see that hallucinations are a part of the illness and not under his control
Listen actively to the patient's family/significant others allowing them to express fears and anxieties about mental illness, giving them support and empathy and emphasizing patient's strengths	Helps family members to respond adaptively to the difficult situation
Educate the patient and family/significant others about the patient's symptoms and importance of medication compliance	This will facilitate learning and improve the knowledge base of patient and family/significant others, ensure patient's continuity of treatment and prevent relapses after discharge

Nursing diagnosis VII

Social isolation related to inability to trust, panic anxiety, delusional thinking evidenced by withdrawal, sad, dull affect, preoccupation with own thoughts, expression of feelings of rejection of aloneness imposed by others.

Objective: Patient will voluntarily spend time with other patients and staff members in group activities on the unit.

Interventions: See **Table 5.10**.

Nursing diagnosis VIII

Impaired verbal communication related to panic anxiety, disordered, unrealistic thinking, evidenced by loosening of associations, echolalia, verbalizations that reflect concrete thinking and poor eye contact.

Objective: Patient will be able to communicate appropriately and comprehensibly by the time of discharge.

Interventions: See **Table 5.11**.

TABLE 5.10: Nursing interventions for withdrawn behavior

Nursing interventions	Rationale
Convey an accepting attitude by making brief, frequent contacts. Show unconditional positive regard	It increases feelings of self-worth and facilitates trust
Offer to be with the patient during group activities that he finds frightening or difficult. Involve the patient gradually in different activities on the unit	The presence of a trusted individual provides emotional security for the patient
Give recognition and positive reinforcement for the patient's voluntary interaction with others	Positive reinforcement enhances self-esteem and encourages repetition of acceptable behavior

TABLE 5.11: Nursing interventions for impaired verbal communication

Nursing interventions	Rationale
Attempt to decode incomprehensible communication pattern. Seek validation and clarification by stating, "Is it what you mean…?" or "I don't understand what you mean by that. Would you please clarify it for me?"	These techniques reveal how the patient is being perceived by others while the responsibility for not understanding is accepted by the nurse
Facilitate trust and understanding by maintaining staff assignments as consistently as possible. The techniques of verbalizing the implied is used with the patient who is mute (either unable or unwilling to speak). For example, 'That must have been a very difficult time for you when your mother left. You must have felt all alone	This approach conveys empathy and encourages the patient to disclose painful issues
Anticipate and fulfill patient's needs until functional communication pattern returns	Self-care ability may be impaired in some patients who may need assistance initially

Nursing diagnosis IX

Ineffective family coping related to highly ambivalent family relationships, impaired family communication evidenced by neglectful care of the patient, extreme denial or prolonged over-concern regarding his illness.

Objective: Family will identify more adaptive coping strategies for dealing with patient's illness and treatment regimen.

Interventions: See **Table 5.12**.

Evaluation

A few questions that may facilitate the process of evaluation can be

❖ Has the patient established trust with at least one staff member?

TABLE 5.12: Nursing interventions to improve family coping skills

Nursing interventions	Rationale
Identify role of the patient in the family and how it is affected by his illness. Identify the level of family functioning. Assess communication patterns, interpersonal relationships between the members, problem solving skills and availability of support systems	These factors will help to identify how successful the family is in dealing with stressful situations and areas where assistance is required

Contd…

Contd...

Nursing interventions	Rationale
Provide information to the family about patient's illness, treatment regimen, long-term prognosis	Knowledge and understanding about what to expect may facilitate the family's ability to successfully integrate the schizophrenic patient into the system
Practice with family members on how to respond to bizarre behavior and communication patterns and when the patient becomes violent	A plan of action will assist the family to respond adaptively in the face of what they may consider to be a crisis situation

- ❖ Is delusional thinking still prevalent?
- ❖ Are hallucinations still evident?
- ❖ Is the patient able to interact with others appropriately?
- ❖ Is the patient able to carry out all activities of daily living independently?

When evaluating the effectiveness of planned interventions, the nurse should look for signs that indicate improved functioning of the patient. These are:

- ❖ Communication with staff and other patients in an appropriate manner, reality based conversation which is an evidence of improved thinking process.
- ❖ Reduction in bizarre and inappropriate behavior which is evidence of improved thinking and perception.
- ❖ Reduced suspiciousness which is evidence of increased willingness to trust staff and other patients.
- ❖ Compliance with taking medications and increased food intake is evidence that the patient has lesser fear of poisoning.
- ❖ Expression of feelings is a positive step as they move towards identification of social support.
- ❖ Involvement in ward activities is a demonstration of their willingness to engage in the company of others.

MOOD DISORDERS

Mood is a state of feeling (emotional) usually temporary resulting from a specific stimulus. The word mood is derived from the ancient English word 'mod' which means 'courage' especially during times of war.

Mood disorders or affect disorders are described by marked disruptions in emotions, severe lows called depression or highs called mania. These are common psychiatric disorders leading to an increase in morbidity and mortality.

Meaning

Mood disorders are characterized by a disturbance of mood accompanied by full or partial manic or depressive syndrome not due to any other physical or mental disorder. In mood disorders people experience extreme changes in mood such as extreme depression or extreme elation. At times both extremes can be observed in the same person.

Prevalence and Incidence

- ❖ The lifetime prevalence of bipolar disorder is about 4%.
- ❖ According to the global burden of disease study 1990–2017, the crude prevalence rate for depressive disorders was 3·3%, depressive disorders are ranked as the single largest contributor to nonfatal health loss affecting 4.4% of global population. In 2017, 45.7 million people suffered from depressive disorders in India. Bipolar disorders had prevalence of 0.6%.
- ❖ The mean age of onset of bipolar disorder is around 25 years. Men typically have an earlier age of onset than women (18 years in men and 20 years in women).
- ❖ Women are more likely to experience many mood episodes in a given year compared to men.
- ❖ Two-thirds of bipolar patients have at least 1 close relative who was also diagnosed with the disease or with unipolar depression.

Manic Episode

❖ Acute mania is the manic phase of bipolar I disorder. It refers to a syndrome in which the central features are mood change (which may be towards elation or irritability), overactivity and self-important ideas.

❖ According to ICD-11 all manic and hypomanic episodes require as defining features lasting at least one week, characterized by euphoria, irritability or expansiveness, mood lability, impulsivity, subjective experience of increased energy, increase in goal-directed activity, rapid or pressured speech, flight of ideas (racy thoughts), distractibility, increased self-esteem or grandiosity, decreased need for sleep, impulsive reckless behavior, increase in sexual drive, sociability or goal-directed activity. Mania must be distinguished from heightened energy and altered functioning that arises from substance use, medical condition or other cause.

❖ The lifetime risk of manic episode is about 0.8–1%. This disorder occurs in episodes lasting usually 3–4 months, followed by complete recovery.

❖ Men and women are equally likely to be affected.

Etiology

The cause is a combination of neurochemical, genetic, psychological and environmental factors **(Figure 5.11)**.

1. Neurochemicals

The neurochemicals serotonin and norepinephrine have an effect on mood. Manic episodes are related to excessive levels of norepinephrine and dopamine, an imbalance between cholinergic and noradrenergic systems or a deficiency in serotonin.

2. Genetic Considerations

There have been multiple studies involving families which show a definite genetic component. The American Psychiatric Association reports that 80–90% of people with bipolar disorder have a relative who is suffering with either depression or bipolar

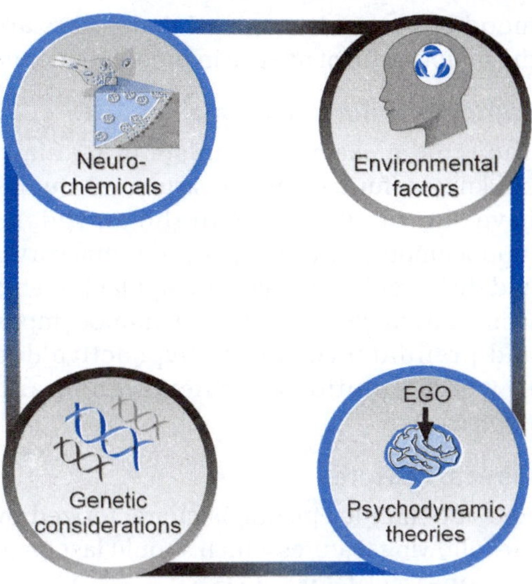

Figure 5.11: Etiology of manic episode

disorder. Factors that influence likelihood of developing bipolar disorder include:

❖ Family history of depression

❖ Family history of schizophrenia

❖ Family members with bipolar disorder
  ○ Monozygotic (identical) twins have a higher concordance rate than normal siblings and other close relatives. Siblings and close relatives have a higher concordance rate of manic-depressive illness than the general population. Cyclothymic characteristics are common among family members of bipolar patients.
  ○ *First degree relative*: 5–10% chance
  ○ *Identical twin with bipolar disorders*: About 40–70% chance

3. Psychodynamic Theories

Developmental theorists have hypothesized that faulty family dynamics during early life are responsible for manic behaviors in later life. Another psychodynamic hypothesis explains manic episodes as a defense against or denial of depression.

4. Environmental Factors

Studies of life events have found that bipolar individuals experience increased stressful events prior to first onset and recurrences of mood episodes. Psychosocial stressors are the major cause of relapse in bipolar patients.

Pathophysiology of Mania

Though the exact mechanism of mania is not known, functional and structural studies have shown alterations in the amygdala, hippocampus, basal ganglia, prefrontal cortex and the anterior cingulate. In bipolar patients while amygdala is hyperactive, hippocampus and prefrontal cortex are hypoactive due to which emotions are heightened and unrestricted.

Clinical Features

An acute manic episode is characterized by the following features which should last for at least one week **(Box 5.17)**:

Elevated, Expansive or Irritable Mood

❖ Elevated mood in mania has four stages depending on the severity of manic episodes: euphoria, elation, exaltation, ecstasy **(Box 5.18)**.

❖ Expansive mood is an extreme expression of emotion which is characterized by inflated self-importance and exaggerated behaviors. Those exhibiting an expansive mood have unending and unselective enthusiasm for interacting with people and surrounding environment. They may act grandiose and superior. Sometimes irritable mood may be

> **BOX 5.17:** Case vignette—Manic episode
>
> Mrs Veena, 35-year-old housewife was admitted to the psychiatric unit with a diagnosis of manic episode. The nurse during admission procedure noted that Mrs Veena was having excessive makeup, eye shadow and lipstick. She wore many necklaces, applied nail polish for all fingers and toes. She was overactive and kept interacting with others. She was cheerful, jovial and unduly happy for no particular reason. Every time the nurse attempted to question her; she responded in a rapid, loud voice. The nurse noted that Mrs Veena was easily distracted and appeared to jump from one idea to another while talking. She also described herself as a MLA for local constituency. She was unable to sleep at night and complete ward activity therapies due to short attention span and distractibility.

> **BOX 5.18:** Four stages of elevated mood
>
> ❑ **Euphoria (Stage I):** Increased sense of psychological well-being and happiness not in keeping with ongoing events
> ❑ **Elation (Stage II):** Moderate elevation of mood with increased psychomotor activity
> ❑ **Exaltation (Stage III):** Intense elevation of mood with delusions of grandeur
> ❑ **Ecstasy (Stage IV):** Severe elevation of mood, intense sense of rapture or blissfulness seen in delirious or stuporous mania

predominant especially when the person is stopped from doing what he wants. There may be rapid, short-lasting shifts from euphoria to irritability or anger.

Psychomotor Activity

There is an increased psychomotor activity ranging from over activeness and restlessness to manic excitement. The individual involves in ceaseless activity with most activities being goal-oriented and based on external environment cues.

Speech and Thought

❖ **Flight of ideas**: Thoughts racing in mind, rapid shifts from one topic to another.

❖ **Pressure of speech**: Speech is forceful, strong and difficult to interrupt. Uses playful language with punning, rhyming, joking, teasing and speaks loudly.

❖ **Clang association**: These are ideas that are related only by similar or rhyming sounds rather than actual meaning.

❖ **Grandiose delusions**: Many patients endorse grandiose delusions believing they are high-level operatives such as members of parliament, IAS officers, etc.

❖ **Other delusions**: Some of the most common delusions are delusions of paranoia with patients believing that people are targeting or following them.

❖ **Distractibility**: In mania selective attention function apparently deteriorates, individual focus on inappropriate and irrelevant stimuli and focus over important data are lost.

Other Features

- During manic phase many patients engage in goal-directed activities that may result in harmful consequences such as spending excessive money, starting businesses, traveling or promiscuity.
- High-risk activities (buying sprees, reckless driving, foolish business investments, distributing money or articles to unknown persons).
- Many patients may involve in property damage or even harm themselves or others through verbal or physical assault.
- Increased sociability
- Impulsive behavior, highly aggressive and agitated
- Disinhibition
- Hypersexual and promiscuous behavior
- Poor judgment
- Dressed up in gaudy and flamboyant clothes although in severe mania, there may be poor self-care
- Decreased need for sleep (<3 hours)
- Decreased food intake due to over-activity
- Decreased attention and concentration
- Absent insight, may not recognize they are behaving out of the norm

Rapid cycling in bipolar disorder is defined as having at least 4 or more mood episodes in a 12-month period. These mood episodes may be mania, hypomania or depressive disorder. These episodes must be separated by periods of partial or full remission of at least 2 months.

Symptoms of Hypomania

Hypomania is a lesser degree of mania. There is a persistent mild elevation of mood and increased sense of psychological well-being and happiness not keeping with ongoing events. In some cases, irritability, conceit, and boorish behavior may take the place of the more usual euphoric sociability.

Concentration and attention may be impaired thus diminishing the ability to settle down to work or to relaxation and leisure. However, this may not prevent the appearance of interests in quite new ventures and activities. In fact, the ability to function becomes better in hypomania, and there is a marked increase in productivity and creativity; many artists and writers have contributed significantly during such periods. Hypomania does not cause a major deficit in social or occupational functioning.

Diagnosis

A psychiatrist usually diagnoses mood disorders through a complete history collection, mental status examination and using psychological tests such as young Mania Rating Scale, mood disorder questionnaire, based on ICD-11 diagnostic criteria and also based on signs and symptoms.

DSM-5 Diagnostic Criteria for Bipolar 1 Disorder

For a diagnosis of bipolar 1 disorder, it is necessary to meet the following criteria for a manic episode. The manic episode may have been preceded by and may be followed by hypomanic or major depressive episode.

1. A distinct period of abnormally and persistently elevated, expansive or irritable mood and abnormally and persistently increased goal-directed activity or energy lasting for at least 1 week and present most of the day.
2. During the period of mood disturbance and increased energy or activity 3 or more of the following symptoms, if mood is irritable 4 of the following symptoms are present to a significant degree and represent a noticeable change from usual behavior.
   a. Inflated self-esteem or grandiosity
   b. Decreased need for sleep
   c. More talkative than usual or pressure to keep talking
   d. Flight of ideas or subjective experience that thoughts are racing
   e. Distractibility
   f. Increase in goal-directed activity or psychomotor agitation
   g. Excessive involvement in activities that have a high potential for painful consequences (e.g., engaging in

unrestrained buying sprees, sexual indiscretions or foolish business investments).
3. The mood disturbance is sufficiently severe to cause marked impairment in social or occupational functioning or to necessitate hospitalization to prevent harm to self or others or marked by psychotic features.
4. The episode is not attributable to the direct physical effects of a substance or any another medical condition.

Treatment Modalities

Mood disorders are often treated with medications, electroconvulsive therapy and psychosocial interventions.

Psychopharmacology

Mania in bipolar I disorder is treated with following medications:

- ❖ **Mood stabilizers**: Most people with bipolar I and II will need mood stabilizers to control mania or hypomanic episodes. Commonly used mood stabilizers are:
  - ❍ *Lithium*: 900–2100 mg/day
  - ❍ *Carbamazepine*: 600–1800 mg/day
  - ❍ *Sodium valproate*: 600–2600 mg/day
  - ❍ *Lamotrigine*: 25–200 mg/day
- ❖ **Antipsychotic drugs**: These may be used to control episodes of depression or mania especially when delusions and hallucinations are occurring. Example, olanzapine, aripiprazole, respiredone, etc.
- ❖ **Other drugs**: Clonazepam, diazepam, lorazepam, calcium channel blockers, etc.

Electroconvulsive Therapy (ECT)

ECT can also be used for acute manic excitement if not adequately responding to antipsychotics and lithium.

Psychosocial Interventions

For bipolar disorders psychological and social interventions are important in addition to continuing on medication. These may include:

- ❖ **Psychoeducation**: Educate patients/carers on symptoms, treatment, compliance, early detection of prodromal symptoms and relapse, lifestyle regularity, etc.
- ❖ **Cognitive behavior therapy**: It is a discrete psychological intervention aimed at making explicit connections between thinking, emotions, and behavior with respect to current or past problems, primarily through behavioral experiments and guided discovery.
- ❖ **Family intervention**: Aims to help families to cope with problems of their next of kin more effectively, provide support and educate the family, reduce levels of distress, improve ways in which the family communicates and negotiates problems to prevent relapses. Family and marital therapy is used to decrease intrafamilial and interpersonal difficulties and reduce or modify stressors. The main purpose is to ensure continuity of treatment and adequate drug compliance.

Prognosis

Prognosis of manic episode is favorable if they adhere to medications and therapy. Some factors associated with poorer outcome are: history of abuse, psychosis, low socio-economic status, comorbid illness or young age of onset.

Nursing Management for Mania

Individuals with manic episode experience intense emotions, grandiose delusions, impulsive behavior, change in sleep pattern and activity level. Nurse should focus on assessment, diagnoses, planning, implementation and evaluation.

Nursing Assessment

Nursing assessment of a manic patient should include assessing the severity of disorder, forming an opinion about the causes, assessing the patient's resources and judging the effects of patient's behavior on other people. As far as possible all relevant data should be collected from the patient as well as from his relatives as the patient may not always recognize the extent of his abnormal behavior.

During assessment the nurse should include mood and affect, thinking and perceptual ability, sleep disturbances, changes in energy level and character of speech patterns. Mood

TABLE 5.13: Objective signs and subjective symptoms of manic patient	
Objective signs	**Subjective symptoms**
• Disturbance of speech • Rapid speech • Loud, pressured speech • Easily distracted • Over activity • Mood lability • Weight changes	• Feelings of joy • Rapid mood swings • Sleep disturbances • Delusions and hallucinations

and affect should be assessed for congruency. Note patterns of verbal speech. The tone of voice, pace at which thoughts are processed and communicated and the rate at which words are spoken are all relevant. Assess for sleeping and eating patterns, energy levels and weight changes **(Table 5.13)**.

Nursing diagnosis I
High-risk for injury related to extreme hyper activity and impulsive behavior evidenced by lack of control over purposeless and potentially injurious movements.

Objective: Patient will not injure self.

Interventions: See **Table 5.14**.

Nursing diagnosis II
High-risk for violence; self-directed or directed at others related to manic excitement, delusional thinking and hallucinations.

Objective: Patient will not harm self or others.

Interventions: See **Table 5.15**.

The following are some guidelines for self-protection when handling an aggressive patient:
❖ Never see a potentially violent person alone.
❖ Keep a comfortable distance away from the patient (arm length).
❖ Be prepared to move, violent patient can strike out suddenly.
❖ Maintain a clear exit route for both the staff and patient.
❖ Be sure that the patient has no weapons in his possession before approaching him

TABLE 5.14: Nursing interventions for hyperactive behavior	
Nursing interventions	**Rationale**
Keep environmental stimuli to a minimum; assign single room; limit interactions with others; keep lighting and noise level low. Keep his room and immediate environment minimally furnished	Patient is extremely distractible and responds to even the slightest stimuli
Remove hazardous objects and substances, caution the patient when there is possibility of an accident	Rationality is impaired and patient may harm self inadvertently
Assist patient to engage in activities such as writing, drawing and other physical exercise	To bring relief from pent up tension and dissipate energy
Stay with the patient as hyperactivity increases	To offer support and provide a feeling of security
Administer medication as prescribed by the physician	To provide rapid relief from symptoms of hyperactivity

TABLE 5.15: Nursing interventions for manic violent behavior	
Nursing interventions	**Rationale**
Maintain low level of stimuli in patient's environment, provide unchallenging environment	To minimize anxiety and suspiciousness
Observe patient's behavior atleast every 15 minutes	Early intervention will ensure patient's and others' safety
Ensure that all sharp objects, glass or mirror items, belts, ties, match boxes have been removed from patient's environment	These may be used to harm self or others
Redirect violent behavior with physical outlet	For relieving pent-up tension and hostility

Contd...

Contd...

Nursing interventions	Rationale
Encourage verbal expression of feelings	-do-
Engage him in physical exercises like aerobics	-do-
Maintain and convey a calm attitude to the patient. Respond matter-of-factly to verbal hostility. Talk to him in low, calm voice, use clear and direct speech	Anxiety is contagious and can be transmitted from staff to patient
Have sufficient staff to indicate a show of strength to patient if necessary. State limitations and expectations	It conveys control over the situation and provides physical security for the staff
Administer tranquilizing medication; if patient refuses, use of restraints may be necessary. In such a case, explain the reason to the patient	Explaining why the restriction is imposed may ensure some control over his behavior
Following application of restraints observe the patient every 15 minutes	To ensure needs for nutrition, hydration and elimination are met
Remove restraints gradually one at a time	To minimize potential for injury to patient and staff

❖ If patient is having a weapon ask him to keep it on the table or the floor rather than fighting with him to take it away.
❖ Keep a pillow, mattress or blanket wrapped around arm between you and the weapon.
❖ Distract the patient momentarily to remove the weapon (throwing water on patient's face, yelling, etc.).
❖ Give prescribed antipsychotic medications.

Nursing diagnosis III
Altered nutrition, less than body requirements related to refusal or inability to sit still long enough to eat evidenced by weight loss, amenorrhea.

Objective: Patient will not exhibit signs and symptoms of malnutrition.

Interventions: See **Table 5.16**.

Nursing diagnosis IV
Impaired social interaction related to egocentric and narcissistic behavior evidenced by inability to develop satisfying relationships and manipulation of others for own desires.

Objective: Patient will interact with others in an appropriate manner.

Interventions: See **Table 5.17**.

Nursing diagnosis V
Self-esteem disturbance related to unmet dependency needs, lack of positive feedback, unrealistic self-expectations.

TABLE 5.16: Nursing interventions to improve nutritional status of manic patient

Nursing interventions	Rationale
Provide high-protein, high caloric, nutritious finger foods and drinks that can be consumed 'on the run'	Patient has difficulty sitting still long enough to eat a meal
Find out patient's likes and dislikes and provide favorite foods	To encourage the patient to eat
Provide 6–8 glasses of fluids per day. Have juice and snacks in the unit at all times	Intake of nutrients is required on regular basis to compensate for increased caloric requirements due to hyperactivity
Maintain accurate record of intake, output and calorie count. Weigh the patient regularly	These are useful data to assess patient's nutritional status
Supplement diet with vitamins and minerals	To improve nutritional status
Walk or sit with patient while he eats	To offer support and encourage the patient to eat

TABLE 5.17: Nursing interventions for manipulative behavior

Nursing interventions	Rationale
Recognize that manipulative behavior helps to reduce feelings of insecurity by increasing feelings of power and control	Understanding the rationale behind the behavior may facilitate greater acceptance of the individual
Set limits on manipulative behavior. Explain the consequences if limits are violated. Terms of the limits must be agreed upon by all the staff who will be working with the patient	Consequences for violation of limits must be consistently administered
Ignore attempts by patient to argue or bargain his way out of the limit setting	Lack of feedback may reduce such behaviors
Give positive reinforcement for non-manipulative behaviors	To enhance self-esteem and promote repetition of desirable behavior
Discuss consequences of patient's behavior and how attempts are made to attribute them to others	Patient must accept responsibility for own behavior before adaptive change can occur
Help patient identify positive aspects about self, recognize accomplishments and feel good about them	As self-esteem increases patient will experience a lesser need to manipulate others for own gratification

TABLE 5.18: Nursing interventions to improve self-esteem among manic patient

Nursing interventions	Rationale
Ask the patient how he would like to be addressed. Avoid approaches that imply different perception of the patient's importance	Grandiosity is thought actually to reflect low self-esteem
Explain rationale for requests related to staff unit routine. Strictly adhere to courteous approaches, matter-of-fact style and friendly attitudes	Nursing approaches should reinforce patient's dignity and worth; understanding reasons enhances co-operation with regimen
Encourage verbalization and identification of feelings related to issues of chronicity, lack of control over-self, etc	Problem solving begins with agreeing on the problem
Offer matter-of-fact feedback regarding unrealistic plans. Help him to set realistic goals for himself	Unrealistic goals will increase failures and lower self-esteem even further
Encourage patient to view life after discharge and identify aspects over which control is possible. Through role play, practice how he will demonstrate that control	Role rehearsal is helpful in returning patient to the level of independent functioning. When the Individual is functioning well, sense of self-esteem is enhanced

Objective: Patient will have realistic expectations about self.

Interventions: See **Table 5.18**.

Nursing diagnosis VI
Altered family processes related to euphoric mood and grandiose ideas, manipulative behavior, refusal to accept responsibility for own actions.

Objective: Family members will demonstrate coping ability in dealing with the patient.

Interventions: See **Table 5.19**.

Evaluation

Evaluation focuses on determining whether improvement has occurred in patient's thought processes, behavior, and overall functioning. Improved communication and social interaction result as thought processes become more rational and reality oriented. As mood states are reduced the patient is able to eat and sleep with little disturbance.

Depressive Episode

Depression is a widespread mental health problem affecting many people. The lifetime risk of depression in males is 8–12% and in

TABLE 5.19: Nursing interventions to improve family coping skills

Nursing interventions	Rationale
Determine individual's situation and feelings of individual family members such as guilt, anger, powerlessness, despair and alienation	Living with a family member having bipolar illness fosters a multitude of feelings and problems that can affect interpersonal relationships which may result in dysfunctional responses and family disintegration
Assess patterns of communication. For example: Are feelings expressed freely? Who makes decisions? How is the interaction between family members?	Provides clues to the degree of problem being experienced by individual family members and coping skills used to handle the crisis
Determine patterns of behavior displayed by patient in his relationship with others, e.g. manipulation of self-esteem of others, limit testing, etc	These behaviors are typically used by the manic individual to manipulate others. The result is alienation, guilt, ambivalence and high rates of divorce
Assess the role of patient in the family such as provider, etc. and how the illness affects the roles of other members	When the role of an ill person is not filled family disintegration can occur
Provide information about behavior patterns and expected course of illness.	Helps the family to understand various aspects of bipolar illness. This may relieve guilt and promote family discussions of the problems and solutions

females 20–26%. Depression occurs twice as frequently in women as in men. Highest incidence of depressive symptoms has been indicated in individuals not having close interpersonal relationships and in persons who are divorced or separated. Prevalence of suicide shows large peak in the spring and a smaller one in October. Major depressive disorders often co-occur with other psychiatric and substance-related disorders. Depression often is associated with a variety of medical conditions.

It is one of the leading causes of disability across the world. The World Health Organization 2006 estimates that depression will rank second only to heart disease by 2020 in terms of global disability. An estimated 3–4% of India's 100 crore plus population suffers from major mental disorders and about 7–10% of the population suffers from minor depressive disorders (Sinha, 2011).

Meaning

Depressive episode is characterized by low or depressed mood, loss of interest in most activities, tiredness, changes in appetite, feelings of worthlessness and recurrent thoughts of death.

Etiology of Depression

There are several factors that contribute to cause of depressive disorder. Various models that explain causes of depression depend on either biological, psychosocial or other factors **(Figure 5.12)**.

Biological Theories

Etiology of depression has been biologically attributed to alterations in neurochemical, genetic, endocrine, circadian rhythm functions and changes in brain anatomy.

❖ **Neurochemical imbalances**: Research findings suggest that depression occurs when there is a reduction in levels of norepinephrine and serotonin, and a dysregulation of acetylcholine and GABA.
❖ **Genetic theories**:
  ○ Major depressive disorders occur more often in first degree relatives than they do in the general population.
  ○ Chances of getting depressed are higher if relatives or siblings are suffering from it.
  ○ Studies of identical twins show that when one twin is diagnosed with major depression, the other twin has a greater than 70% chance of developing it.

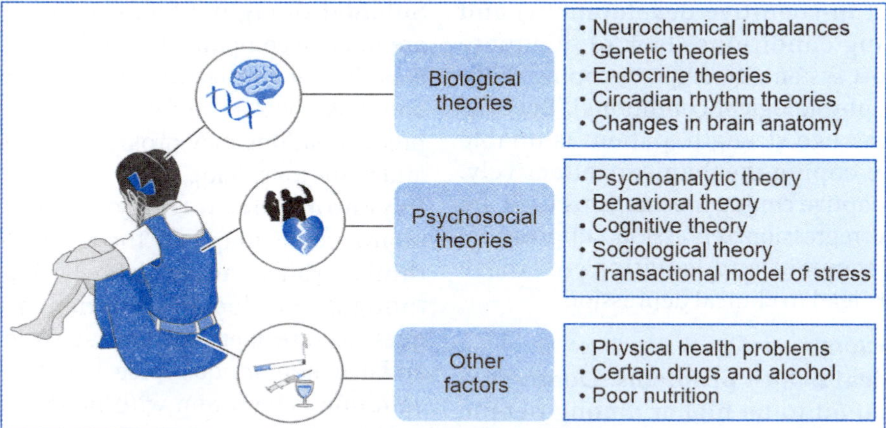

Figure 5.12: Etiology of depression

* **Endocrine theories**: Normally, the hypothalamic-pituitary-adrenal (HPA) axis is a system that mediates the stress response. However, in some depressed people this system malfunctions and creates cortisol, thyroid and hormonal abnormalities.

* **Circadian rhythm theories**: Circadian rhythms are responsible for the daily regulation of wake-sleep cycles, arousal and activity patterns, and hormonal secretions. Individuals experiencing circadian rhythm changes are at an increased risk for developing depressive symptoms and other mood symptoms. These changes might be caused by medications, nutritional deficiencies, physical or psychological illnesses, hormonal fluctuations.

* **Changes in brain anatomy**: Loss of neurons in the frontal lobes, cerebellum and basal ganglia has been identified in depression.

Psychosocial Theories

Psychoanalytic, behavioral, cognitive and social theories explained psychosocial causes of depression.

* **Psychoanalytic theory**: According to Freud (1957) depression results due to loss of a 'loved object', and fixation in the oral sadistic phase of development.

* **Behavioral theory**: This theory of depression connects depressive phenomena to the experience of uncontrollable events.

According to this model, depression is conditioned by repeated losses in the past. Grief can be from the death or loss of a loved one, losing a job or income, getting divorced or retiring, past physical, sexual or emotional abuse.

* **Cognitive theory**: According to this theory, depression is due to negative cognitions which includes:
  - Negative expectations of the environment
  - Negative expectations of the self
  - Negative expectations of the future

  These cognitive distortions arise out of a defect in cognitive development and cause the individual to feel inadequate, worthless and rejected by others.

* **Sociological theory**: Stressful life events, e.g., death, marriage, financial loss before the onset of the disease or a relapse probably have a formative effect. Stressful life events overwhelm a person's ability to cope leading to depression. High levels of cortisol hormone secreted during periods of stress may affect the neurotransmitter serotonin and contribute to depression.

* **Transactional model of stress/adaptation:** According to transactional model of stress/adaptation, depression occurs as a combination of predisposing factors (family history and biochemical alterations), past experiences (object loss in infancy,

defect in cognitive development) and existing conditions (lack of adequate support system, inadequate coping skills, other physiological conditions). Because of weak ego strength, patient is unable to use coping mechanisms effectively. Maladaptive coping mechanisms used are denial, regression, repression, suppression, displacement and isolation. All these factors lead to clinical depression.

Other Factors

- ❖ **Physical health problems**: Depression rates tend to be higher among people who have chronic pain, diabetes, multiple sclerosis, cancer, sleep disorder, thyroid condition, liver disorders, etc.
- ❖ **Certain drugs and alcohol**: Drugs and alcohol can contribute to depressive disorders. Some of the prescription drugs linked to depression are anticonvulsants, statins, stimulants, benzodiazepines, corticosteroids, and beta-blockers.
- ❖ **Poor nutrition**: A poor diet can contribute to depression. Nutrient deficiencies of B-complex vitamins, Vitamin C and D, magnesium, potassium, manganese, zinc, iron, selenium and calcium are involved in depression. Some studies have found that diets either low in omega-3 fatty acids or with an imbalanced ratio of omega-6 to omega-3 are associated with increased rates of depression.

Clinical Features

A typical depressive episode is characterized by the following features which should last for at least two weeks in order to make a diagnosis:

Depressed mood: Sadness of mood or loss of interest and loss of pleasure in almost all activities (pervasive sadness), present throughout the day (persistent sadness).

Depressive cognitions: Hopelessness (a feeling of 'no hope in future' due to pessimism), helplessness (the patient feels that no help is possible), worthlessness (a feeling of inadequacy and inferiority), unreasonable guilt and self-blame over trivial matters in the past.

Suicidal thoughts: Ideas of hopelessness are often accompanied by a thought that life is no longer worth living and that death had come as a welcome release. These gloomy preoccupations may progress to thoughts of and plans for suicide.

Psychomotor activity: Psychomotor retardation is frequent. The retarded patient thinks, walks and acts slowly. Slowing of thought is reflected in patient's speech; questions are often answered after a long delay and in a monotonous voice. In older patients, agitation is common with marked anxiety, restlessness and feelings of uneasiness.

Psychotic features: Some patients have delusions and hallucinations (the disorder may then be termed as psychotic depression); these are often mood congruent, i.e., they are related to depressive themes and reflect the patient's dysphoric mood. For example, nihilistic delusions (beliefs about the non-existence of some person or thing), delusions of guilt, delusions of poverty, etc. may be present.

Some patients experience delusions and hallucinations that are not clearly related to depressive themes (mood incongruent), e.g., delusion of control. The prognosis then appears to be much worse.

Somatic symptoms of depression are also termed as 'melancholic features' in DSMIV **(Box 5.19)**.

Other Features

- ❖ Difficulties in thinking and concentration
- ❖ Subjective poor memory

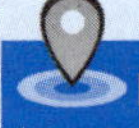

> **BOX 5.19:** Somatic symptoms of depression
>
> - ❑ Significant decrease in appetite or weight
> - ❑ Early morning awakening, at least 2 or more hours before the usual time of waking up
> - ❑ Diurnal variation, with depression being worst in the morning
> - ❑ Pervasive lack of interest and lack of reactivity to pleasurable stimuli
> - ❑ Psychomotor agitation or retardation

TABLE 5.20: Symptoms of depression

Common symptoms	Other symptoms
• Apathy	• Fatigue
• Sadness	• Thoughts of death
• Sleep disturbances	• Decreased libido
• Hopelessness	• Dependency
• Helplessness	• Spontaneous crying
• Worthlessness	• Passiveness
• Guilt	
• Anger	

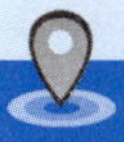

BOX 5.20: Case vignette—Depressive episode

Mrs Beena, a 25-year-old nursing officer complained of fatigue while doing her job, not enjoying her work, has no interest in socializing with her peers and family members. She reported loss of appetite for the last one month during which she lost 5 kg of weight. On observation she looks sad, exhibited no hope for the future, decreased sleep and says she is of no use for her family. She had a few episodes of headache and body pain during the last two weeks. Psychiatrist diagnosed it as depression without psychotic symptoms. She was prescribed antidepressants, and provided supportive psychotherapy.

❖ Menstrual or sexual disturbances
❖ Vague physical symptoms such as fatigue, aching discomfort, constipation, etc. (**Table 5.20 and Box 5.20**).

Diagnosis

❖ Psychological tests: Beck depression inventory (BDI), Hamilton rating scale for depression (HRSD) to assess severity and prognosis.
❖ Dexamethasone suppression test showing failure to suppress cortisol secretions in depressed patients.
❖ Toxicology screening suggesting drug-induced depression.

DSM-5 Criteria

DSM-5 outlines the following criteria to make a diagnosis of depression. The individual must be experiencing five or more symptoms during the same 2-week period and at least one of the symptoms should be either depressed mood or loss of interest or pleasure.

❖ Depressed mood for most of the day, nearly everyday.
❖ Markedly diminished interest or pleasure in all or almost all activities for most of the day, nearly everyday.
❖ Significant weight loss when not dieting or weight gain, or decrease or increase in appetite nearly everyday.
❖ Slowing down of thought and a reduction in physical movement (observable by others, not merely subjective feelings of restlessness or being slowed down).
❖ Fatigue or loss of energy nearly everyday.
❖ Feelings of worthlessness or excessive or inappropriate guilt nearly everyday.
❖ Diminished ability to think or concentrate, or indecisiveness, nearly everyday.
❖ Recurrent thoughts of death, recurrent suicidal ideation without a specific plan, or a suicide attempt or a specific plan for committing suicide.

To receive a diagnosis of depression these symptoms must cause the individual clinically significant distress or impairment in social, occupational, or other important areas of functioning. The symptoms must also not be a result of substance abuse or other medical condition.

Treatment Modalities

Many types of treatment modalities are available to treat depression. Some of the important ones are presented in **Figure 5.13**:

I. Antidepressants

Antidepressants establish a blockade for the reuptake of norepinephrine and serotonin into their specific nerve terminals. This permits them to linger longer in synapses and to be more available to postsynaptic receptors. Antidepressants also increase the sensitivity of the postsynaptic receptor sites. SSRIs act by inhibiting the reuptake of serotonin and increasing its levels at the receptor site. Tricyclic antidepressants mode of action is by blocking the reuptake of norepinephrine (NE) and/or serotonin (5-HT) at the nerve terminals, thus increasing the NE and 5-HT levels at the receptor site.

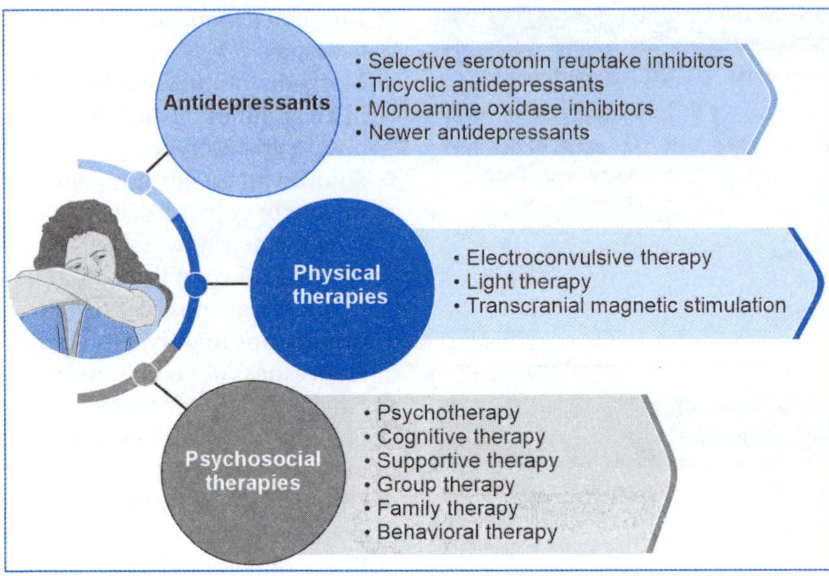

Figure 5.13: Treatment modalities for depression

MAOIs are responsible for the degradation of catecholamines after reuptake. The final effect is the same, a functional increase in the NE and 5-HT levels at the receptor site. Atypical antidepressants modestly inhibit the reuptake of norepinephrine and dopamine.

Major categories of antidepressants

1. **Selective serotonin reuptake inhibitors (SSRIs)**
   - Citalopram (Celexa), Fluoxetine (Prozac), Sertraline (Zoloft)
2. **Tricyclic antidepressants (TCAs)**
   - Amitriptyline (Elavil), Clomipramine (Anafranil), Imipramine (Tofranil), Doxepin (Adapin, Sinequan)
3. **Monoamine oxidase inhibitors (MAOIs)**
   - Isocarboxazid (Morplan), Phenelzine (Nardil)
4. **Other Newer Antidepressant drugs such as Bupropion, Maprotiline**

II. Physical Therapies

❖ **Electroconvulsive therapy (ECT):** Severe depression with suicidal risk is the most important indication for ECT.

❖ **Light therapy:** Sometimes called photo therapy, it involves exposing the patient to an artificial light source during winter months to relieve seasonal depression. The light source must be very bright, full-spectrum light, usually 2500 lux. The patient is instructed to sit in front of the light at a distance of about 3 feet. The duration of administration is 1 to 2 hours daily.

❖ **Repetitive transcranial magnetic stimulation (RTMS) and vagus nerve stimulation (VNS)** directly affect brain function by stimulating the nerves that are direct extensions of the brain. RTMS increases the release of neurotransmitters and downregulates beta adrenergic receptors, thus ameliorating depressive symptoms and other disorders.

III. Psychosocial Treatment

❖ **Psychotherapy:** Psychotherapy based on psychoanalytic interventions emphasizes helping patients gain insight into the cause of their depression.

❖ **Cognitive therapy:** It aims at correcting the depressive negative cognitions like hopelessness, worthlessness, helplessness and pessimistic ideas, and replacing them with new cognitive and behavioral responses.

❖ **Supportive psychotherapy**: Various techniques are employed to support the patient. They are reassurance, ventilation, occupational therapy, relaxation and other activity therapies.

❖ **Group therapy**: Group therapy is useful for mild cases of depression. It not only helps in recognition of negative feelings such as anxiety, anger, guilt and despair but also aids in emotional growth through expression of feelings.

❖ **Family therapy**: Family therapy is used to mitigate intrafamilial and interpersonal difficulties and reduce or modify stressors thereby helping in faster and more complete recovery.

❖ **Behavioral therapy**: It includes social skills training, problem solving techniques, assertiveness training, self-control therapy, activity scheduling and decision-making techniques.

Nursing Management of Major Depressive Episode

Nursing management for a patient with depressive episode should include assessment, diagnosis, planning care, implementation and evaluation of nursing care.

Nursing Assessment

Nursing assessment should focus on judging the severity of the disorder including the risk of suicide, identifying the possible causes, social resources available to the patient, and the effects of the disorder on other people. Although there is a risk of suicide in every depressed patient, the risk is much more in the presence of following factors:

❖ Presence of marked helplessness
❖ Male sex
❖ More than 40 years of age
❖ Unmarried, widowed or divorced
❖ Written or verbal communication of suicidal intent or plan
❖ Early stages of depression

❖ Recovery from depression (at the peak of depression the patient is usually either too depressed or too retarded to commit suicide)
❖ Period of three months from recovery. The nurse should routinely enquire about patient's work, finances, family life, social activities, general living conditions and physical health. It is also important to consider whether the patient could endanger other people particularly if there are depressive delusions as the patient may act on them.
❖ Observe for mood, affect, thinking, perceptual ability, somatic complaints, sleep disturbances, and changes in energy level.
❖ Determine the amount of assistance required for personal hygiene, and elimination needs.
❖ Assess for any suicidal ideation and whether a plan has been devised.
❖ Assess for objective signs and subjective symptoms **(Table 5.21)**.

Nursing diagnosis I
High-risk of self-directed violence related to depressed mood, feelings of worthlessness and anger directed inward on the self.
Objective: Patient will not harm self.
Interventions: See **Table 5.22**.

Nursing diagnosis II
Dysfunctional grieving related to real or perceived loss, bereavement, evidenced by denial of loss, inappropriate expression of anger, inability to carryout activities of daily living.

Objective: Patient will be able to verbalize normal behaviors associated with grieving.

Interventions: See **Table 5.23**.

TABLE 5.21: Objective signs and subjective symptoms of depression	
Objective signs	**Subjective symptoms**
• Alterations of activity • Poor personal hygiene • Apathy • Altered social interactions • Impairment of cognition • Somatic symptoms • Delusions and hallucinations	• Anhedonia • Worthlessness • Hopelessness • Helplessness • Suicidal ideas

TABLE 5.22: Nursing interventions for suicidal behavior

Nursing interventions	Rationale
Ask the patient directly, "Have you thought about harming yourself in anyway? If so, what do you plan to do? Do you have the means to carry out this plan?"	The risk of suicide is greatly increased if the patient has developed a plan and if means exist for the patient to execute the plan
Create a safe environment for the patient. Remove all potentially harmful objects from patient's vicinity, for example—sharp objects, straps, belts, glass items, alcohol, etc. Supervise closely during meals and medication administration	Patient's safety is nursing priority
Formulate a short-term verbal or written contract that the patient will not harm self. Secure a promise that the patient will seek out staff when feeling suicidal	A degree of the responsibility for his safety is given to the patient. Increased feelings of self-worth may be experienced when patient feels accepted unconditionally regardless of behavior
It may be desirable to place the patient near the nursing station. Do not leave the patient alone. Observe for passive suicide—the patient may starve or fall asleep in the bath-tub or sink	Patient's safety is nursing priority
Close observation is mostly required when the patient is recovering from the disease	At the peak of depression the patient is usually too retarded to carry out his suicidal plans
Do not allow the patient to put the bolt on his side of the door of bathroom or toilet	Patient's safety is nursing priority
If the patient suddenly becomes unusually happy or gives any other clues of suicide, special observation may be necessary	-do-
Encourage the patient to express his feelings including anger	Depression and suicidal behavior may be viewed as anger turned inward on the self. If the anger can be verbalized in a non-threatening environment, the patient may be able to eventually resolve these feelings

TABLE 5.23: Nursing interventions for grief reaction

Nursing interventions	Rationale
Assess stage of fixation in grief process	Accurate baseline data is required to plan accurate care
Be accepting of patient and spend time with him. Show empathy, care and unconditional positive regard	These interventions provide the basis for a therapeutic relationship
Explore feelings of anger and help patient direct them towards the intended object or person	Until patient can recognize and accept personal feelings regarding the loss, grief work cannot progress
Provide simple activities which can be easily and quickly accomplished. Gradually, increase the amount and complexity of activities	Physical activities are safe and an effective way of relieving anger

Nursing diagnosis III
Powerlessness related to dysfunctional grieving process, lifestyle of helplessness evidenced by feelings of lack of control over life situations, over-dependence on others to fulfill needs.

Objective: The patient will be able to take control of life situations.

Interventions: See **Table 5.24**.

Nursing diagnosis IV
Self-esteem disturbance related to learned helplessness, impaired cognition, negative view of self, evidenced by expression of worthlessness, sensitivity to criticism, negative and pessimistic outlook.

Objective: Patient will be able to verbalize positive aspects about self and attempt new activities without fear of failure.

Interventions: See **Table 5.25**.

Nursing diagnosis V
Altered communication process related to depressive cognitions evidenced by being unable to interact with others, withdrawn, expressing fear of failure or rejection.

Objective: Patient will communicate or interact with staff or other patients in the unit.

Interventions: See **Table 5.26**.

TABLE 5.24: Nursing interventions for over dependence behavior

Interventions	Rationale
Allow the patient to take decisions regarding self-care	Providing the patient with choices will enhance his feeling of control
Ensure that goals are realistic and that patient is able to identify life situations that are realistically under his control	To avoid repeated failures which usually amplify a sense of powerlessness
Encourage the patient to verbalize feelings about areas that are not in his ability to control	Verbalization of unresolved issues may help the patient to accept what cannot be changed

TABLE 5.25: Nursing interventions to improve self-esteem in depressed patients

Nursing interventions	Rationale
Be accepting of patient and spend time with him, even though pessimism and negativism may seem objectionable	These interventions contribute towards feeling of self-worth
Focus on strengths and accomplishments and minimize failures	-do-
Provide him with simple and easily achievable activity. Encourage the patient to perform his activities without assistance	Success and independence promote feelings of self-worth
Encourage patient to recognize areas of change and provide assistance toward this effort	This will facilitate problem solving
Teach assertiveness and coping skills	Their use can serve to enhance self-esteem

TABLE 5.26: Nursing interventions to improve communication skills in depressed patients

Nursing interventions	Rationale
Observe for nonverbal communication. The patient may say that he is happy but looks sad. Point out this discrepancy in what he is saying and actually feeling	To facilitate better response and communication
Use short sentences. Ask questions in such a way that the patient will have to answer in more than one word	-do-
Use silence appropriately without communicating anxiety or discomfort in doing so	Using silence when the situation demands as it can be therapeutic
Introduce the patient to another patient who is quiet and possibly convalescing from depression	There is less anxiety in relating to a person other than staff
As he improves, take him to other patients and see that he is actually included as part of the group	Group support is important in facilitating communication

Nursing diagnosis VI

Altered sleep and rest related to depressed mood and depressive cognitions evidenced by difficulty in falling asleep, early morning awakening, verbal complaints of not feeling well-rested.

Objective: Patient will sleep adequately during the night.

Interventions: See **Table 5.27**.

Nursing diagnosis VII

Altered nutrition, less than body requirements related to depressed mood, lack of appetite or lack of interest in food evidenced by weight loss, poor muscle tone, pale conjunctiva, poor skin turgor.

Objective: Patient's nutritional status will improve.

Interventions: See **Table 5.28**.

Nursing diagnosis VIII

Self-care deficit related to depressed mood, feelings of worthlessness evidenced by poor personal hygiene and grooming.

TABLE 5.28: Nursing interventions to improve nutritional status in depressive patients

Nursing interventions	Rationale
Closely monitor the patient's food and fluid intake; maintain intake and output chart	These are useful data for assessing nutritional status
Record patient's weight regularly	–do–
Find out the likes and dislikes of the person before he was sick and serve the best preferred food	To encourage eating and improve nutritional status
Serve small amounts of light or liquid diet frequently that is nourishing	-do-
Record the patient's pattern of bowel elimination	To assess for constipation
Encourage more fluid intake, roughage diet and green leafy vegetables	For relief of constipation if present

Objective: Patient will maintain adequate personal hygiene.

Interventions: See **Table 5.29**.

TABLE 5.27: Nursing interventions to improve sleeping pattern

Nursing interventions	Rationale
Plan daytime activities according to patient's interests, do not allow him to sit idle	To improve the quality of sleep at night
Ensure a quiet and peaceful environment when the patient is preparing for sleep	-do-
Provide comfort measures (backrub, tipid bath, warm milk, etc.)	-do-
Do not allow the patient to sleep for long-time during the day	-do-
Give prn sedatives as prescribed	-do-
Talk to the patient for a brief period at bed time. Do not enter into lengthy conversations	Talking to the patient helps to relieve his anxiety, but engaging in long talks may prolong depressive thinking

TABLE 5.29: Nursing interventions to improve self-care for depressed patients

Nursing interventions	Rationale
Ensure that he takes his bath regularly	Depressive patient will not have any interest for self-care and may need assistance
Do not ask patient's permission for a wash or bath. For instance, do not ask "Do you want to have a bath?" Instead lead the patient to the action with positive suggestions. For example, "The water is ready, let me take you for a bath."	Positive suggestions will usually enhance patient's co-operation
When the patient has taken care of himself, express realistic appreciation	Positive reinforcement will improve desirable behavior

TABLE 5.30: Bipolar disorder: Good and poor prognostic factors	
Good prognostic factors	**Poor prognostic factors**
◆ Abrupt or acute onset ◆ Severe depression ◆ Typical clinical features ◆ Well-adjusted premorbid personality ◆ Good response to treatment	◆ Double depression ◆ Comorbid physical disease, personality disorders or alcohol dependence ◆ Chronic ongoing stress ◆ Poor drug compliance ◆ Marked hypochondriacal features or mood-incongruent psychotic features

Evaluation

Evaluation will focus on determining whether improvement has occurred in patient's thought processes, behavior and overall functioning. Interest and participation in self-care and hygiene show an elevation in self-appreciation. Increased hope and worth relieves the acute need for self-destruction. As depression reduces, the patient is able to eat and sleep with fewer disturbances.

Evaluation is facilitated by using following types of questions:

* Has self-harm to the individual been avoided?
* Have suicidal ideations subsided?
* Does patient set realistic goals for self?
* Is he able to verbalize positive aspects about self, past accomplishments and future prospects?

Course and Prognosis of Mood Disorders

While an average manic episode lasts for 3–4 months, a depressive episode lasts for 4–9 months. The prognosis of mood disorders depends on several factors. These are presented in **Table 5.30.**

NEUROTIC DISORDERS

Neurotic disorder (neurosis) is a less severe form of psychiatric disorder where patients show either excessive or prolonged emotional reaction to any given stress. These disorders are not caused by organic disease of the brain and do not involve hallucinations and delusions. The neuroses term is no longer used in the current scientific literature.

ANXIETY OR FEAR-RELATED DISORDERS

Anxiety is a normal phenomenon which is characterized by a state of apprehension or uneasiness arising out of anticipation of danger. Normal anxiety becomes pathological when it causes significant subject distress and impairment in the normal functioning of the individual.

Anxiety and fear related disorders are characterized by excessive fear, anxiety and related behavioral disturbances with symptoms that are severe enough to result in significant distress or impairment in personal, family, social, educational, occupational or other important areas of functioning which are not caused by organic brain disease or any other psychiatric disorder.

Prevalence and Incidence of Anxiety Disorders

* According to the global burden of disease study 1990–2017, the crude prevalence rate for anxiety disorders was 3.3% (3.0–3.5). In 2017, 44.9 million people had anxiety disorders in India.
* The disorder has a prevalence of 2–5% and is twice as more common in females as compared to males.
* Onset is usually in 20s, although persons of any age can be affected.
* The disorder is more commonly seen in primary care settings wherein individuals seek help from general practitioners or cardiologists or gastroenterologists.
* Childhood, adolescence, and early adulthood are considered high-risk periods for the onset of anxiety disorders.

Etiology of Anxiety Disorders

The exact cause of anxiety disorders is currently unknown as it involves a combination of genetic, environmental, psychological and developmental factors **(Table 5.31).**

TABLE 5.31: Etiology of anxiety disorders

Genetic theory	• Genetic predisposition • Family history
Biochemical factors	• Imbalance in neurotransmitters • Alteration in GABA
Psychodynamic theory	• Defense mechanisms • Repression
Behavioral theory	• Classical conditioning • Unconditional inherent response
Cognitive theory	• Faulty cognitions • Negative automatic thoughts
Other factors	• Certain personality traits • Physical health issues • Stressful life events

❖ **Genetic theory**: Anxiety disorder can run in families having genetic predisposition. An increased likelihood of anxiety disorders can be observed in individuals with a family history of anxiety. About 15–20% of the first-degree relatives of patients with anxiety disorder exhibit anxiety disorders themselves. The concordance rate in monozygotic twins of patients with panic disorder is 80%.

❖ **Biochemical factors**: An imbalance in neurotransmitters is responsible for regulating mood and emotions. Alteration in GABA levels may lead to production of clinical anxiety.

❖ **Psychodynamic theory**: According to this theory, anxiety is usually dealt with repression. When repression fails to function adequately, other secondary defense mechanisms of ego come into action. In anxiety, repression fails to function adequately and the secondary defense mechanisms are not activated. Hence, anxiety comes to the forefront. In phobia, the secondary defense mechanism is displacement. By displacement anxiety is transferred from a really dangerous or frightening object to a neutral object. These two objects are connected by symbolic association. In contrast to the frightening object, the neutral object (chosen unconsciously) can be easily avoided in day-to-day activities.

❖ **Behavioral theory**: Anxiety is viewed as an unconditional inherent response of the individual to a painful stimulus. According to classical conditioning a stressful stimulus produces an unconditioned response—fear. When the stressful stimulus is repeatedly paired with a harmless object, eventually the harmless object alone produces the fear which is now a conditioned response. If the person avoids the harmless object to avoid fear, the fear becomes a phobia.

❖ **Cognitive theory**: According to this theory, anxiety is related to cognitive distortions and negative automatic thoughts. Anxiety is the product of faulty cognitions or anxiety-inducing self-instructions. Cognitive theorists believe that some individuals engage in negative and irrational thinking that produce anxiety reactions. The individual begins to seek out avoidance behaviors to prevent anxiety reactions resulting in phobias.

❖ **Other factors**: Certain personality traits such as being shy or perfectionistic are more susceptible to developing an anxiety disorder. Life events or stressful experiences such as abuse, violence, loss or illness can trigger or exacerbate anxiety disorders. In some individuals' positive life events such as marriage, having a baby or starting a new job can induce anxiety. Certain physical health issues such as diabetes, heart disease, thyroid problems or hormonal imbalances can contribute to the onset or manifestation of anxiety symptoms.

Generalized Anxiety Disorder

Generalized anxiety disorders are those in which anxiety is unrealistic, excessive, which is generalized and persistent, present all the time and not restricted to certain situations or exposure to certain objects.

According to ICD-11, generalized anxiety disorder is characterized by marked symptoms of anxiety that persist for at least several months, manifested by either general apprehension (free-floating anxiety) or excessive worrying focused on multiple everyday events, mostly concerning family, health, finances, school and work. Additional symptoms include muscular tension, autonomic hyperactivity symptoms.

Clinical Features

Generalized anxiety disorder (GAD) is manifested by psychological, autonomic and motor symptoms **(Figure 5.14 and Box 5.21)**

1. **Psychological symptoms:**
   - General apprehensiveness that is not restricted to any particular environmental circumstances
   - Excessive worry or apprehension
   - Subjective experience of nervousness, restlessness, difficulty in concentrating, irritability, sleep disturbances, forgetfulness

2. **Autonomic hyperactivity:** It is evidenced by frequent gastro intestinal symptoms such as nausea and abdominal distress, shortness of breath, palpitations, sweating, trembling, shaking, dry mouth, dizziness, light-headedness, hot flushes or chills,

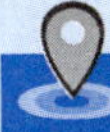

> **BOX 5.21:** Case vignette—Generalized anxiety disorders
>
> Mr James, a 30-year-old man visited psychiatric OPD with complaints of excessive worrying for everything, restlessness, dizziness, burning sensation in the stomach, insomnia, irritability, difficulty focusing on work, significant back and muscle tension and more frequency in urination. On examination Mr James had cold and clammy hands, increased radial pulse, looked tense, was fidgeting with his clothes. Psychiatrist diagnosed it as generalized anxiety disorder and put him on anxiolytics.

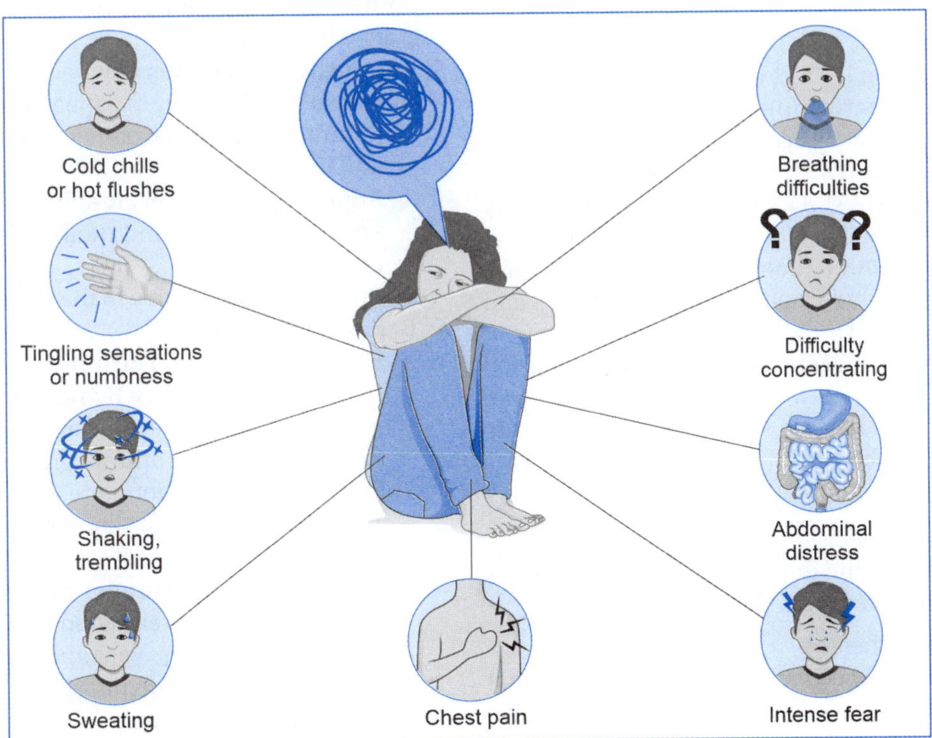

Figure 5.14: Clinical features of generalized anxiety disorder (GAD)

frequent urination, trouble in swallowing or lump on throat

3. **Motor symptoms:** Muscle tension or motor restlessness which can lead to symptoms like tremulousness, feeling shaky, muscle tension, generalized aches, pain in the chest, back pain, pain in the extremities, muscle soreness, easy fatigability, etc.

Symptoms should persist for at least several months, not related to another medical condition (e.g., hyperthyroidism) and are not due to the effects of substance or medication on the central nervous system. The symptoms result in significant distress or significant impairment in personal, family, social, educational, occupational or other important areas of functioning.

Course

❖ Insidious onset in the early-to-mid 30s with a chronic course

❖ Early onset of symptoms is associated with greater impairment of functioning and presence of co-occurring mental disorders

❖ Full remission of symptoms is uncommon

Diagnosis

❖ Based on ICD-11 criteria

❖ Use of screening tools to assess anxiety such as Generalized Anxiety Disorder Scale (GAD-7), Hamilton Anxiety Rating Scale (HAM-A), Zung Self-Rating Anxiety Scale (SAS), Depression Anxiety Stress Scale (DASS-21 and 42), Revised Children's Anxiety and Depression Scale (RCADS and RCADS-P)

❖ Anxiety is a central feature of many mental disorders, psychiatric evaluation to rule out phobias, OCD, depression and acute schizophrenia

Treatment Modalities

Treatment decisions are based on the severity, persistence and impact of symptoms as well as patient preferences (**Figure 5.15**).

Pharmacotherapy

Commonly used medications for the treatment of anxiety disorders are antianxiety agents, antidepressants and beta-blockers.

Pharmacotherapy	Psychological therapies
• Antianxiety agents • Antidepressants • Betablockers	• Supportive psychotherapy • Behavior therapy • Cognitive therapy

Figure 5.15: Treatment modalities for generalized anxiety disorders

❖ **Antianxiety agents**: Benzodiazepines (alprazolam, clonazepam). These drugs reduce anxiety by decreasing vigilance, easing somatic symptoms.

❖ **Antidepressants**: Tricyclic antidepressants (imipramine, buspirone), selective serotonin reuptake inhibitors (sertraline, escitalopram).

❖ **Beta-blockers**: Propranolol to control severe palpitations that have not responded to anxiolytics.

❖ Treatment is usually continued for 9–12 months after symptom remission and gradually phased out as recommended.

Psychological therapies

Commonly used psychological therapies are supportive psychotherapy, behavioral and cognitive therapy.

❖ **Supportive psychotherapy:**
  o Empathetic listening to patient problems
  o Identifying stressors, patients' strengths and limitations
  o Appreciating and encouraging patient's positive strengths and qualities by the therapist
  o Providing reassurance to the patient

❖ **Behavior therapy:**
  o Biofeedback to reduce physical symptoms of anxiety by teaching the patient on how to become aware of and then consciously control various body functions such as blood pressure, heart and respiratory rates, skin temperature and perspiration.
  o Relaxation techniques: Jacobson's progressive muscle relaxation technique, breathing exercises, yoga, pranayama, meditation and self-hypnosis.
  o Lifestyle modification
  o Supportive psychotherapy

❖ **Cognitive therapy:**
  ○ To reduce cognitive distortions by teaching the patient on how to restructure his thoughts and view worries more realistically.
  ○ In one approach, patient is taught to record anxiety levels and list evidence that justifies or contradicts each one. Patient learns that 'worrying about worry' maintains anxiety; avoidance and procrastination are ineffective problem-solving techniques.

Panic Disorder

Panic disorder is characterized by anxiety which is intermittent and unrelated to particular circumstances (unlike phobic anxiety disorders where though anxiety is intermittent, it occurs only in particular situations). The central feature is the occurrence of panic attacks, i.e., sudden attacks of anxiety in which physical symptoms predominate and are accompanied by fear of a serious consequence such as a heart attack.

Prevalence and Incidence

The lifetime prevalence of panic disorder is 1.5–2%. It is seen 2 to 3 times more often in females.

Clinical Features

Recurrent panic attacks which are discrete episodes of intense fear or apprehension characterized by **(Box 5.22):**
❖ Palpitations or increased heart rate
❖ Sweating
❖ Trembling
❖ Shortness of breath
❖ Feeling of choking
❖ Chest pain
❖ Nausea or abdominal distress
❖ Feeling of dizziness or light-headedness
❖ Chills or hot flushes
❖ Tingling or lack of sensation in extremities
❖ Depersonalization or derealization
❖ Fear of losing control or going mad
❖ Fear of imminent death
❖ Panic attacks followed by persistent concern or worry about their recurrence

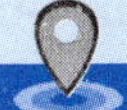

BOX 5.22: Case vignette—Panic attacks

Ms C, a 26-year-old software engineer is recently engaged to a business man from Mumbai. Two weeks after the engagement, Ms C experienced episodes of dizziness, fainting, fatigue, chest pain, increased heart rate, tremors of hands, tightness in chest, sweating and chocking sensations on four separate occasions. Initially she felt intense fear that reached a peak within few minutes. During the last episode, she was convinced that she had a heart attack and that she would die if emergency medical treatment was not given. She persistently worried about an impending attack which might lead to sudden death. As a result, she began avoiding unfamiliar places and people as it would be difficult to get timely help in the event of another attack. She took an appointment with the physician to discuss her symptoms. A detailed physical and cardiac assessment revealed no medical problems. Physician referred her to a psychiatrist who diagnosed it as a typical case of panic attacks.

❖ Significant impairment in personal, family, social, educational, occupational or other important areas of functioning
❖ Symptoms that are not a manifestation of an alternate medical condition and are not due to the effect of a substance or medication on the central nervous system.

Course

❖ The onset is usually in early third decade with often a chronic course.
❖ It occurs recurrently every few days. Some individuals experience episodic symptom outbreaks with long periods of remission while others experience persistent severe symptoms.
❖ The episode is usually sudden in onset and lasts for a few minutes. More than 95% of those diagnosed with agoraphobia have an accompanying diagnosis of panic disorder. Up to two-thirds of those with this disorder also experience depression or engage in substance abuse to cope with anxiety.

Diagnosis

❖ Tests to rule out organic or pharmacologic basis for symptoms (some physical conditions and drug effects can mimic panic disorder)

- Serum glucose measurements to rule out hypoglycemia
- Thyroid function tests to rule out hyperthyroidism
- Urine and serum toxicology tests to rule out presence of psychoactive substances such as barbiturates, caffeine and amphetamines
- Based on ICD-11 criteria

Treatment Modalities

Treatment of panic disorder includes combination of medications and psychological treatment **(Figure 5.16)**.

Medications

- Benzodiazepines (e.g., alprazolam, clonazepam)
- Selective serotonin reuptake inhibitors (e.g., fluoxetine, sertraline, escitalopram)
- Beta-blockers to control severe palpitations that have not responded to anxiolytics (for example, propranolol)

Behavioral therapies

- Relaxation techniques to help the patient cope with a panic attack by easing physical symptoms and directing attention elsewhere.
- Deep breathing exercises which also reduce the risk of hyperventilation.
- Progressive relaxation which involves conscious tightening and relaxation of the skeletal muscles in a sequential fashion.
- Positive verbalization or guided imagery in which the patient elicits peaceful mental images or some other purposeful thought or action thereby promoting feelings of relaxation, renewed hope and a sense of being in control of a stressful situation.
- Listening to calming music

Cognitive therapy

- Cognitive techniques have been found to be more effective in long-term maintenance of cure. They help in identifying the catastrophic thoughts in the individual which develop into automatic thoughts that unconsciously result in the panic attack. The individual is helped to identify the triggering cues and take a realistic view.
- Teaches the patient to replace negative thoughts with more realistic and positive ways of viewing the attacks.
- Helps the patient to identify possible triggers for the panic attacks such as a particular thought or situation or even a slight change in heartbeat.
- Helps the patient to identify and evaluate the catastrophic thoughts that precede anxiety and then restructure them to gain a more realistic perception.

The patient and the family members need to be reassured that the illness is not physical, is not serious and the episodes remit spontaneously after a short period of

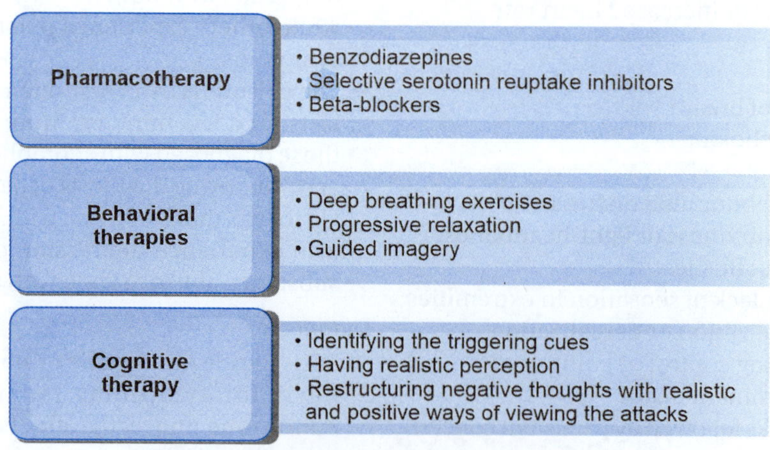

Figure 5.16: Treatment modalities for panic disorder

15–30 minutes. The patient should not avoid situations where such an episode has occurred. A little rest is sufficient with no immediate need to rush to a doctor or a hospital.

Phobic Anxiety Disorder

A phobia is an unreasonable fear of a specific object, activity or situation. This irrational fear is characterized by various features **(Box 5.23)**. In phobic anxiety disorders, the individual experiences intermittent anxiety which arises in particular circumstances, i.e., in response to the phobic object or situation.

Types of Phobias

There are three main groups of phobias: simple/specific phobia, agoraphobia, and social phobia/social anxiety disorder **(Figure 5.17)**.

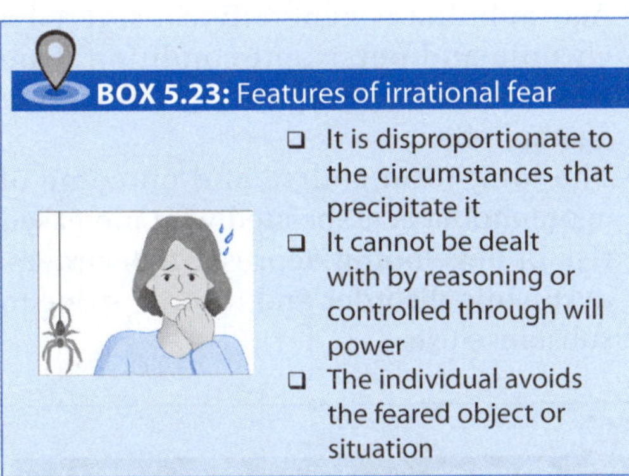

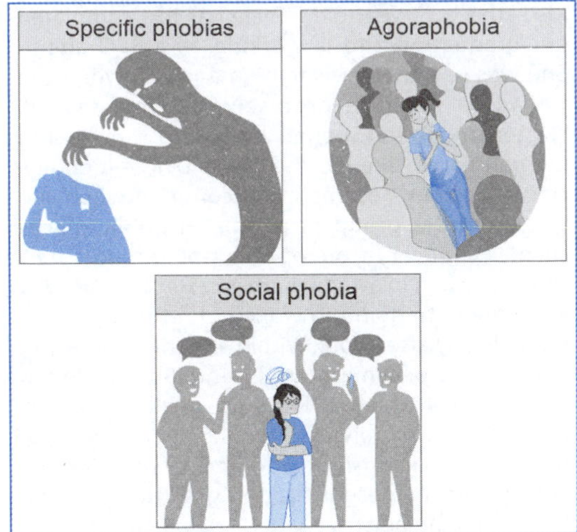

Figure 5.17: Types of phobias

1. Specific phobia (simple phobia)

It refers to irrational fear of a specific object or stimulus. Simple phobias are common in childhood. By early teenage though most of these fears are lost, a few persist till adult life. Sometimes they may reappear after a symptom-free period. Exposure to the phobic object often results in panic attacks **(Box 5.24)**.

According to ICD-11 specific phobia is characterized by a marked and excessive fear or anxiety that consistently occurs upon exposure or anticipation of exposure to one or more specific objects or situations such as proximity to certain animals, flying, heights, closed spaces, sight of blood or injury that is out of proportion to actual danger. The phobic objects or situations are avoided or else endured with intense fear or anxiety. Symptoms persist for at least several months and are sufficiently severe to result in significant distress or impairment in personal, family, social, educational, occupational or other important areas of functioning.

Signs and symptoms of specific phobia

- ❖ Irrational and persistent fear of an object or situation
- ❖ Immediate anxiety on contact with feared object or situation
- ❖ Loss of control, fainting or panic response
- ❖ Avoidance of activities involving feared stimulus
- ❖ Anxiety when thinking about stimulus
- ❖ Worry with anticipatory anxiety
- ❖ Possible impaired social or work functioning

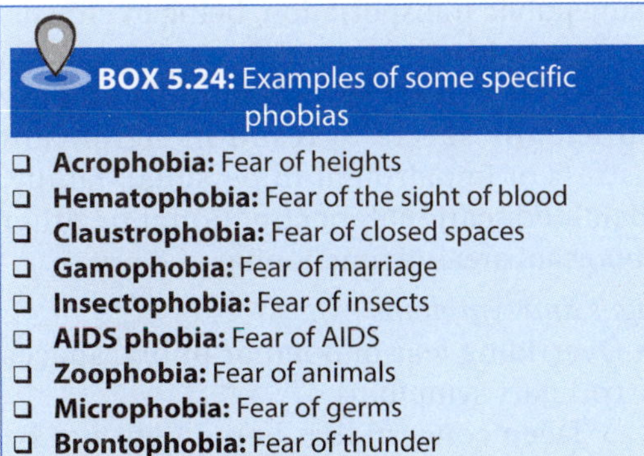

- ❑ **Acrophobia:** Fear of heights
- ❑ **Hematophobia:** Fear of the sight of blood
- ❑ **Claustrophobia:** Fear of closed spaces
- ❑ **Gamophobia:** Fear of marriage
- ❑ **Insectophobia:** Fear of insects
- ❑ **AIDS phobia:** Fear of AIDS
- ❑ **Zoophobia:** Fear of animals
- ❑ **Microphobia:** Fear of germs
- ❑ **Brontophobia:** Fear of thunder
- ❑ **Algophobia:** Fear of pain

❖ The most common phobias are for particular animals (animal phobias), heights (acrophobia), enclosed spaces (claustrophobia), sight of blood or injury, flying, driving, storms, darkness and medical/dental procedures, etc.

❖ While phobic stimuli may result in significant physiological arousal, individuals who fear the sight of blood, invasive medical procedures may experience a vasovagal response that can result in a fainting spell.

Course

❖ Onset is more common during early childhood (7–10 years of age).

❖ Individuals with specific phobias report high life-time rates of co-occurring disorders particularly depressive disorders and other anxiety or fear related disorders.

❖ Specific phobias that persist from childhood into adolescence and adulthood rarely remit spontaneously.

2. Agoraphobia

It is characterized by an irrational fear of being in places away from the familiar setting of home, in crowds, or in situations that the patient cannot leave easily. As the agoraphobia increases in severity, there is a gradual restriction in normal day-to-day activities. The activity may become so severely restricted that the person becomes self-imprisoned at home. According to ICD-11, agoraphobia is characterized by marked and excessive fear or anxiety that occurs in response to multiple situations where escape might be difficult or help might not be available such as using public transportation, being in crowds, being outside the home alone. Symptoms persist for at least several months and are sufficiently severe to result in significant distress or impairment in personal, family, social, educational, occupational or other important areas of functioning.

Signs and symptoms

❖ Overriding fear of open or public spaces (primary symptom)
  ○ Deep concern that help might not be available in such places

  ○ Avoidance of public places and confinement to home

❖ The individual is consistently fearful or anxious about these situations due to fear of specific negative outcomes such as panic attacks.

❖ When accompanied by panic disorder, fear that having panic attack in public will lead to embarrassment or inability to escape (for symptoms of a panic attack).

❖ Experiences feared by individuals with agoraphobia may include symptoms of a panic attack as described in panic disorder.

❖ Individuals with agoraphobia may employ a variety of different behavioral strategies which include avoiding leaving their homes or participating in activities outside their comfort zone **(Box 5.25)**.

Course

❖ Agoraphobia is generally considered a chronic and persistent condition. Late adolescence is the typical age for onset of agoraphobia.

❖ The long-term course and outcome of agoraphobia is associated with increased risk of developing depressive disorders, dysthymic disorder and disorders due to substance use.

BOX 5.25: Case vignette—Agoraphobia

Ms Latha, a 24-year-old female has just completed her graduation and is working as a BPO agent. She was in a theater watching a movie when she began to perspire profusely, became fearful, started trembling, began breathing rapidly and felt nauseated. She left the movie before it ended. Her symptoms became more common when she was around a group of people in public places such as a grocery store or a shopping center. As a result, she began avoiding crowds. Her daily activity was limited to going to work and returning home immediately after work. Within a month, Latha quit her job and became housebound. She consulted a psychiatrist to relive her of the anxiety. She was placed on an anxiolytic to reduce her anxiety. She participated in insight-oriented psychotherapy and systematic desensitization with the help of a behavioral therapist.

❖ Greater symptom severity and co-occurring disorders are associated with poorer prognosis.

3. Social phobia/social anxiety disorder

It is an irrational fear of performing activities in the presence of other people or interacting with others. The patient is afraid of his own actions being viewed by others critically, resulting in embarrassment or humiliation. A person with social phobia often suffers from social anxiety disorder.

According to ICD-11, social anxiety disorder is characterized by marked and excessive fear or anxiety that consistently occurs in one or more social situations such as social interactions. For example, having a conversation or doing something while feeling observed, eating or drinking in the presence of others or giving a speech. The symptoms persist for at least several months and are sufficiently severe to result in significant distress or impairment in personal, family, social, educational, occupational or other important areas of functioning.

Signs and symptoms of social anxiety disorder

❖ Unjustified or excessive fear of being in social situations. Exposing to such situations or activities leads to intense fear or anxiety.

❖ Symptoms of intense fear or anxiety are hyperventilation, sweating, cold and clammy hands, blushing, palpitations, confusion, gastrointestinal symptoms, trembling hands and voice, urinary urgency, muscle tension.

❖ Having difficulty meeting new people, maintaining friendships, etc.

❖ Avoiding interaction with others, giving speeches or presentations at work, staying back home rather than going out with friends and family members.

❖ Experiencing significant distress and impairment in their ability to function in day-to-day life.

❖ Extreme self-consciousness and intense fear of negative evaluation by others may make the individual worrisome about others imagining them to be stupid, boring or unlikable, or acting awkward or embarrassing themselves even when they are not actually doing anything wrong. All these result in avoidance of social situations and cause significant distress.

❖ Anticipatory anxiety occurs well in advance of a particular situation such as a public speech or social event. This leads to thoughts of dread leading up to the event. The added anxiety results in actual or perceived failure in the situation, leading to embarrassment and further anxiety. This pattern sets up a vicious cycle of persistent discomfort that can be incapacitating. Many people who have social phobia are under-achievers because of test anxiety, poor job performance, or poor communication skills. They may have few or no friends, limited support system, and poor interpersonal relationships **(Box 5.26)**.

Course

❖ Typically occurs during childhood and adolescence.

❖ Onset can be gradual, occurs subsequent to a stressful or humiliating social experience and course is chronic.

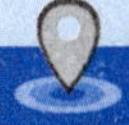

BOX 5.26: Case vignette—Social anxiety disorder

Mr James a 20-year-old college studying boy was referred to a private psychiatric clinic. Clinical interview revealed that he avoids most social situations as they make him too anxious and panicky. He considers himself unattractive, ugly and a loser. During social interactions he assumes that he may not interact well, feels that everybody is looking at him and laughing at him. He has a fear of negative evaluation and is concerned about how others view him. When he loses his concentration he stutters, starts to sweat and feels uneasy. According to James, the problem of social anxiety began when he was in class 7. He had difficulty conversing in English due to which his classmates made fun of him. This event caused him a lot of embarrassment and it is since then that he has become afraid of speaking in public. As this progressed, he slowly started avoiding social gatherings, meeting others and his relatives.

- Later onset, less severe level of impairment and absence of co-occurring disorders have been associated with spontaneous remission.
- Poorer prognosis associated with greater symptom severity and co-occurring disorders such as alcohol misuse, personality disorder and other anxiety disorders.

Separation Anxiety

It is characterized by an excessive and persistent fear of separation from a loved one, such as parent or caregiver. In children and adolescents, separation anxiety typically focuses on caregivers, parents or other family members and the fear or anxiety is beyond what would be considered developmentally normative. In adults the focus is typically a romantic partner or children. It typically begins in childhood but can also occur in adults. The symptoms persist for at least several months and are sufficiently severe to result in significant distress or impairment in personal, family, social, educational, occupational or other important areas of functioning.

Signs and Symptoms

- Excessive fear or anxiety about separation from specific attachment figures.
- It may include thoughts of harm or untoward events befalling the attachment figure.
- It can also include physical symptoms such as sweating, heart palpitations and stomach upset.
- May avoid leaving home or reluctance to go to school or work or social events.
- Recurrent excessive distress upon separation.
- Reluctance or refusal to sleep away from the attachment figure and recurrent nightmares about separation. They may also have difficulty sleeping away from home or sleeping alone **(Box 5.27)**.

Selective Mutism

It is characterized by consistent selectivity in speaking. For example, a child demonstrating adequate language competence in specific

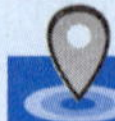

BOX 5.27: Case vignette—Separation anxiety

A 15-year-old girl by name Mary came to psychiatric OPD with a history of anxiety in relation to sleeping away from home specially being away from her mother. She expressed her anxiety as a fear that something would happen to her mother. During such instances she experienced fear, worry, trembling of hands, sweating, difficulty in falling asleep and stomach discomfort. History revealed that during preschool period she was very clingy and that she would not separate from her mother when dropped off at school. The patient would attach herself to her mother, and the teacher would have to meddle her off to create a physical separation. Between the ages of 5–10 years, the patient recalled having a nightmare in which her mother died and she was unable to help her. At age of 11 years, the patient experienced homesickness while away on a NCC camp which produced high level of distress. As the staff were unable to console her, the parents were notified and advised to take her back. She was diagnosed with separation anxiety disorder and recommended to consult clinical psychologist for therapy.

social situations, typically at home but consistently failing to speak at school.

Signs and Symptoms

- Consistent selectivity in speaking
- Duration of disturbance is at least 1 month but not limited to the first month of school
- Associated with severe impairment in academic and social functioning **(Box 5.28)**

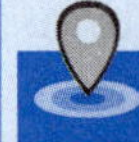

BOX 5.28: Case vignette—Selective mutism

A 10-year-old girl was brought to child psychiatric OPD with the complaint of refusing to talk to outsiders and being unable to speak in social situations. She interacts only with her family members at home. She has since been communicating with her classmates and teachers using gestures and facial expressions or nodding of head. History revealed no significant stressors or problems related to speech development. On examination she was making adequate eye contact and communicating by nodding. She exhibited normal level of intelligence, good academic record, regular sleep and appetite. She was diagnosed with selective mutism and referred for psychological interventions.

Diagnosis

❖ No specific diagnostic test. Diagnosis confirmed if ICD-11 criteria is met.
❖ History of anxiety when exposed to or anticipating specific entity or situation.

Treatment for Anxiety Disorders

The two main treatments for anxiety disorders are medications, behavior therapy and psychotherapy **(Figure 5.18)**.

Medications

❖ Benzodiazepines (e.g., alprazolam, clonazepam, lorazepam, diazepam)
❖ Antidepressants (e.g., imipramine, sertraline, phenelzine)

Behavior Therapy

❖ Desensitization therapy to gradually reintroduce the feared situation while coaching the patient on relaxation techniques (progressive muscle relaxation, deep-breathing exercises, listening to calming music)
❖ Role-playing in guided imagery to allow the patient rehearse ways to relax while confronting a feared object or situation.
❖ Assertive training to help the patient become assertive in interpersonal interactions.
❖ Modeling behavior: Patient observes someone modeling or demonstrating appropriate behavior when confronted with the feared situation.
❖ Cognitive behavioral technique called negative thought stopping to reduce the frequency and duration of disturbing thoughts by interrupting them and substituting competing thoughts:
  ○ Teaches patient to recognize negative thoughts
  ○ Uses an intense distracting stimulus such as snapping a rubber band around the wrist to stop the thought
  ○ With practice, allows patient to control thoughts without using distracting stimulus

Psychotherapy

Supportive psychotherapy is a helpful adjunct to behavior therapy and drug treatment.

Nursing Management for Anxiety or Fear-related Disorders

Nursing management includes symptom assessment, providing emotional support, teaching relaxation techniques and promoting overall well-being.

Nursing Assessment

Assessment should focus on collection of physical, psychological and social data. It should focus on physical symptoms, precipitating factors, avoidance behavior associated with phobia, impact of anxiety on physical functioning, normal coping ability, thought content and social support systems. The nurse should be particularly aware of the fact that major physical symptoms are often associated with autonomic nervous system stimulation. Specific symptoms should be

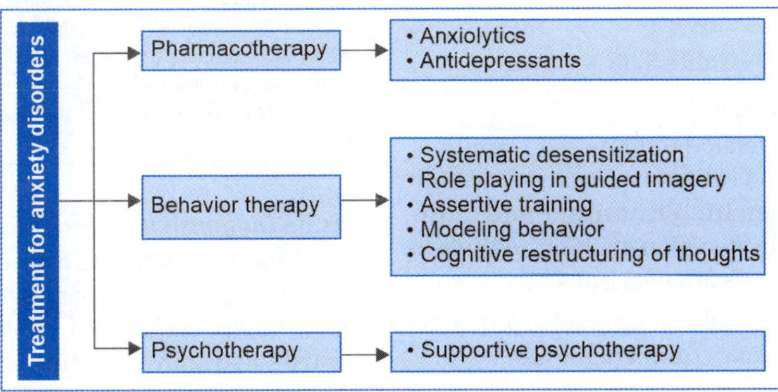

Figure 5.18: Treatment of anxiety disorders

noted along with statements made by the patient about subjective distress. The nurse must use clinical judgment to determine the level of anxiety being experienced by the patient.

History and Mental Status Examination

❖ During assessment of patients with high levels of anxiety the nurse should make observations of thought processes, affect, communication, psychomotor, and physiological responses.

❖ The nurse should use directive questions to elicit subjective information about how the patient is currently feeling and what happened before the onset of symptoms.

❖ Ask the patient about other somatic symptoms such as fatigue, muscle aches, eating patterns, bowel habits, sleeping patterns and non-verbal fatigue.

❖ Assess the patient for communication pattern

❖ Observe patient's ability to perform and complete tasks.

❖ Particular attention should be given to specific anxiety-reducing behaviors. For example, leaving group therapy, going to bathroom, avoiding an activity, etc.

❖ Assess for social support system.

Nursing Diagnosis I

Panic anxiety related to real or perceived threat to biological integrity or self-concept evidenced by various physical and psychological manifestations.

Objective: Patient will be able to recognize symptoms of onset on anxiety and intervene before reaching panic level.

Interventions: See **Table 5.32**.

Nursing Diagnosis II

Powerlessness related to impaired cognition, evidenced by verbal expression of lack of control over life situations and non-participation in decision-making related to own care or significant life issues.

Objective: Patient will be able to solve problems effectively and take control of his life.

Interventions: See **Table 5.33**.

TABLE 5.32: Nursing interventions to reduce panic anxiety

Nursing interventions	Rationale
Stay with the patient and offer reassurance of safety and security	Presence of trusted individual provides feeling of security and assurance of personal safety
Maintain a calm, non-threatening matter-of-fact approach	Anxiety is contagious and may be transferred from staff to patient or vice-versa
Use simple words and brief messages, spoken calmly and clearly to explain hospital experiences	In an intensely anxious situation, patient is unable to comprehend anything but the most elementary communication
Keep immediate surroundings low in stimuli (dim lighting, few people)	A stimulating environment may result in increase of anxiety level
Administer tranquilizing medication as prescribed by the physician. Assess for effectiveness and side-effects	Antianxiety medication provides relief from the immobilizing effects of anxiety
When level of anxiety has been reduced, explore possible reasons for occurrence	Recognition of precipitating factors is the first step in teaching patient to interrupt escalating anxiety
Teach signs and symptoms of escalating anxiety and ways to interrupt its progression using relaxation techniques, deep-breathing exercises and meditation, or physical exercise like brisk walks and jogging	The first three of these activities result in physiologic response opposite of the anxiety response, i.e., a sense of calm, slowed heart rate, etc. The latter activities discharge energy in a healthy manner

Nursing Diagnosis III

Fear related to a specific stimulus (simple phobia), or causing embarrassment to self in front of others, evidenced by behavior directed towards avoidance of the feared object/situation.

TABLE 5.33: Nursing interventions to improve self-control in anxious patients

Nursing interventions	Rationale
Allow patient to take as much responsibility as possible for self-care activities, provide positive feedback for decisions made	Providing choices will enhance patient's feeling of control
Assist patient to set realistic goals	Unrealistic goals set the patient up for failure and reinforce feelings of powerlessness
Help identify life situations that are within patient's control	Patient's emotional condition interferes with the ability to solve problems
Help patient identify areas of life situation that are not within his ability to control. Encourage verbalization of feelings related to this inability	Assistance is required to perceive the benefits and consequences of available alternatives accurately, to deal with unresolved issues and accept what cannot be changed

Objective: Patient will be able to function in the presence of a phobic object or situation without experiencing panic anxiety.

Interventions: See **Table 5.34**.

Nursing Diagnosis IV

Social isolation related to fear of being in a place from which one is unable to escape evidenced by staying alone, refusing to leave the room/home.

Objective: Patient will voluntarily participate in group activities with peers.

Interventions: See **Table 5.35**.

TABLE 5.34: Nursing interventions to reduce fear

Nursing interventions	Rationale
Reassure the patient that he is safe	At the panic level of anxiety patient may fear for his own life
Explore patient's perception of the threat to physical integrity or threat to self-concept	It is important to understand patient's perception of the phobic object or situation to assist with the desensitization process
Include patient in making decisions related to selection of alternative coping strategies (for example, patient may choose either to avoid the phobic stimulus or attempt to eliminate the fear associated with it)	Allowing the patient to choose provides a measure of control and serves to increase feelings of self-worth
If the patient elects to work on eliminating the fear, techniques of desensitization or implosion therapy may be employed	Fear reduces as the physical and psychological sensations diminish in response to repeated exposure to the phobic stimulus under non-threatening conditions
Encourage patient to explore underlying feelings that may be contributing to irrational fears	Facing these feelings rather than suppressing them may result in more adaptive coping abilities

TABLE 5.35: Nursing interventions to reduce social isolation behavior in anxious patients

Nursing interventions	Rationale
Convey an accepting attitude and unconditional positive regard. Make brief, frequent contacts. Be honest and keep all promises	These interventions enhance feelings of self-worth and facilitate a trusting relationship
Attend group activities with the patient that may be frightening for him	Presence of a trusted individual provides emotional security
Administer anti-anxiety medications as ordered by the physician, monitor for effectiveness and adverse effects	Antianxiety medications help to reduce the level of anxiety in most individuals thereby facilitating interactions with others
Discuss with the patient signs and symptoms of increasing anxiety and techniques to interrupt the response (e.g., relaxation exercises, thought stopping)	Maladaptive behavior such as withdrawal and suspiciousness are manifested during times of increased anxiety
Give recognition and positive reinforcement for voluntary interactions with others	To enhance self-esteem, encourage repetition of acceptable behaviors

Evaluation

Effectiveness of planned interventions is demonstrated in the patient's ability to recognize and deal with the anxiety-producing factors. Relaxed participation in unit activities and reports of longer periods of restful sleep indicate reduced anxiety. Reassessment is conducted to determine if the nursing interventions have been successful in achieving the objectives of care. Following questions are helpful in evaluation:

- Is the patient experiencing a reduced level of anxiety?
- Does the patient recognize symptoms as anxiety-related?
- Is the patient able to use newly learned behavior to manage anxiety?
- Does the patient face phobic object/situation without anxiety?
- Does the patient voluntarily participate in group activities?
- Is the patient able to demonstrate techniques that he may use to prevent anxiety from escalating to panic level?

Obsessive-Compulsive Disorder

Obsessive-compulsive disorder (OCD) is a chronic mental health condition that involves obsessions (uncontrollable and recurring thoughts), compulsions (repetitive behaviors) or both.

- **Obsessions:** These are an unwanted and unpleasant thoughts, images or urges that repeatedly enter the mind causing feelings of anxiety, disgust or unease. The individual attempts to suppress such thoughts, urges or images with some other thought or action.
- **Compulsions:** These are repetitive behaviors or mental acts that the person feels driven to perform in response to an obsession. The behaviors or mental acts aim at reducing anxiety or distress or preventing some dreaded situation.

According to ICD-11 obsessive-compulsive disorder is characterized by the presence of persistent obsessions or compulsions, or most commonly both. Obsessions are repetitive and persistent thoughts, images, or impulses/urges that are intrusive, unwanted and commonly associated with anxiety. The individual attempts to ignore or suppress obsessions or neutralize them by performing compulsions. Compulsions are repetitive behaviors including repetitive mental acts that the individual feels driven to perform in response to an obsession, according to rigid rules, or to achieve a sense of 'completeness'. In order for obsessive-compulsive disorder to be diagnosed, obsessions and compulsions must be time consuming (e.g., taking more than an hour per day) or result in significant distress or significant impairment in personal, family, social, educational, occupational or other important areas of functioning **(Box 5.29).**

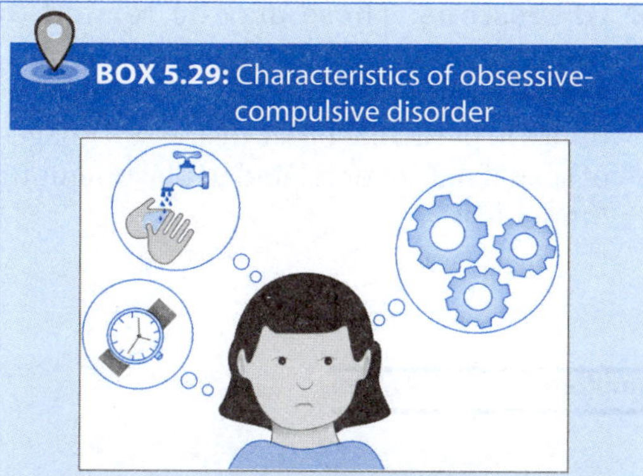

BOX 5.29: Characteristics of obsessive-compulsive disorder

- They are recurrent and persistent ideas, doubts, ruminations, impulses or images which intrude into conscious awareness repeatedly
- They are recognized as the individual's own thoughts or impulses and not attributed to others
- They are unpleasant and anxiety provoking
- Patient tries to resist them but is unable to do so
- Failure to resist leads to marked distress
- Rituals/compulsions are the motor counterpart of obsessions, performed with a sense of subjective compulsion (urge to act)
- These are recurrent behaviors such as counting, checking, washing, touching or avoiding
- They are aimed at either preventing or neutralizing the distress or fear arising out of obsessions
- Not performing the behaviors commonly causes great distress often attached to a specific fear of dire consequences
- Thoughts or compulsions are time consuming (more than one hour a day) which can significantly interfere with a person's daily activities and social interaction
- Both obsessions and compulsions are recognized as irrational or senseless, unnecessary and excessive. Client is not able to ignore or control it.

OCD has a life time prevalence of about 3%. The disorder may begin in childhood but more often begins in adolescence or early adulthood. It is equally common among men and women. The course is usually chronic. Many OCD sufferers also have major depressive disorder, panic disorder, social phobia, specific phobia, eating disorder, substance abuse or personality disorders.

Etiology

The exact cause of obsessive-compulsive disorder though unknown is most likely multifactorial **(Figure 5.19)**.

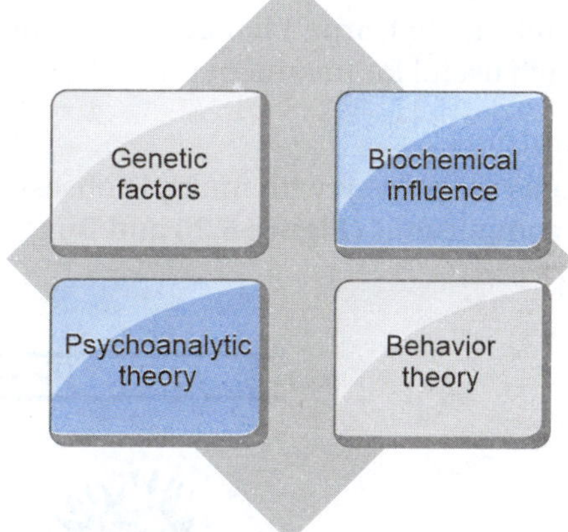

Figure 5.19: Etiology for obsessive compulsive disorder

Genetic Factors

Twin studies have consistently found a significantly higher concordance rate for monozygotic twins than for dizygotic twins. Family studies of these patients have shown that 35% of the first-degree relatives of obsessive-compulsive disorder patients are also affected with the disorder.

Biochemical Influences

A number of studies suggest that the neurotransmitter serotonin (5-HT) may be abnormal in individuals with obsessive-compulsive disorder.

Psychoanalytic Theory

The psychoanalytic concept (Freud) views patients with obsessive-compulsive disorder (OCD) as having regressed to developmentally earlier stages of the infantile superego whose harsh exacting punitive characteristics now reappear as part of the psychopathology.

Freud also proposed that regression to the pre-oedipal anal-sadistic phase combined with the use of specific ego defense mechanisms like isolation, undoing, displacement and reaction information, may lead to OCD.

Behavior Theory

This theory explains obsessions as a conditioned stimulus to anxiety. Compulsions have been described as learned behavior that reduces the anxiety associated with obsessions. This reduction in anxiety positively reinforces the compulsive acts and they become stable learned behavior. This theory is much useful for treatment purposes.

Symptoms

Patients are present with multiple obsessions and compulsions **(Figure 5.20 and Box 5.30)**

❖ **Obsessions**: These may be related to contamination with dirt, repetitive doubts, aggressive impulses, excessive need to have things in particular order, distressful images of sexual nature or related to blasphemous thoughts.

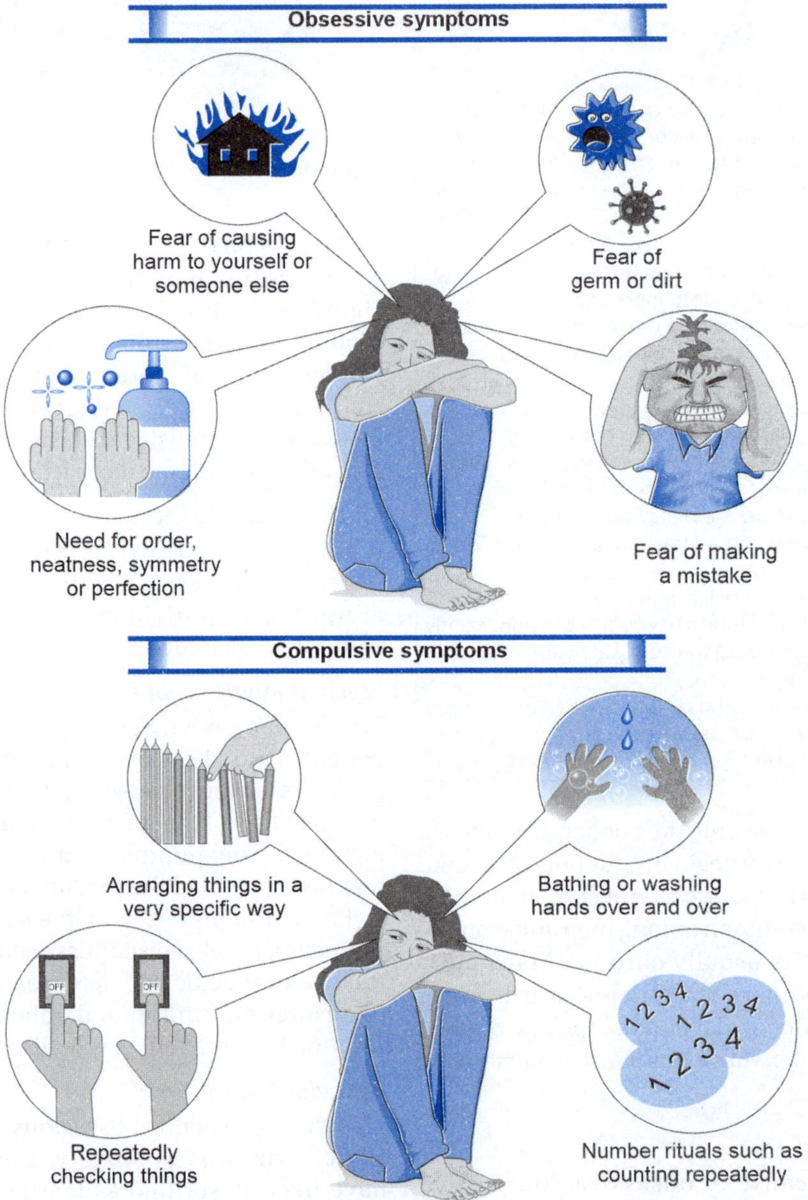

Figure 5.20: Symptoms of obsessive compulsive disorder

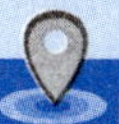

BOX 5.30: Case vignette—Obsessive compulsive disorder

A 25-year-old woman visited psychiatric OPD with following complaints: Feeling compelled to wash hands, cleaning door handles, drawer handles, etc. These activities are performed in response to an obsession that she might contract a dreadful disease due to contamination. Though she knew that the idea was strange and silly, she could not stop thinking about it. These behaviors turned out to be very time consuming and cumbersome. Also at home, the rules and functioning imposed led to a significant burden on family members. At assessment recurrent intrusive thoughts of contamination were reported. She was diagnosed with obsessive-compulsive disorder and put on escitalopram 10 mg daily. She was later referred for cognitive behavioral therapy.

❖ **Obsessional thoughts**: These are words, ideas and beliefs that intrude forcibly into the patient's mind. They are usually unpleasant and shocking to the patient and may be obscene or blasphemous.

❖ **Obsessional images**: These are vividly imagined scenes often of a violent or disgusting kind involving abnormal sexual practices.

❖ **Obsessional ruminations**: These involve internal debates in which arguments for and against even the simplest everyday actions are reviewed endlessly.

❖ **Obsessional doubts**: These may concern actions that may not have been completed adequately. The obsession often implies some danger such as forgetting to turn off the stove or not locking a door. It may be followed by a compulsive act such as the person making multiple trips back into the house to check if the stove has been turned off. Sometimes these may take the form of doubting the very fundamentals of beliefs such as, doubting the existence of God and so on.

❖ **Obsessional impulses**: These are urges to perform acts usually of a violent or embarrassing kind such as injuring a child, shouting in church, etc.

❖ **Obsessional rituals**: These may include both mental activities such as counting repeatedly in a special way or repeating a certain form of words, and repeated but senseless behaviors such as washing hands 20 or more times a day. Sometimes such compulsive acts may be preceded by obsessional thoughts; for example, repeated handwashing may be preceded by thoughts of contamination. These patients usually believe that contamination is spread from object to object or person to person even by slight contact and may literally rub the skin off their hands by excessive hand washing.

❖ **Obsessive slowness**: Severe obsessive ideas or extensive compulsive rituals characterize obsessional slowness in the relative absence of manifested anxiety. This leads to marked slowness in daily activities.

❖ **Compulsions**: These may include excessive hand washing, bathing, repetitive checking of doors, locks or taps, etc.

❖ Patients often suffer with secondary depression, disinterest, hopelessness, helplessness, disturbed sleep.

Course and Prognosis

Course is usually long and fluctuating. About two-thirds of patients improve by the end of a year. A good prognosis is indicated by good social and occupational adjustment, the presence of a precipitating event and an episodic nature of symptom.

Prognosis appears to be worse when the onset is in childhood, the personality is obsessional, symptoms are severe, compulsions are bizarre, or there is a coexisting major depressive disorder.

Treatment

Treatment of OCD includes behavior therapy and medications.

Pharmacotherapy

❖ Antidepressants (e.g., fluvoxamine, sertraline)

❖ Anxiolytics (e.g., benzodiazepines)

Behavior Therapy

- **Exposure and response prevention (ERP):** This is vivo exposure procedure combined with response prevention techniques. The basic principle of ERP is that the patient is exposed to the obsessional stimuli and not allowed to perform neutralizing behaviors. For example, compulsive hand washers are encouraged to touch contaminated objects and then refrain from washing in order to break the negative reinforcement chain.
- **Thought stoppage:** Thought stopping is a technique that helps an individual to learn to stop thinking unwanted thoughts. Following are the steps in thought stopping:
  - Sit in a comfortable chair bringing to mind the unwanted thought, concentrating on only one thought per procedure.
  - As soon as the thought forms, give the command 'Stop!' Follow this with calm and deliberate relaxation of muscles and diversion of thought to something pleasant.
  - Repeat the procedure to bring the unwanted thought under control.
- **Relaxation technique:** It includes deep breathing exercise, progressive muscle relaxation, meditation, imagery and music.

Other Therapies

- Supportive psychotherapy
- ECT—for patients' refractory to other forms of treatment

Nursing Management

Nursing care for patients with OCD involves implementing the interventions based on assessment data and evaluating the outcomes.

Nursing Assessment

Assessment should focus on the collection of physical, psychological and social data. The nurse should be particularly aware of the impact of obsessions and compulsions on physical functioning, mood, self-esteem and normal coping ability. The defense mechanisms used, thought content or process

potential for suicide, ability to function and social support systems available should also be noted.

Nursing diagnosis I
Ineffective individual coping related to underdeveloped ego, punitive superego, avoidance learning, possible biochemical changes evidenced by ritualistic behavior or obsessive thoughts.

Objective: Patient will demonstrate ability to cope effectively without resorting to obsessive-compulsive behaviors.

Interventions: See **Table 5.36.**

TABLE 5.36: Nursing interventions to reduce obsessive compulsive behavior	
Nursing interventions	**Rationale**
Work with patient to determine types of situations that increase anxiety and result in ritualistic behaviors	Recognition of precipitating factors is the first step in teaching the patient to interrupt escalating anxiety
Initially meet the patient's dependency needs. Encourage independence and give positive reinforcement for independent behaviors	Sudden and complete elimination of all avenues for dependency would create intense anxiety on the part of the patient. Positive reinforcement enhances self-esteem and encourages repetition of desired behaviors
In the early phase of treatment, allow plenty of time for rituals. Do not be judgmental or verbalize disapproval of the behavior	Denying patient this activity may precipitate panic anxiety
Support patient's efforts to explore the meaning and purpose of the behavior	Patient may be unaware of the relationship between emotional problems and compulsive behaviors. Recognition is important before change can occur

Contd...

Contd...

Nursing interventions	Rationale
Provide structured schedule of activities for patient including adequate time for completion of rituals	Structure provides a feeling of security for the anxious patient
Gradually begin to limit amount of time allotted for ritualistic behavior as patient becomes more involved in unit activities	Anxiety is minimized when patient is able to replace ritualistic behaviors with more adaptive ones
Give positive reinforcement for non-ritualistic behaviors	Positive reinforcement encourages repetition of desired behaviors
Help patient learn ways of interrupting obsessive thoughts and ritualistic behavior with techniques such as thought stopping, relaxation and exercise	These activities help in interruption of obsessive thoughts

Nursing diagnosis II

Altered role performance related to the need to perform rituals evidenced by inability to fulfill usual patterns of responsibility.

Objective: Patient will be able to resume role-related responsibilities.

Interventions: See **Table 5.37**.

Evaluation

Evaluation of patient with obsessive-compulsive disorder may be done by asking the following questions:

❖ Does the patient continue to display obsessive-compulsive symptoms?

❖ Is the patient able to use newly learned behaviors to manage anxiety?

❖ Can the patient adequately perform self-care activities?

Post-traumatic Stress Disorder

Post-traumatic stress disorder (PTSD) is a psychological condition which may develop following exposure to one or more traumatic events. Exposure may be direct experiencing or

TABLE 5.37: Nursing interventions to improve role-related responsibilities in OCD patients

Nursing interventions	Rationale
Determine patient's previous role within the family and the extent to which this role is altered by the illness. Identify roles of other family members	This is important assessment data for formulating an appropriate plan of care
Encourage patient to discuss conflicts evident within the family system. Identify how patient and other family members have responded to this conflict	Identifying specific stressors as well as adaptive and maladaptive responses within the system is necessary before assistance can be provided in an effort to facilitate change
Explore available options for changes or adjustments in role. Practice through role play	Planning and rehearsal of potential role transitions can reduce anxiety
Provide the patient lots of positive reinforcement enabling him to resume his role responsibilities by limiting the need for ritualistic behaviors	Positive reinforcement enhances self-esteem and promotes repetition of desired behaviors

witnessing of the traumatic event as it occurred to others. The lifetime prevalence of PTSD is approximately 8% with female adults and adolescents being more likely to be diagnosed than males.

According to ICD-11, PTSD is characterized by re-experiencing the traumatic event, avoidance of thoughts and memories of the event/events and hypervigilance state. In ICD-11, it is classified under disorders specifically associated with stress (6B40).

Causes

The risk factors are preexisting genetic factors, severe traumatic experience, childhood adversities, pre-existing mental illness, low socio-economic status, poor education, lack of social support. PTSD can develop after a stressful, frightening or distressing event or after a prolonged traumatic experience. The traumatic events may include following:

- ❖ Physical or sexual assault
- ❖ Abuse including childhood or domestic abuse
- ❖ Terrorist attacks, natural disasters
- ❖ Serious accidents
- ❖ Death of someone with close association
- ❖ Acute life-threatening illness
- ❖ War or conflict
- ❖ Torture
- ❖ Witnessing the threatened or actual injury or death of others in a sudden, unexpected or violent manner, etc.

Signs and Symptoms

The four important features of PTSD are **(Figure 5.21 and Box 5.31)**:

1. **Re-experiencing the traumatic event in the present**: It is not just remembering but is experienced as occurring again in the here and now. This typically occurs in the form of vivid intrusive memories or images; flashbacks or repetitive dreams/nightmares. Re-experiencing may occur in one or more sensory modalities, is typically accompanied by strong overwhelming emotions such as fear or horror and strong physical sensation. These are hard to control and intrude into everyday life.
   - ○ Memories or disturbing thoughts can be prompted by smell, sound, words or other triggers.
   - ○ Reminders of the trauma cause extreme distress.

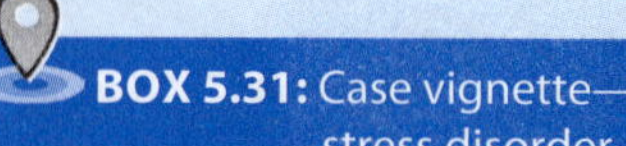

BOX 5.31: Case vignette—Post-traumatic stress disorder

Mrs Vimala, 35-year-old software engineer came to psychiatric clinic with the following complaints: difficulty in sleeping, irritable, unable to concentrate at work, overly alert, low mood, fearful, demotivated, not interacting with others and not going to work for the last 15 days. History revealed that 3 months ago while driving back home from work, she lost control of her car while negotiating a bend in the road. The car spun and came to a halt after hitting a wall. She was taken to the hospital and treated for injuries. Vimala had no memory of the event after losing control of the car. The above symptoms began manifesting 3 months after the occurrence of said incidence. On mental status examination she was found to be having intrusive memories of the accident everyday in which she saw the car spinning. Vimala had flashbacks when she drove her car which happened several times a week. As she felt hot and sweaty in these situations, she gradually began avoiding places that reminded her of the trauma. She often woke up with nightmares of the accident.

2. **Deliberate avoidance of reminders**: This may include either of active internal avoidance of thoughts and memories related to the events or external avoidance of people, conversation, activities or situations reminiscent of the event. These include:
   - ○ Staying away from places, people or objects that may trigger memories of the traumatic event
   - ○ Changing a normal routine to avoid triggering memories

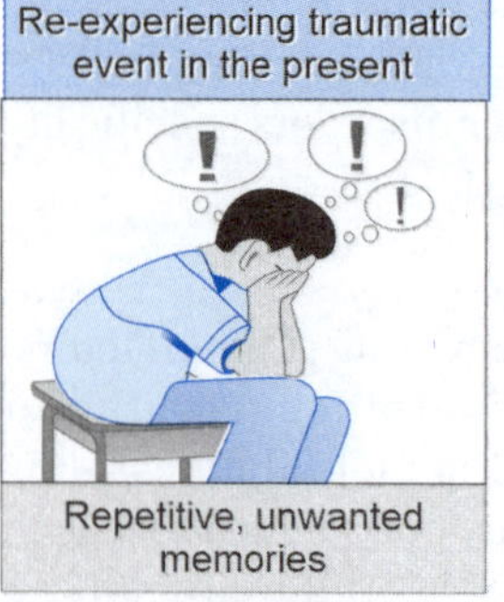

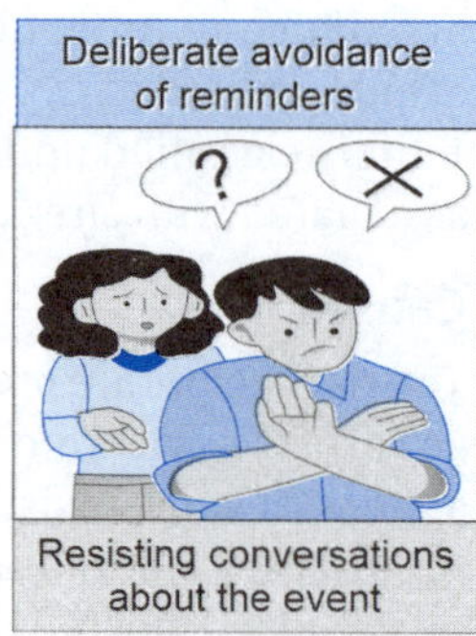

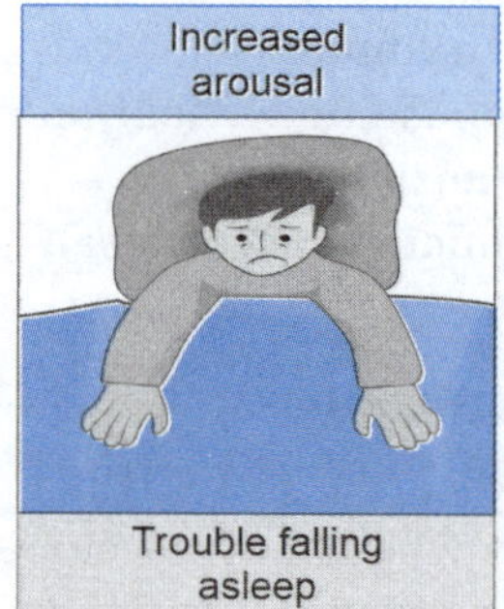

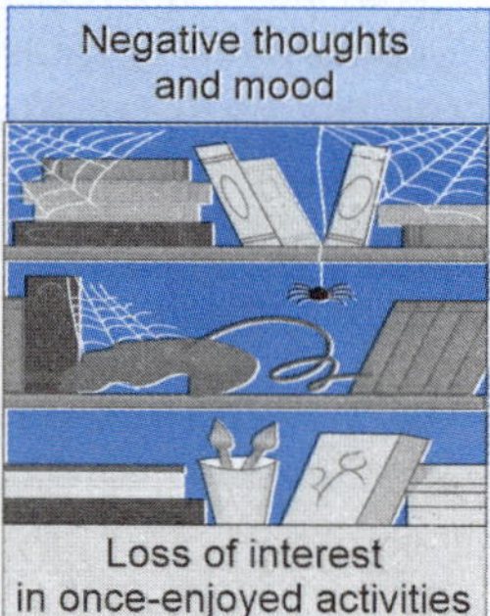

Figure 5.21: Signs and symptoms of PTSD

- ○ Not wanting to talk about or think about the event
- ○ Feeling numb
3. **Increased arousal:** This is persistent perception of heightened current threat, for example:
   - ○ Constant excessive alertness
   - ○ Scanning the environment for signs of danger
   - ○ Being easily startled
   - ○ Irritable or aggressive behavior
   - ○ Difficulty in sleeping
   - ○ Poor concentration
4. **Negative thoughts and mood:** This may include negative beliefs about self and others.
   - ○ Hopelessness about the future
   - ○ Blaming self or others
   - ○ Intense worry, depression, anger or guilt
   - ○ Loss of interest in once enjoyed activities
   - ○ Emotionally detached from others
   - ○ Not being able to experience positive emotions

The above disturbance results in significant impairment in personal, family, social, educational, occupational or other important areas of functioning. The symptoms must persist for more than 1 month for a diagnosis to be made.

Course and Prognosis

Onset of PTSD symptoms typically occurs within three months following exposure to a traumatic event. Symptoms may appear even years after exposure to a traumatic event. Course may vary from person to person. Recurrence of symptoms may occur after the exposure to reminders of the traumatic event. Nearly one half of individuals diagnosed with PTSD experience complete recovery within 3 months of its onset.

Treatment

Treatment of PTSD includes medications and psychological therapies.

Medications

- ❖ **Antidepressants**: Used to reduce depression and anxiety symptoms, and improve sleep problems and concentration. Selective serotonin reuptake inhibitors such as sertraline and paroxetine are approved by food and drug administration for PTSD.
- ❖ **Antianxiety medication**: Used to relieve severe anxiety and related symptoms.

Psychological Therapies

- ❖ **Cognitive behavior therapy**: Helps to recognize relationship among thoughts, feelings and behaviors. It teaches the patient on how to modify and challenge negative thoughts.
- ❖ **Exposure therapy**: Helps to overcome flashbacks and nightmares. It exposes the individual to trauma-related memories, feelings and situations through imagination or virtual reality program in a gradual manner. The patient presumably learns that the trauma-related memories and cues are not dangerous and do not need to be avoided.
- ❖ **Eye movement desensitization and reprocessing (EMDR) therapy**: A structured therapy which encourages the patient to briefly focus on the trauma memory while simultaneously experiencing bilateral stimulation (typically eye movements) which is associated with a reduction in the vividness and emotion associated with the trauma memories.

Nursing Interventions

Nursing care for patients with PTSD involves implementing the interventions based on assessment data and evaluating the outcomes.

Nursing Assessment

Nurse should employ open-ended questions to assess the internal and external presentation of fear, determine the patient's anxiety level, assess the patient's degree of fear or perceived threat and find out how the patient has coped in the past with fear.

Nursing Diagnoses

1. Fear related to perceived threat or danger secondary to PTSD as evidenced by verbalization of fearful feelings, agitation.

2. Anxiety related to anticipation of harm secondary to PTSD as evidenced by increased anxiety.
3. Insomnia related to difficulty maintaining normal sleep secondary to PTSD as evidenced by sleep deprivation.

Outcome
- ❖ The patient will demonstrate effective coping behavior.
- ❖ The patient will verbalize feelings of anxiety effectively.
- ❖ The patient will get adequate amount of sleep.

Nursing Interventions
- ❖ Establish rapport to gain trusting relationship.
- ❖ Encourage the patient to express grief and complete the mourning process.
- ❖ Ensure that the patient is in a calm and safe environment and reassure him repeatedly that he is safe.
- ❖ Evaluate patient's coping strategies and encourage the implementation of positive ones.
- ❖ Assist the patient in identifying sources of emotions.
- ❖ Administer prescribed medications as needed.
- ❖ Some healthy ways to cope during a fearful situation are positive self-talk, listening to music and use of other relaxation techniques. Encourage them to try various methods and see which is most helpful. Relaxation techniques include deep breathing, yoga and meditation.
- ❖ Reassure the patient that feelings of fear after a traumatic event are normal and valid.
- ❖ Show compassion.
- ❖ Assess the severity of anxiety, stimulants for anxiety.
- ❖ Encourage the patient to express emotions openly, use silence and active listening to portray a caring attitude.
- ❖ Assist in regaining control over angry outbursts by identifying how anger escalates.
- ❖ Encourage move from physical to verbal expressions of anger.

- ❖ Educate the patient about medications and their adverse effects, and advise him not to discontinue medication without physician consultation.

Evaluation
During the evaluation process, assess for reduction in anxiety and fearfulness, improvement in level of functioning. The patient must also come to an understanding of the relationship between the fear state and the increased anxiety that is felt as repressed past trauma is triggered by environmental factors.

Dissociative Disorders
Dissociative disorders involve experiencing a loss of connection between thoughts, memories, feelings, behavior and identity. People with dissociative disorder are not aware that they have a disorder until it is brought to their attention. The common features of dissociative disorders are presented in **Box 5.32.**

According to ICD-11, dissociative disorders are characterized by involuntary disruption or discontinuity in the normal integration of one or more of the following: identity, sensations, perceptions, affect, thoughts, memories, control over bodily movements or behavior.

Etiology
- ❖ According to psychodynamic theory, dissociation is the result of overuse of the defense mechanism of dissociation.

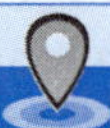

BOX 5.32: Common features of dissociative disorder

- ❑ Disturbance in the normal integrated functions of consciousness, identity and or memory
- ❑ Disturbance may be sudden or gradual, is usually temporary, recovery often abrupt
- ❑ These disorders tend to occur in response to severe trauma or abuse. A frequent stressful situation is an ongoing war
- ❑ Significant impairment in general and social functioning
- ❑ Detailed physical examination and investigations do not reveal any abnormality that can explain the symptoms adequately

❖ According to behavioral theory, symptoms are learnt from the surrounding environment. These symptoms bring about psychological relief by avoidance of stress.

❖ According to the American Psychological Association, people who have experienced sexual or physical abuse in childhood are at an increased risk of developing dissociative identity disorder.

❖ These disorders usually arise as a reaction to shocking, distressing or painful events and help push away difficult memories.

❖ These symptoms can worsen during stressful situations.

Dissociative Neurological Symptom Disorder

According to ICD-11, dissociative neurological symptom disorder is characterized by the presentation of motor, sensory, or cognitive symptoms that imply an involuntary discontinuity in the normal integration of motor, sensory, or cognitive functions and are not consistent with a recognized disease of the nervous system, other mental or behavioral disorder, or other medical condition. These include dissociative neurological symptom disorder with auditory disturbance, with vertigo or dizziness, with sensory disturbance, with non-epileptic seizures, with speech disturbances, with paresis or weakness, with gait disturbances.

Dissociative Motor Disorders

It is characterized by motor disturbances like paralysis or abnormal movements. Paralysis may be a monoplegia, paraplegia or quadriplegia. The abnormal movement may be tremors, choreiform movements or gait disturbances which increase when attention is directed towards them. Examination reveals normal tone and reflexes.

Dissociative Convulsions (Hysterical Fits or Pseudo-seizures)

It is characterized by convulsive movements and partial loss of consciousness. Differential diagnosis with true seizures is important **(Table 5.38 and Box 5.33)**.

TABLE 5.38: Differences between epileptic seizures and dissociative convulsions

Characteristics	Epileptic seizures	Dissociative convulsions
Aura (warning)	Usual	Unusual
Attack pattern	Stereotyped	Purposive body movements
Clinical pattern	Present	Absence of any established pattern
Tongue bite	Present	Absent
Incontinence of urine and feces	Can occur	Very rare
Injury	Can occur	Very rare
Duration	Usually about 30–70 sec	20–800 sec (prolonged)
Amnesia	Complete	Partial
Time of day	Anytime; can occur during sleep also	Never occurs during sleep
Place of occurrence	Anywhere	Usually indoors or in safe places
Postictal confusion	Present	Absent
Neurological signs	Present	Absent

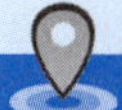 **BOX 5.33:** Case vignette—Dissociative convulsions

A 45-year-old female came to neurology OPD with complaint of seizures. A close relative who is a healthcare professional witnessed the episode and described as follows: there was abnormal violent shaking of both upper and lower limbs lasting for five minutes. Patient was conscious and able to communicate throughout the event, did not experience bowel or bladder incontinence, no evidence of tongue bite. Each episode was followed by a brief period of reduced responsiveness. This reduced responsiveness lasted for about 3 minutes after which he was fully responsive and mobile. The patient reported being aware of his surroundings during the episode and recalled what was happening around him. Most of the episodes occurred when she was in a group, and never occurred when alone. Neurological examination revealed the patient to be normal. She was referred to psychiatric OPD.

Dissociative Sensory Loss and Anesthesia

It is characterized by sensory disturbances like hemianesthesia, blindness, deafness and glove and stocking anesthesia (absence of sensations at wrists and ankles). The disturbance is usually based on patient's knowledge of that particular illness whose symptoms are produced. A detailed examination does not reveal any abnormalities.

Dissociative Amnesia

Most often, dissociative amnesia follows a traumatic or stressful life situation. There is a sudden inability to recall important personal information particularly concerning the stressful life event. The extent of the disturbance is too great to be explained by ordinary forgetfulness. The amnesia may be localized, generalized, selective or continuing in nature.

Dissociative Fugue

Dissociative (psychogenic) fugue is a sudden, unexpected travel away from home or workplace with the assumption of a new identity and an inability to recall the past. The onset is sudden, often in the presence of severe stress. Following recovery there is no recollection of the events that took place during the fugue. The course is typically a few hours to days and sometimes months.

Possession and Trance Disorders

This disorder is very common in India. It is characterized by a temporary loss of both the sense of personal identity and full awareness of the person's surroundings. When the condition is induced by religious rituals, the person may feel taken over by a deity or spirit. The focus of attention is narrowed to a few aspects of the immediate environment, and there is often a limited but repeated set of movements, postures and utterances.

Dissociative Identity Disorder (Multiple Personality Disorder)

In this disorder, the person is dominated by two or more personalities of which only one is manifest at a time. Usually, one personality is not aware of the existence of the other personalities. Each personality has a full range of higher mental functions and performs complex behavior patterns. Transition from one personality to another is sudden, and the behavior usually contrasts strikingly with the patient's normal state.

Depersonalization and Derealization Disorders

Depersonalization is characterized by experiencing the self as strange or unreal. It is a feeling of being outside yourself and observing your actions, feelings or thoughts from a distance. Derealization on the other hand is characterized by experiencing other persons, objects or the world as strange or unusual. People and things around may seem 'lifeless' or 'foggy'. The symptoms result in significant distress or impairment in personal, family, social, educational, occupational or other important areas of functioning.

Diagnosis

- ❖ Rule out physical disorders and substance abuse
- ❖ Standard tests including the Dissociative Experiences Scale (DES) and the Dissociative Disorders Interview schedule (DDIS) to demonstrate presence of dissociation
- ❖ ICD-11 criteria

Treatment Modalities

With appropriate treatment many people recover from illness and improve their ability to function and live a productive and fulfilling life. Medications have a very limited role which may be limited to treating related conditions like anxiety and depression, for example, antidepressants and anxiolytics. Treatment typically involves psychological therapies such as cognitive behavioral therapy, dialectical behavioral therapy, hypnosis, abreaction therapy, supportive psychotherapy.

Nursing Management

Nursing care for patients with dissociative disorder involves implementing the interventions based on assessment data and evaluating the outcomes.

Nursing Assessment

During the assessment process, any physical condition that could produce symptoms of amnesia and dissociation must be ruled out. Psychological tests are used to further evaluate the authenticity of the symptoms. Collect information related to childhood or adult trauma. Along with physical assessment, a baseline psychosocial assessment is done to determine behavioral alterations such as disorientation, level of anxiety, amnesia, depression and level of functioning.

Nursing Diagnoses

- Altered thought process related to memory loss and repressed trauma.
- Self-care deficit related to trance like state or aimless wandering.
- Ineffective individual coping related to repressed memories and issues, loss of identity or travel away from home.
- Personality identity disturbance related to childhood trauma or more than one personality state.
- Anxiety related to repressed traumatic events or loss of identity.

Nursing Interventions

The nurse must first establish a trusting and supportive therapeutic relationship with the patient. It is important to use active listening and communication techniques that encourage verbalization of feelings, conflicts and information regarding the traumatic events that led to the current dissociative state. Patients need encouragement and support to achieve control over their anxiety and previous dissociative response to those situations that trigger the symptoms.

- Monitor physician's ongoing assessments, laboratory reports and other data to rule out organic pathology.
- Identify primary and secondary gains.
- Do not focus on the disability, encourage the patient to perform self-care activities as independently as possible, intervene only when patient requires assistance.
- Do not allow the patient to use disability as a manipulative tool to avoid participating in therapeutic activities.

- Withdraw attention if the patient continues to focus on physical limitations.
- Encourage the patient to verbalize fears and anxieties.
- Provide positive reinforcement for identification or demonstration of alternative adaptive coping strategies.
- Identify specific conflicts that remain unresolved and assist the patient in recognizing possible solutions.
- Assist the patient to set realistic goals for the future.
- Help the patient to identify areas of life situation that are not within his ability to control.
- Encourage verbalization of feelings related to this inability.
- Promote a safe environment.
- Identify environmental stressors that trigger the dissociative symptoms and decrease anxiety producing stimuli.
- Assist the patient to identify alternatives to self-injury such as physical exercise, written method of expression or creative art and task-oriented activities which provide a means of non-verbal expression of thoughts.
- Encourage the patient to keep a daily diary of thoughts and feelings.

Evaluation

During the evaluation process assess for reduction in dissociative episodes and improvement in level of functioning. The patient must also come to an understanding of the relationship between the dissociative state and the increased anxiety that is felt as repressed past trauma is triggered by environmental factors.

Somatoform Disorders

Somatoform disorder or somatic symptoms disorder or somatization is a form of mental illness characterized by repeated presentation with physical symptoms which do not have any physical basis, and a persistent request for investigations and treatment despite repeated assurance by the treating doctors. In these disorders, manifestation of physical symptoms is caused by psychological distress.

The characteristics of these disorders are presented in **Box 5.34**.

Signs and Symptoms

- ❖ Multiple somatic complaints unexplained by medical findings
- ❖ The symptoms are vague, presented in a dramatic manner and involve multiple organ systems
- ❖ Complaints of pain in atleast four different locations: two gastrointestinal, one sexual or reproductive and one neurologic symptom
- ❖ Moderate to severe anxiety
- ❖ Inability to voluntarily control the symptoms

- ❖ Dependency with demanding, attention getting behaviors
- ❖ Secondary gain
- ❖ Significant distress or impairment in social or occupational areas **(Box 5.35)**

Diagnoses

- ❖ Physical work up to rule out medical and neurologic conditions
- ❖ Complete patient history with emphasis on current psychological stressors
- ❖ Tests to rule out underlying organic disease

Treatment Modalities

The main goal of treatment is to help control symptoms and allow the person to function as normal as possible. Physician can offer support and reassurance, monitor health and symptoms and avoid unnecessary tests and treatments.

Medications

Antidepressants and anxiolytics are helpful if the person is experiencing significant depression and anxiety.

Psychological Treatment

Psychological therapies can help the individual to change his thinking and behavior and learn ways to cope with pain or other symptoms, deal with stress and improve the level of functioning. Commonly used therapies are cognitive behavioral therapy, supportive psychotherapy and relaxation interventions.

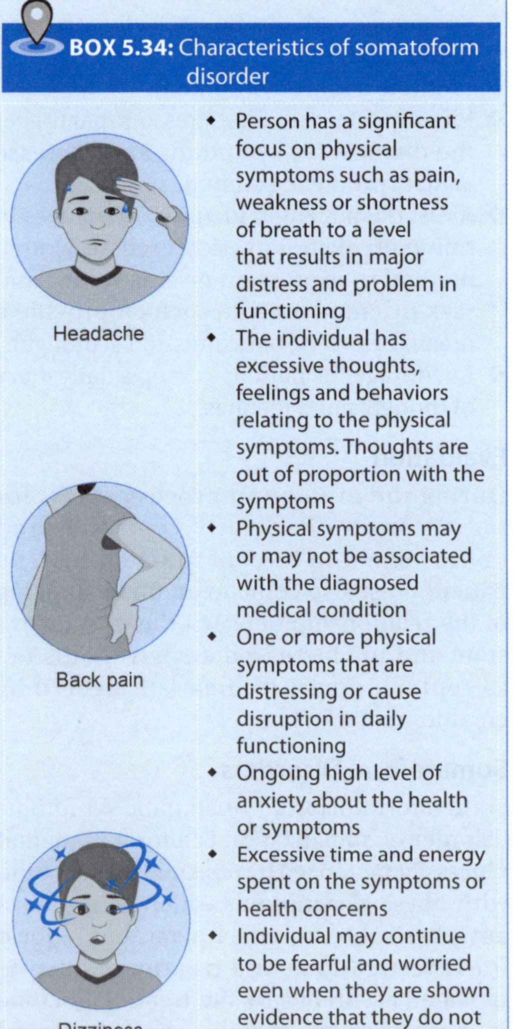

BOX 5.34: Characteristics of somatoform disorder

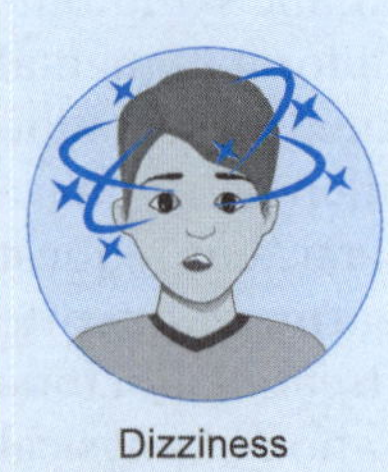

- ◆ Person has a significant focus on physical symptoms such as pain, weakness or shortness of breath to a level that results in major distress and problem in functioning
- ◆ The individual has excessive thoughts, feelings and behaviors relating to the physical symptoms. Thoughts are out of proportion with the symptoms
- ◆ Physical symptoms may or may not be associated with the diagnosed medical condition
- ◆ One or more physical symptoms that are distressing or cause disruption in daily functioning
- ◆ Ongoing high level of anxiety about the health or symptoms
- ◆ Excessive time and energy spent on the symptoms or health concerns
- ◆ Individual may continue to be fearful and worried even when they are shown evidence that they do not have a serious condition

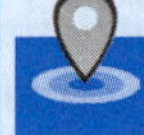

BOX 5.35: Case vignette—Somatoform disorders

A 40-year-old married woman visited psychiatric clinic with multiple complaints. She presented with abdominal pain as sharp and stabbing in nature, radiating down her left leg, abdominal discomfort, bloating, retching, poor appetite, poor sleep, headache, diplopia for 3 months. Patient reported to be suffering from a 10-year history of upper and lower gastrointestinal symptoms. All investigations including CT scans, endoscopies and barium meal were normal. No organic cause was found for her abdominal pain. She was prescribed antidepressants and referred for psychological therapy.

Nursing Interventions

- ❖ Before a somatoform determination, a physical examination and diagnostic testing are necessary to rule out any underlying pathology.
- ❖ Create an accepting, safe and supportive atmosphere that allows open communication with the patient.
- ❖ Focus on the whole person including psychological, social and family factors in addition to the physical symptoms.
- ❖ It must be remembered that they are not consciously trying to be sick or avoid responsibilities.
- ❖ Respond to patient with understanding and patience.
- ❖ Identify types of primary and secondary gains achieved by symptoms.
- ❖ Minimize time and attention given to physical symptoms.
- ❖ Encourage patient to keep a diary of daily happenings and feelings along with physical symptoms.
- ❖ Encourage the patient to take decisions and responsibility for situations related to them.
- ❖ Help the patient to identify more effective coping mechanisms rather than focus on somatic symptoms.

SUBSTANCE USE DISORDERS

Substance use disorder (SUD) is a complex condition in which there is uncontrolled use of substance despite harmful consequences. People with SUD have an intense focus on using a certain substance such as alcohol, tobacco or illicit drugs to the point where the person's ability to function in day-to-day life becomes impaired.

Terminology

- ❖ **Substance**: A term used in reference to any drug, medication or toxin that shares the potential for abuse.
- ❖ **Addiction**: It refers to the physiologic and psychologic dependence on alcohol or other drugs of abuse that affect the central nervous system in such a way that withdrawal symptoms are experienced when the substance is discontinued.
- ❖ **Abuse**: It refers to maladaptive pattern of substance use that impairs health in a broad sense.
- ❖ **Dependence**: It refers to certain physiological and psychological phenomena induced by the repeated taking of a substance.
- ❖ **Tolerance**: It is a state in which after repeated administration, either a drug produces a decreased effect or increasing doses are required to produce the same effect. It is the need for increased amounts of substance to attain the desired effect.
- ❖ **Withdrawal state**: A group of signs and symptoms recurring for a limited time when a drug is withdrawn or reduced in amount. The nature of the withdrawal state is related to the class of substance used.
- ❖ **Poly substance use**: The use of more than one substance at the same time.

Meaning

- ❖ **Substance use disorder** (SUD) is a mental disorder that affects a person's brain and behavior leading to his inability to control the use of substances like legal or illegal drugs, alcohol or medications.
- ❖ **Disorders due to substance use and addictive behaviors** are mental and behavioral disorders that develop due to use of predominantly psychoactive substances including medications or specific repetitive, rewarding and reinforcing behaviors.
- ❖ **Substance abuse**: It is an addictive disorder that describes a pattern of substance use leading to significant problems or distress such as failure to attend occupational activities, substance use in dangerous situations, substance-related legal problems or continued substance use that interferes with friendships or family relationships.
- ❖ **Substance dependence**: It is an addictive disorder that describes continued use of drugs or alcohol even when significant problems related to their use have developed. Signs include increased tolerance; withdrawal symptoms with decreased use, unsuccessful efforts to decrease use; increased time spent in activities to obtain

the substance; withdrawal from social and recreational activities and continued use of the substance even with awareness of the physical or psychological problems encountered by the extent of substance use.

Commonly Abused Substances

Both legal and illegal substances are commonly abused. Most of these substances can alter a person's thinking and judgment, lead to health risks including addiction, drugged driving, infectious diseases and adverse effects on pregnancy. Most commonly used substances are presented in **Table 5.39**.

Etiological Factors for Substance Use Disorders

Substance use disorders are caused by multiple factors. These include biological, psychological and social factors **(Figure 5.22)**.

Biological Factors

❖ **Genetic vulnerability**: Family history of substance use disorder. For example, twin studies suggest that genetic mechanisms might account for alcohol consumption. Research suggests that alcohol dependence and other substance addictions may be associated with genetic variations in 51 different chromosomal regions.

❖ **Biochemical factors**: For example, role of dopamine and norepinephrine have been implicated in cocaine, ethanol and opioid dependence. Abnormalities in alcohol dehydrogenase or in the neurotransmitter mechanism are thought to play a role in alcohol dependence.

❖ **Neurobiological theories**: Drug addicts may have an inborn deficiency of endomorphins. According to another neurobiological theory, enzymes produced by a given gene might influence hormones and neurotransmitters thereby contributing to the development of a personality that is more sensitive to peer pressure.

❖ Withdrawal and reinforcing effects of drugs (they serve as maintaining factors).

TABLE 5.39: Commonly abused substances		
Name of the substance	**Commercial and street name**	**Mode of consumption**
Alcohol (ethyl alcohol)	✦ Beer, wine, toddy, spirits	✦ Swallowed
Opioids ✦ Heroin ✦ Opium	 ✦ Smack, horse, brown sugar ✦ Black stuff, block, hop	 ✦ Injected, smoked, snorted ✦ Swallowed, smoked
Cannabinoids (Marijuana and Hashish)	✦ *Ganja, bhang, charas,* hemp	✦ Smoked, swallowed
Stimulants ✦ Cocaine ✦ Amphetamines ✦ Methamphetamine	 ✦ Crack, rock ✦ Biphetamine ✦ Crystal, glass, fire	 ✦ Snorted, smoked, injected ✦ Swallowed, snorted, smoked, injected ✦ Swallowed, snorted, smoked, injected
Hallucinogens	✦ LSD, phencyclidine	✦ Swallowed, smoked
Sedatives and hypnotics	✦ Alprazolam, nitrazepam	✦ Swallowed
Inhalants	✦ Volatile solvents, Glues, Ink eraser fluid, Petrol	✦ Inhaled through nose or mouth
Nicotine (tobacco)	✦ Cigarettes, *beedi, gutka,* smokeless tobacco (snuff, chewing, etc.)	✦ Smoked, snorted, chewed
Ketamine	✦ K-special, cat valium	✦ Injected, sorted, smoked

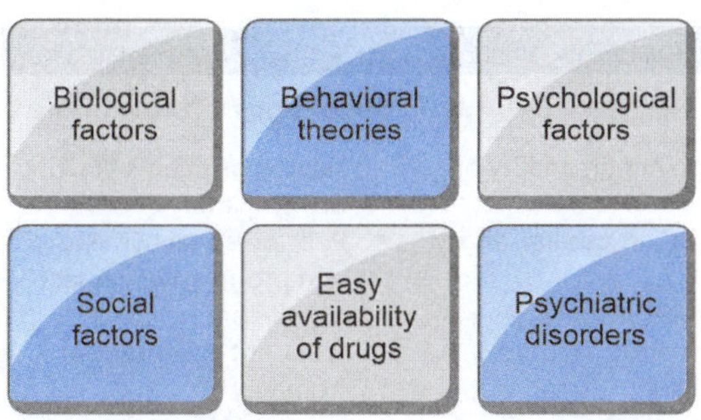

Figure 5.22: Etiological factors for substance abuse

❖ Comorbid medical disorder (for example, to control chronic pain).

Behavioral Theories

❖ Behavioral scientists view drug abuse as the result of conditioning or cumulative reinforcement from drug use.
❖ Drug use causes euphoric experience perceived as rewarding, thereby motivating user to keep taking the drug (which then serves as a biological reward).
❖ Stimuli and settings associated with drug use may themselves become reinforcing or may trigger drug craving that can lead to relapse (many recovering addicts change their environment to eliminate cues that could promote drug use).

Psychological Factors

❖ Individual personality characteristics: General rebelliousness, sense of inferiority, poor impulse control, low self-esteem, inability to cope with the pressures of living and society (poor stress management skills), desire to escape from reality, desire to experiment, a sense of adventure, pleasure-seeking behavior, machoism
❖ Sexual immaturity
❖ Loneliness, unmet needs

Social Factors

❖ Religious reasons
❖ Peer pressure
❖ Effects of television and other mass media
❖ Urbanization
❖ Extended periods of education
❖ Unemployment

❖ Overcrowding
❖ Poor social support

Easy Availability of Drugs

❖ Taking drugs prescribed by doctors (for example, benzodiazepine dependence)
❖ Taking drugs that can be bought legally without prescription (e.g., nicotine, opioids)
❖ Taking drugs that can be obtained from illicit sources (e.g., street drugs)

Psychiatric Disorders

Substance use disorders are more common in depression, anxiety disorders (particularly social phobias), personality disorders (especially antisocial personality) and occasionally in organic brain disease and schizophrenia.

Risk Factors for Substance Dependence

Some of the common risk factors for substance abuse are:

Age

The earlier a person begins drinking, the greater the risk for dependence. People with a history of abuse, family violence, family history of alcoholism, depression and stressful life events are at a high risk for early drinking.

Gender

Studies suggest that women are more vulnerable than men to many of long-term consequences of alcoholism like alcohol hepatitis, cirrhosis of liver and brain cell damage by alcohol.

History of Abuse

Individuals who are victims of physical, sexual or psychological abuse are not only at a higher risk for substance abuse but also exhibit poor response to treatment than those without such a history.

Other Factors

Physically disabled adolescents, certain occupations such as in chefs, barmen, executives, salesmen, actors, entertainers, army personnel, journalists, medical personnel, etc.

TABLE 5.40: Signs of substance abuse

Physical signs	Psychological signs	Social signs
• Changes in sleeping and eating pattern • Injection marks on the skin • Trembling or sweating, slurred speech or impaired coordination • Bloodshot eyes, pupils larger or smaller than usual • Usually smells on breath, body or clothing or impaired co-ordination	• Unexplained change in personality or attitude • Sudden mood swings, irritability, angry outbursts, etc. • Lack of interest in routine activities • Sudden change in friends, favorite hangouts and hobbies • Spending more time alone • Inability to stop drug taking behavior • Lot of time spent on seeking substances or dealing with their after effects • Problems with relationships • Trouble managing responsibilities • Increase in risk taking behavior such as rash driving, having unprotected sex • Engaging in secretive or suspicious behavior • Appearing fearful, anxious or paranoid with no reason	• Having problems at work or with family • Poor personal hygiene and progressive neglect of self-care • Frequent absenteeism from work • Legal trouble such as arrests for disorderly conduct, driving under the influence of drugs

Signs of a Substance Abuse

Recognizing the signs of addiction is the first step to help or guide others. The nurse should understand the signs of abuse. These are physical, psychological and social signs **(Table 5.40)**.

Consequences of Substance Abuse

❖ Substance abuse commonly leads to physical dependence, psychological dependence or both.
❖ It may cause unhealthy lifestyles and behaviors such as poor diet.
❖ Chronic substance abuse impairs social and occupational functioning, creating personal, professional, financial, and legal problems (drug seeking is commonly associated with illegal activities such as robbery or assault).
❖ Drug use beginning in early adolescence may lead to emotional and behavioral problems including depression, problems with family relationships, problems with or failure to complete school, and chronic substance abuse problems.
❖ In pregnant women, substance abuse jeopardizes fetal well-being.
❖ IV drug abuse may lead to life-threatening complications.
❖ Psychoactive substances produce negative outcomes in many patients including maladaptive behavior, "bad trips," and even long-term psychosis.
❖ Illicit street drugs pose added dangers; materials used to dilute them can cause toxic or allergic reactions.

Disorders Due to Use of Alcohol

Moderate consumption of alcohol is safe but heavier use can lead to problems. Since alcohol is a depressant, heavier use can impair brain function and motor skills. It can also affect every organ in the body.

❖ Alcoholism refers to the use of alcoholic beverages to the point of causing damage to the individual, society or both.
❖ Alcohol use disorder is a medical condition, involves heavy or frequent alcohol drinking even when it causes problems, emotional distress or physical harm.

❖ Alcohol use disorder is "an impaired ability to stop or control alcohol use despite adverse social, occupational or health consequences".—**The National Institute on Alcohol Abuse and Alcoholism (NIAAA)**

❖ Alcohol dependency is characterized by craving, tolerance, preoccupation and continuation of consumption despite harmful consequences.

Properties of Alcohol

Alcohol is a clear colored liquid with a strong burning taste. More specifically termed as ethyl alcohol or ethanol it is produced by fermentation of sugars. There are various varieties of alcohol drinks with alcohol concentrations typically ranging from 1.5% to 60%. It is a central nervous system depressant with an ability to produce alcohol intoxication and dependence producing properties. The rate of absorption of alcohol into the bloodstream is more rapid than its elimination. Absorption of alcohol into the bloodstream is slower when food is present in the stomach. A small amount is excreted through urine and a small amount exhaled.

A concentration of 80–100 mg of alcohol per 100 mL of blood is considered intoxication. A person with 200–250 mg will be toxic, sleepy, confused and his thought process altered. If blood level is 300 mg/100 mL of blood the person may lose consciousness. A concentration of 500 mg/100 mL is fatal. The above symptoms can change according to tolerance of the individual.

Prevalence and Incidence

Alcohol use is a public health problem in India. About 14.6% of the Indian population between the ages of 10 and 75 years consumes alcohol. Of the 160 million alcohol consumers in the country, 50.7 million are affected with alcohol dependence. Every third alcohol user in India requires medical help for alcohol related problems (Ambekar et al., 2019).

1. **Episode of harmful use of alcohol**: An episode of use of alcohol that has caused clinically significant damage to a person's physical health or mental health or has resulted in behavior leading to harm to the health of others.

2. **Harmful pattern of use of alcohol**: A pattern of alcohol use that has caused damage to a person's physical or mental health or has resulted in behavior leading to harm to the health of others.

3. **Alcohol dependence**: The characteristic feature is a strong desire to take alcohol, which is manifested by impaired ability to control use, a physiological withdrawal state, development of tolerance, progressive neglect of alternative pleasures or interests persisting with substance use despite clear evidence of harmful consequences **(Box 5.36 and Figure 5.23)**.

4. **Alcohol intoxication:** Acute intoxication develops during or shortly after alcohol ingestion. It is characterized by disturbances in consciousness, cognition, perception, affect, behavior or coordination. These disturbances are related to amount of alcohol consumption. These are time-limited and decrease as alcohol is cleared from the body. The features are impaired attention, aggressive behavior, poor

> **BOX 5.36:** Case vignette—Alcohol dependence
>
> Mr A, is a 35-year-old laborer, married for 10 years, hails from urban area, belongs to middle socio-economic background. He lives with his wife and two children. He began drinking alcohol along with his friends at the age of 20 years. He started with 30 mL of brandy but then gradually increased it to 3–4 quarters of vodka (540–720 mL) per day due to his heavy work schedule. He has now started drinking in the morning. If he does not, then his hands start to shake, also he is unable to sleep well. He gets aggressive towards his wife when 'drunk' leading to a strained marriage. Others have suggested him to stop consumption of alcohol. He promises, but is unable to keep up his word. Mr A has continued to drink despite having pain in the stomach which increases with alcohol consumption. He is hardly able to contribute financially to household expenses. Other relatives have begun avoiding Mr A due to his habit of alcohol consumption.

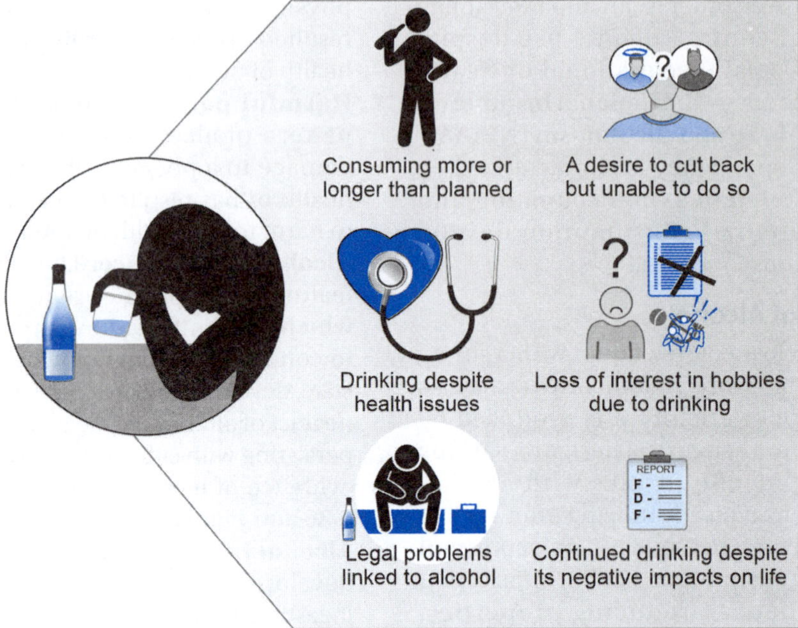

Figure 5.23: Signs of alcohol use disorder

coordination, unsteady gait, nystagmus, inappropriate sexual behavior, mood lability, impaired judgment, slurred speech and impaired memory. Severe intoxication may finally result in stupor or coma.

5. **Alcohol withdrawal:** In persons who have been drinking heavily over a prolonged period of time, any rapid decrease in the amount of alcohol in the body is likely to produce withdrawal symptoms. Withdrawal symptoms begin within 6–48 hours and peak about 24–35 hours after the last drink. During this period, the inhibition of brain activity caused by alcohol is abruptly reversed. Stress hormones are overproduced and the central nervous system becomes overexcited.

   o *Simple withdrawal syndrome*: It is characterized by mild tremors, nausea, vomiting, weakness, irritability, insomnia and anxiety, psychomotor agitation, depressed or dysphoric mood, transient visual, tactile or auditory illusions or hallucination.

6. **Alcohol-induced delirium**: The withdrawal state may progress to a very severe form of delirium. It occurs usually within 2–4 days of complete or significant abstinence from heavy alcohol drinking. The course is short with recovery occurring within 3–7 days. It is characterized by:

   o A dramatic and rapidly changing picture of disordered mental activity with clouding of consciousness and disorientation in time and place
   o Poor attention span
   o Vivid hallucinations which are usually visual; tactile hallucinations can also occur
   o Severe psychomotor agitation, shouting and evident fear
   o Delusions
   o Grossly tremulous hands which some times pick up imaginary objects; truncal ataxia
   o Autonomic disturbances such as sweating, fever, tachycardia, raised blood pressure, pupillary dilatation
   o Dehydration with electrolyte imbalances
   o Reversal of sleep wake pattern or insomnia

○ Blood tests reveal leukocytosis and impaired liver function

○ Death may occur due to cardiovascular collapse, infection, hyperthermia or self inflicted injury

7. **Alcohol-induced psychotic disorder**: It is characterized by psychotic symptoms such as delusions, hallucinations and disordered behavior. These develop during or soon after intoxication with or withdrawal from alcohol.

8. **Other alcohol-induced disorders:** This includes alcohol-induced mood disorders and anxiety disorders.

Complications of Alcohol Abuse

Alcoholism reduces life expectancy by about 10–12 years. The earlier people begin drinking heavily, the greater their chance of developing serious illnesses later on. Alcohol damages body tissues by irritating them directly, through changes that occur during its metabolism, by interacting with other drugs, by aggravating existing disease, or through accidents brought on by intoxication. Tissue damage can lead to a host of complications **(Figure 5.24)**.

Alcohol abusers who require surgery are at an increased risk for postoperative complications including infections, bleeding, insufficient heart and lung functions and propels with wound healing. Alcohol withdrawal symptoms after surgery may impose further stress on the patient and hinder recuperation.

Alcohol interacts with many drugs used by people with diabetes. It interferes with drugs that prevent seizures or blood clotting. It increases the risk for gastrointestinal bleeding in people taking aspirin or other nonsteroidal inflammatory drugs (NSAIDs) including ibuprofen and naproxen.

Diagnosis

❖ Blood tests reveal very recent consumption of alcohol. They cannot tell whether a person has been drinking heavily for a long time.

❖ Carbohydrate deficient transferrin (CDT) is a marker for heavy drinking and can be helpful in monitoring patients for progress towards abstinence. It is the only biologic

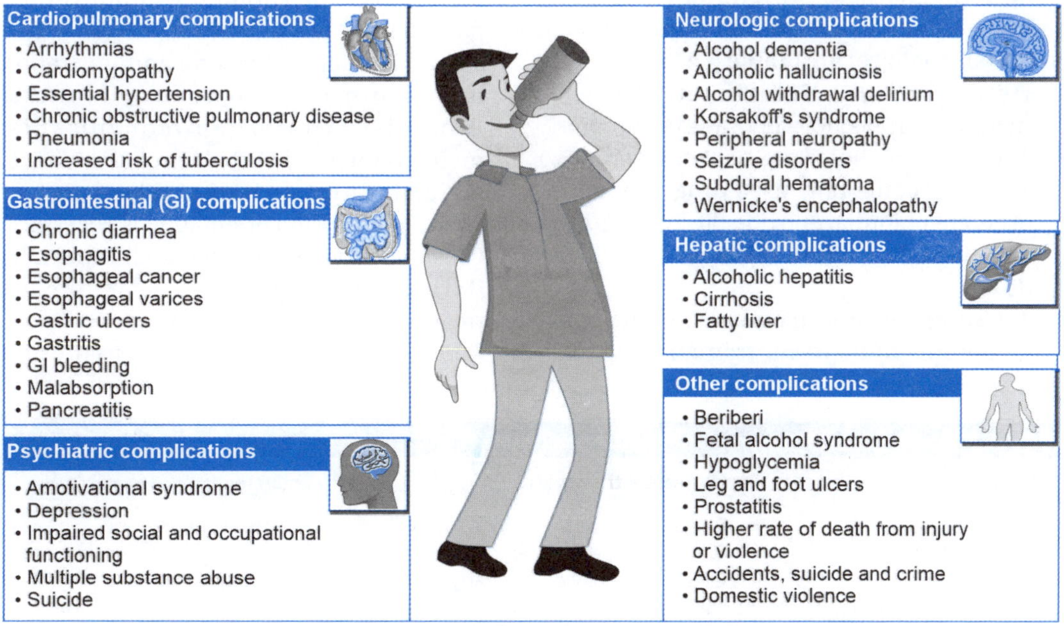

Figure 5.24: Complications of alcohol abuse

marker approved by the FDA to help detect chronic heavy drinking.

❖ Gamma glutamyl transferase (GGT), a liver enzyme is very sensitive to alcohol and can be elevated after moderate alcohol intake and in chronic alcoholism.

❖ Testosterone is a male hormone. Its levels are low in men with alcoholism.

❖ Estimation of mean corpuscular volume (MCV), a blood test measures the size of red blood cells which increase in alcoholics with vitamin deficiencies.

❖ Urine toxicology to reveal use of other drugs.

❖ Serum electrolyte analysis revealing electrolyte abnormalities associated with alcohol use.

❖ Liver function studies demonstrating alcohol related liver damage.

❖ Hematologic work-up possibly revealing anemia, thrombocytopenia.

❖ Echocardiography and electrocardiography (ECG) demonstrating cardiac problems.

Treatment

The initial goal of treatment is detoxification and stabilizing the patient, medical management for craving, and psychiatric comorbidity. Long-term goals are prevention of relapse, re-integration into society and improvement in overall quality of life (**Table 5.41**).

a. **Detoxification:** Detoxification is the treatment for alcohol withdrawal symptoms. The drugs of choice are benzodiazepines. The most commonly used drugs from this class are chlordiazepoxide 80–200 mg/day and diazepam 40–80 mg/day, in divided doses.

b. **Treating delirium tremens:** People with symptoms of delirium tremens must be treated immediately. Untreated delirium tremens has a fatality rate that can be as high as 20%. Treatment usually involves intravenous administration of antianxiety medications and IV fluids. Restraints may be necessary to prevent injury to the patient or to others.

c. **Treating seizures:** Seizures are usually self limited and treated with a benzodiazepine. Intravenous phenytoin (dilantin) along with a benzodiazepine may be used in patients who have a history of seizures, who have epilepsy, or in those with ongoing seizures. Because phenytoin may lower blood pressure, the patient's blood pressure should be monitored during treatment.

d. **Treating psychosis:** For hallucinations or extremely aggressive behavior, antipsychotic drugs particularly haloperidol (haldol) may be administered. Korsakoff's psychosis (Wernicke-Korsakoff syndrome) is caused by severe vitamin B_1 (thiamine) deficiencies, which cannot be replaced orally. Rapid and immediate injection of the B vitamin thiamin is necessary.

e. **Others:** For vitamin B deficiency a preparation of vitamin B containing 100 mg of thiamine should be administered parenterally, twice daily for 3–5 days. This should be followed by oral administration of vitamin B for at least 6 months. Administration of anticonvulsants, maintaining fluid and electrolyte balance, strict monitoring of vitals, level of consciousness and orientation is necessary. Close observation is essential, especially during the first five days. Symptomatic treatment may involve respiratory support, fluid replacement, IV glucose to prevent

TABLE 5.41: Treatment for disorders due to use of alcohol

Medications	Psychological therapies	Agencies
• Naltrexone • Acamprosate • Disulfiram • Antidepressants	• Brief intervention • Motivational enhancement therapy • Cognitive behavioral therapy • Family intervention • Relapse prevention techniques	• Alcohol anonymous • Office of Indian alcohol and substance abuse • National action plan for drug demand reduction

hypoglycemia, correction of hypothermia or acidosis, and emergency measures for trauma, infection or GI bleeding.

Inpatient versus outpatient treatment: Inpatient treatment may be performed in a general or psychiatric hospital or in a de-addiction center. Factors that indicate a need for inpatient treatment are:

- Delirium tremens
- Potential harm to self or others
- Failure to respond to conservative treatments
- Coexisting medical or psychiatric disorder
- Disruptive home environment

Inpatient treatment includes:

- A physical examination and other tests to uncover medical problems
- Psychiatric work up for any mental disorders
- Detoxification—involves initiating abstinence, managing withdrawal symptoms and complications
- On going treatment with medications in some cases
- Psychotherapy, usually cognitive behavioral therapy
- An introduction to AA

  People with mild-to-moderate withdrawal symptoms are usually treated as outpatients.

Outpatient treatment includes:

- Medications
- Psychotherapy or counseling
- Social support groups such as AA
- Involvement of family and other significant people in patient's life

Medications

Three drugs are specifically approved to treat alcohol dependence:

1. Naltrexone (ReVia, Vivitrol) (anticraving drug)
2. Acamprosate (Campral) (anticraving drug)
3. Disulfiram (Antabuse)

   Other types of medications such as anti-depressants may also be used to treat patients with alcoholism

Anticraving Medications

Anticraving drugs are opioid antagonists. These drugs reduce the intoxicating effects of alcohol and the urge to drink.

- Naltrexone is available in oral (ReVia, Vivitrol) and injectable (Vivitrol) forms. This helps reduce alcohol dependence in the short-term for people with moderate-to-severe alcohol dependency. While ReVia, a pill is taken daily by mouth, Vivitrol is injected once a month. This drug should be prescribed along with psychotherapy or other supportive medical management. The common side effects are nausea, vomiting, headache, fatigue and stomach pain which are usually mild and temporary. Some patients suffer adverse injection site reactions such as spreading of skin infections and abscesses. Patients should be monitored for pain, swelling, tenderness, bruising or redness at injection site. If symptoms do not improve within 2 weeks, a physician is to be approached. High doses can cause liver damage. The drug should not be administered if narcotics have been used within the last 7–10 days.
- Acamprosate (campral) calms the brain and reduces cravings by inhibiting the transmission of neurotransmitter gamma aminobutyric acid (GABA). Studies indicate that it reduces the frequency of drinking and in combination with psychotherapy improves quality of life even in patients with severe alcohol dependence. The drug may cause occasional diarrhea, headache and impair certain memory functions though it does not alter short-term working memory or mood. People with kidney problems should use acamprosate cautiously. For some patients, combination therapy with naltrexone or disulfiram may provide greater benefit than acamprosate alone.

Aversion Medications (Disulfiram)

Some drugs have properties that interact with alcohol to produce distressing side effects. Disulfiram (antabuse) causes flushing, headache, nausea, and vomiting if a person consumes alcohol while taking the drug. The symptoms may trigger after drinking half a glass of wine or half a shot of liquor and may last from half an hour to 2 hours depending on the dosage of drug and the amount of alcohol consumed. One dose of disulfiram is usually effective for 1–2 weeks. Overdose can be dangerous, causing low blood pressure, chest pain, shortness of breath and even death.

Other Drugs

Topiramate (Topamax) is an anti seizure drug used to treat epilepsy. It also helps control impulsivity. Studies indicate that it may help treat alcohol dependence. Side effects included burning and itching skin sensations, change in taste sensation, loss of appetite, and difficulty concentrating. Baclofen (lioresal) is a muscle relaxant and antispasmodic drug. It is being investigated for its benefits in helping maintain abstinence particularly in patients with alcoholic cirrhosis.

Psychological Therapies

Commonly used psychological therapies are brief interventions, motivational enhancement therapy, cognitive behavioral therapy, drink refusal skills, family therapy, aversive conditioning, relapse prevention techniques, cue exposure technique, etc.

1. **Brief intervention**: It is a structured patient centered therapy conducted by a trained therapist. It uses 1 to 4 face-to-face interactive sessions of short duration. Main goal is harm reduction and a drop in alcohol consumption. This intervention is used to raise awareness of the effects of substance use with a careful emphasis on the harm that can occur. It is based on the principles of motivational interviewing which uses techniques such as FRAMES (feedback, responsibility, advice, menu, empathy and self-efficacy). FRAMES counseling approach is as follows:

   o *Feedback*: Providing personally relevant feedback regarding alcohol consumption by use of CAGE or AUDIT questionnaire. For example: "You have scored 16 on the Audit questionnaire which indicates that you are at high risk for harm from your current pattern of drinking".

   o *Responsibility*: Encourage the client to take up the responsibility of stopping from drinking. For example, "On a scale of one to ten how important is it to make a change in your current heavy use of alcohol?"

   o *Advice*: Simple suggestion. For example, "The best way for you to reduce the risk is to cut down or stop drinking completely".

   o *Menu of options*: Self-management options. For example: Identify high risk situations and cope with substitute activities (4 Ds-Delay, Distract, Drink water, Deep breathing).

   o *Express empathy:* Validation of emotions. For example: "I know your states of uncertainty about the recovery process. Let us see if we can solve this together".

   o *Support self-efficacy*: Fostering self-confidence. For example: "I am sure you can also do it because many people have done it".

2. **Motivational enhancement therapy (MET) or motivational interviewing (MI):** This therapy focuses on enhancement of motivation and commitment to change. The therapist helps the patient to explore and resolve their ambivalence about their substance use. Delivered in 1 to 4 sessions, it builds on the stages of change helping people move from thinking about making a change to actively working toward it. The principles of MI include expressing empathy through reflective listening, developing discrepancy between patients' goals or their current behaviors, avoid argument and direct confrontation, supporting self-efficacy and optimism.

3. **Cognitive behavioral therapy (CBT):** It uses a structured teaching approach wherein patients are given instructions and homework assignments intended to improve their ability to cope with basic living situations, control behavior and change the way they think about drinking. For example, patients might detail on their drinking experiences and describe what they consider to be risky situations. They are then assigned activities to help them cope when exposed to 'cues' (situations or places that trigger their desire to drink).

Patients may also be given tasks that are designed to replace drinking. CBT may be effective when used in combination with opioid antagonist such as naltrexone.

4. **Combined behavioral interventions:** This therapy combines elements from cognitive behavioral therapy, motivational enhancement therapy, and a 12 step program wherein patients are taught on how to cope with drinking triggers, learn strategies for refusing alcohol so as to achieve and maintain abstinence.

5. **Family intervention:** Among the various treatment modalities, family intervention is the most notable current advance in the area of psychosocial treatment of alcoholism. Ingredients of family intervention include:
   - Increasing cohesion within the family members
   - Highlighting the positive aspects in marriage
   - Enhancing communication and conflict resolution skills within the family
   - Reducing adverse family atmosphere
   - Enhancing problem solving capacity of family members
   - Maintaining reasonable expectations for patient performance
   - Achieving changes in family members' behavior and belief system

6. **Group therapy:** Group therapy enables the patients to observe their own problems mirrored in others and to work out better ways of coping with them.

7. **Relapse prevention technique:** This technique helps the patient to identify high risk relapse factors and develop strategies to deal with them. It also enables the patient to learn methods to cope with cognitive distortions.

8. **12-step program:** This is a support group program where individuals share their experiences and techniques that help other individuals to quit substance abuse. Support groups give the individual a sense of support, help the individual to structure his life and avoid temptations of the substance.

9. **Other therapies** include assertiveness training, behavior counseling, supportive psychotherapy and individual psycho therapy.

Agencies Concerned with Disorders Due to Alcohol Use

There are many resources available both for clients suffering from alcohol use disorder and care givers trying to support them.

Alcoholics Anonymous (AA)

- This is a recovery support group where people dealing with alcoholism can come together to seek support and guidance.
- This self-help organization was founded in the USA by two alcoholic men, Dr Bob Smith and Bill Wilson, a stockbroker on the 10th of June, 1935. It has since then spread to many countries in the world.
- AA considers alcoholism as a physical, mental and spiritual disease, a progressive one which can be arrested but not cured.
- It remains the most well-known program for helping people with alcoholism. AA offers a very strong support network using group meetings open 7 days a week in locations all over the world.
- A companion system, group understanding of alcoholism, and forgiveness for relapses are AA's standard methods for building self-worth and alleviating feelings of isolation.
- Each member is assigned a support person from whom he may seek help when the temptation to drink occurs. In crisis he can obtain immediate help by telephone. Once sobriety is achieved, he is expected to help others.
- The organization works on the firm belief that abstinence must be complete. The only requirement for membership is a desire to stop drinking. There is no authority but only a fellowship of imperfect alcoholics whose strength is formed out of weakness.
- Their primary purpose is to help each other stay sober and also help other alcoholics to achieve sobriety. This support group provides an opportunity for the individual

to build a new sober support network, help others and find purpose.

❖ AA is founded on the 12 steps, which are guiding principles for recovery.

❖ Research has found that attending AA can help people achieve sobriety, develop confidence in their recovery and improve relationships.

Al-Anon

Al-Anon is a group started by Mrs Anne, wife of Dr Bob to support the spouses of alcoholics.

Al-Ateen

Provides support to their teenage children.

Hostels

These are intended mainly for those rendered homeless due to alcohol-related problems. They provide rehabilitation and counseling. Usually, abstinence is a condition of residence.

Other resources are Office of Indian alcohol and substance abuse, National Action Plan for Drug Demand Reduction.

Nursing Management

Nurses provide support and care to patients suffering from alcohol use disorder by treating physical symptoms, offering resources, and managing psychosocial distress. Nurses working in de-addiction centers can make positive contributions by delivering a range of nursing interventions.

Nursing Assessment

1. **Recognition of alcohol abuse:** The CAGE questionnaire may be adopted for this purpose:

   C: Have you ever felt you ought to CUT down on your drinking?

   A: Have people ANNOYED you by criticizing your drinking?

   G: Have you ever felt GUILTY about your drinking?

   E: Have you ever had a drink first thing in the morning (an EYE-OPENER) to steady your nerves or get rid of a hangover?

2. **Be suspicious about 'at-risk' factors:** Problems in the marriage and family, at work, with finances or with the law; at risk occupations; withdrawal symptoms after admission; alcohol-related physical disorders; repeated accidents; deliberate self harm.

3. If at-risk factors raise suspicion, the next step is to ask tactful but persistent questions to confirm the diagnosis.

4. **Certain clinical signs lead to the suspicion that drugs are being injected:** Needle tracks and thrombosed veins, wearing garments with long sleeves, etc. IV use should be suspected in any patient who presents with subcutaneous abscesses or hepatitis.

5. **Behavioral changes:** Absence from school or work, negligence of appearance, minor criminal offences, isolation from former friends and adoption of new friends in a drug culture.

6. **Laboratory tests:**
   - Raised gamma-glutamyl transferase (GGT)
   - Raised mean corpuscular volume
   - Blood alcohol concentration
   - Most drugs can be detected in urine with notable exception being LSD

7. **Nervous system:**
   - Orientation
   - Level of consciousness
   - Co-ordination, gait
   - Memory (short and long-term)
   - Signs of depression or anxiety
   - Tremors or decreased reflexes
   - Pupils (constricted or dilated)

8. **Cardiovascular and respiratory:**
   - Vital signs
   - Peripheral pulses
   - Dyspnea on exertion
   - Abnormal breath sounds
   - Arrhythmias
   - Fatigue
   - Peripheral edema

9. **Gastrointestinal:**
   - Nausea/vomiting
   - Changes in weight or appetite
   - Signs of malnutrition
   - Color and consistency of stool

10. **Integumentary:**
    - Skin lesions
    - Needle tracks on scarring on arms, legs, fingers, toes, under the tongue or between gums and lips
11. **Emotional behavior:**
    - Affect
    - Rate of speech
    - Suspiciousness, anger, agitation
    - Occurrence of hallucinations, blackouts
    - History of violent episodes
    - Support system

When assessing the patient who abuses substances it is first important to remember that underneath the surface of denial and rationalization are the feelings of fear, insecurity, anxiety and low self-esteem.

- ❖ Identify the type of substance the person has been using, amount, frequency, method of administration and the length of time the substance has been abused.
- ❖ Note for suicidal ideation or intent with drained symptoms.
- ❖ Assess for level of motivation for treatment.
- ❖ Identify reason for admission.
- ❖ A baseline physical and emotional nursing assessment is done to determine admission status and seek a reference point from which to determine progress towards an expected outcome.

TABLE 5.42: Nursing interventions during acute intoxication

Nursing interventions	Rationale
Place the patient in a room near the nurse's station or where the staff can observe the patient closely.	Patient's safety is nursing priority.
Monitor patient's sleep pattern; he may need to be restrained at night if confused or wanders or attempts to climb out of bed.	- do -
Decrease environmental stimuli (bright lights, television, visitors) when the patient is restless, irritable or tremulous.	Too many stimuli in the environment may increase misperceptions and restlessness.
Institute seizure precautions (padded tongue blade and airway at bedside, raised side-rails, etc.).	Seizures can occur during withdrawal; precautions can minimize chances of injury.
Reorient the patient to person, time, place and situation as needed.	The patient is often confused and needs to be reoriented.
Talk to the patient in simple, direct, concrete language.	Patient's ability to deal with complex or abstract ideas is limited.

Nursing diagnosis I

Risk for injury related to hallucinosis, acute intoxication evidenced by confusion, disorientation, inability to identify potentially harmful situations.

Objective: Patient will not harm self.

Interventions: See **Table 5.42.**

Nursing diagnosis II

Altered health maintenance related to inability to identify, manage or seek out help to maintain health, evidenced by various physical symptoms, exhaustion, sleep disturbances, etc.

Objective: The patient will maintain optimum health status.

Interventions: See **Table 5.43.**

Nursing diagnosis III

Ineffective denial related to weak, under developed ego, evidenced by lack of insight, rationalization of problems, blaming others, failure to accept responsibility for his behavior.

Objective: Patient will understand the effect of his behavior on others and verbalize acceptance of responsibility and desire for change.

Interventions: See **Table 5.44.**

Nursing diagnosis IV

Ineffective individual coping related to impairment of adaptive behavior and problem-solving abilities, evidenced by use of substances as coping mechanisms.

TABLE 5.43: Nursing interventions to improve health status of alcoholics

Nursing interventions	Rationale
Monitor the patient's health status. Administer medications as prescribed by physician. Observe the patient for any behavioral changes and inform physician when necessary	To evaluate the patient's progress accurately
Maintain fluid and electrolyte balance	Patients with alcohol abuse are at high risk for fluid and electrolyte imbalances
Provide food or nourishing fluids as soon as the patient can tolerate eating (bland food usually is tolerated best at first)	Many patients who use alcohol heavily experience gastritis, anorexia and so forth. Therefore, bland foods are tolerated most easily. It is important to re-establish nutritional intake as soon as possible
Ensure that amount of protein in the diet is correct for individual patient condition	Diseased liver may be incapable of metabolizing proteins properly resulting in accumulation of ammonia in the blood that circulates to the brain which in turn can lead to altered consciousness
Provide small frequent feedings of patient's favorite foods. Supplement with vitamins and minerals	To correct malnutrition
Assist the patient in self-care activities; it may be necessary to provide complete physical care depending on the severity of patient's withdrawal	The level of patient independence is determined by the severity of withdrawal symptoms. Patient's needs should be met with the greatest degree of independence he can attain

TABLE 5.44: Nursing interventions to improve adaptive behavior

Nursing interventions	Rationale
Develop trust, convey an attitude of acceptance. Ensure that patient understands it is not him but his behavior that is unacceptable.	Unconditional acceptance promotes dignity and self-worth.
Identify recent maladaptive behaviors or situations that have occurred in the patient's life and discuss how use of drugs/alcohol may be a contributing factor.	The first step in limiting denial and rationalization is for patient to see the relationship between substance use and personal problems.
Do not allow the patient to rationalize or blame others for behaviors associated with substance use.	This only serves to prolong the denial.
Provide positive reinforcement when the patient shows insight into his behavior.	It enhances repetition of desirable behavior.

Objective: Patient will be able to use adaptive coping mechanisms instead of abusing drugs/alcohol in response to stress.

Interventions: See **Table 5.45.**

Evaluation

The following questions can be useful in evaluating the nursing care:

❖ Has detoxification occurred without complications?

❖ Has a correlation been made between personal problems and the use of subtances?

❖ Does he accept responsibility for own behavior?

Acute withdrawal outcomes are achieved when the patient no longer exhibits any signs or symptoms of substance intoxication or withdrawal. As the patient gains insight into the illness he expresses willingness to admit and take responsibility for his own substance problem.

TABLE 5.45: Nursing interventions to improve adaptive coping skills among alcoholics

Nursing interventions	Rationale
Encourage patient to explore options available to deal with stress, rather than resorting to substance use. Practice these techniques	To develop desirable ways of coping with stress
Give positive reinforcement for ability to delay gratification and respond to stress with adaptive coping strategies	Because of weak ego, patient needs a lot of positive feedback to enhance self-esteem
Teach patient and family that alcoholism is a disease that requires long-term treatment and follow-up. Refer to AA, Al-Anon and other support groups as indicated	Family and significant others are also affected by the patient's substance use and need help
Teach the patient about prevention of HIV transmission	Patients with alcohol/drug use may involve in high-risk behaviors which increase the risk of HIV transmission
Maintain frequent contact with the patient, even if it is only by a brief telephone call	Patient will not feel left alone to deal with his problems
If drinking occurs, discuss the events that led to the incident with the patient in a non-judgmental manner. Discuss ways to avoid similar circumstances in the future	The patient may be able to see the relatedness of the event or a pattern of behavior while discussing the situation. Anticipatory planning may prepare the patient to avoid similar circumstances in future
Assist the patient to plan weekly, or even daily, schedules of purposeful activities, such as appointments, talking, walks, etc	Scheduled events provide the patient with something to look forward to

Disorders Due to Use of Cannabis

It is the most commonly abused illegal drug. This mild hallucinogen is derived from *Cannabis sativa* plant. The dried leaves and flowering tops are often referred to as ganja or marijuana. The resin of the plant is referred to as hashish. Bhang is a drink made from cannabis. It is smoked or taken in liquid form. It is a central nervous system depressant, stimulant and hallucinogen. It has dependence-producing properties resulting in cannabis dependence. Marijuana abuse can lead to distorted perceptions, impaired coordination and difficulty with thinking, problem solving, learning and memory. Higher doses speed up heart rate and raise blood pressure.

Acute Intoxication

Mild intoxication is characterized by mild impairment of consciousness and orientation, tachycardia, a sense of floating in the air, euphoria, dream like states, 'flashback' phenomena, alteration in psychomotor activity, tremors, photophobia, lacrimation, dry mouth and increased appetite. Severe intoxication causes perceptual disturbances like depersonalization, derealization, synesthesia and hallucinations.

Withdrawal Symptoms

They are mostly found in the first 72–96 hours and include increased salivation, hyperthermia, insomnia, decreased appetite and loss of weight.

Complications

❖ Transient or short-lasting psychiatric disorders such as acute anxiety, paranoid psychosis, hysterical fugue-like states, hypomania, schizophrenia like state.
❖ A motivational syndrome
❖ Memory impairment

Treatment

❖ Anxiolytics, antipsychotics, antidepressants.
❖ Contingency management gives patients tangible rewards for positive behaviors

while cognitive behavior therapy helps to identify and modify faulty thinking and behavior.

Disorders Due to Use of Opioids

In the last few decades the use of opioids has increased markedly world over. India, surrounded on both sides by routes of illicit transport namely Golden Triangle (Burma, Thailand, Laos) and Golden Crescent (Iran, Afghanistan, Pakistan) is particularly affected. The most important dependence producing derivatives are morphine and heroin.

Commonly abused opioids (narcotics) in our country are heroin (*brown sugar, smack*) and synthetic preparations like pethidine, fortwin (pentazocine) and tidigesic (buprenorphine). Drugs injected through a needle are heroin, buprenorphine and pentazocine. Though most opiate users had begun chasing (inhaling the smoke or *chasing the dragon*) heroin they gradually shifted to needle use. These injecting drug users have become a high-risk group for HIV infection.

Opioids act on the body's central nervous system by stimulating the brain's reward center. It produces a euphoric feeling and clouded thinking followed by drowsy state. Heroin abuse is one of the hardest drug addictions to beat.

Acute Intoxication

It is characterized by apathy, bradycardia, hypotension, respiratory depression, subnormal temperature and pinpoint pupils. Later delayed reflexes, thready pulse and coma can occur.

Withdrawal Syndrome

Narcotic withdrawal rarely produces a life threatening situation. Common symptoms include watery eyes, running nose, yawning, loss of appetite, irritability, tremors, sweating, stomach cramps, muscle twisting, tachycardia hypertension, nausea, diarrhea, insomnia, raised body temperature, piloerection and anorexia. Withdrawal symptoms may appear as early as 4 hours after the last dose of heroin, peak within 48–72 hours and subside after about a week.

Complications

- ❖ **Complications due to illicit drug use**: Parkinsonism, peripheral neuropathy, transverse myelitis
- ❖ **Complications due to intravenous use**: Skin infection, thrombophlebitis, pulmonary embolism, endocarditis, septicemia, AIDS, viral hepatitis and tetanus
- ❖ Involvement in criminal activities

Treatment

- ❖ **Treatment of opioid overdose**: Opioid overdose can be treated with narcotic antagonists, for example, naloxone, naltrexone.
- ❖ **Detoxification**: Withdrawal symptoms can be managed by methadone, clonidine, naltrexone, buprenorphine, etc.
- ❖ **Maintenance therapy**: After the detoxification phase is over the patient is maintained on one of the following regimens:
  - ○ Methadone maintenance
  - ○ Opioid antagonists
  - ○ Psychological methods like individual psychotherapy, behavior therapy, group therapy and family therapy

Disorders Due to Use of Sedatives, Hypnotics or Anxiolytics

Sedatives, hypnotics or anxiolytics cause physical dependence. Withdrawal occurs when abuse is reduced or stopped suddenly. These drugs reduce arousal and stimulation in various areas of the brain. As a result, the user may experience a sense of calm or sedation, sleep. Higher doses may cause respiratory depression or coma which can be very dangerous. The commonly abused barbiturates are secobarbital, pentobarbital and amobarbital.

Intoxication

Acute intoxication is characterized by irritability, lability of mood, disinhibited behavior, slurring of speech, incoordination, attention and memory impairment.

Complications

Intravenous use can lead to skin abscesses, cellulitis, infections, embolism and hyper sensitivity reactions.

Withdrawal Syndrome

It is characterized by marked restlessness, tremors, and seizures in severe cases resembling delirium tremens.

Treatment

If the patient is conscious, induction of vomiting and use of activated charcoal can reduce the absorption. Treatment is symptomatic.

Disorders Due to Use of Cocaine

It is a white crystalline powder with the properties of being a powerful addictive stimulant. It is derived from coca leaves and popularly known by its common street name 'crack'. It can be administered orally, intranasally (snorted) or smoking or parenterally. It gives a euphoric feeling when ingested. Cocaine abuse can lead to addiction, severe health problems and even death.

Acute Intoxication

Characterized by pupillary dilatation, tachycardia, hypertension, sweating and nausea and hypomanic picture.

Withdrawal Syndrome

Agitation, depression, anorexia, fatigue and sleepiness.

Complications

Acute anxiety reaction, uncontrolled compulsive behavior, seizures, respiratory depression, cardiac arrhythmias.

Treatment

❖ **Management of intoxication**: Amyl nitrite is an antidote; diazepam or propranolol is also used.
❖ **For withdrawal symptoms**: Anti-depressants (imipramine or amitriptyline) and psychotherapy.

Disorders Due to Use of Stimulants Including Amphetamines

Amphetamines are powerful CNS stimulants with peripheral sympathomimetic effects. Commonly used amphetamines are pemoline and methylphenidate. Methamphetamine is a white powder that is smoked, snorted or injected. It is highly addictive and a powerful central nervous stimulant with peripheral sympathomimetic effects. It can produce long-term wakefulness. It may also increase physical activity which can result in increased performance. When used over a long period of time it can cause anxiety, insomnia and even psychotic symptoms.

Acute Intoxication

Characterized by tachycardia, hypertension, cardiac failure, seizures, tremors, hyper pyrexia, pupillary dilation, panic, insomnia, restlessness, irritability, paranoid hallucinatory syndrome and amphetamine induced psychosis.

Withdrawal Syndrome

Characterized by depression, apathy, fatigue, hypersomnia or insomnia, agitation and hyperphagia

Complications

Seizures, delirium, arrhythmias, aggressive behavior, coma

Treatment

Ammonium chloride, antipsychotics, tricyclic antidepressants, diazepam or propranolol

Disorders Due to Use of Caffeine

It is a natural chemical with stimulant effects. It is found in coffee, tea, chocolate, cola, cocoa, etc. It works by stimulating the central nervous system, heart, muscles and the centers that control blood pressure. As a stimulant, caffeine can cause the heart to beat faster and hasten the effects of cold temperatures on the body. It is most commonly used for mental alertness and to relieve headache. Coffee and other caffeinated products can create physical dependence leading to chemical changes in the brain. Daily consumption can quickly lead to caffeine addiction characterized by cravings and withdrawal symptoms if intake is reduced or ceased.

Intoxication

Overuse can lead to intoxication. Symptoms include restlessness, nervousness, excitement, insomnia, increased urine production, GI upset, tachycardia, muscle twitching, etc.

Withdrawal Symptoms

Withdrawal symptoms usually begin 12–24 hours after the last dose and peak after 24–48 hours of abstinence. These can last up to nine days. Withdrawal symptoms include headache, fatigue, drowsiness, low mood, difficulty in concentration, muscle pain, etc.

Treatment

Gradual reduction of caffeine intake (weaning method) can reduce withdrawal symptoms.

Disorders Due to Use of Synthetic Cathinones

Synthetic cathinones are central nervous system stimulants known as new psychoactive substances, marketed as bath salts. They produce similar effects as other stimulants like methamphetamine or MDMA. These are white or brown powders or crystals or capsules, usually snorted, swallowed or injected.

Intoxication

With small doses the person experiences intense pleasure, energy, muscle tension, blurred vision, distorted sense of time, dry mouth, sweating, memory loss and reduced speech. These effects may be experienced and may last for approximately 2–4 hours. Higher doses cause anxiety, paranoia, hallucinations, agitation, seizures, panic attacks, increased sex drive, irregular heartbeat, chest pain, tremors, convulsions and death.

Withdrawal Symptoms

The drug triggers intense, uncontrollable urges (strong compulsion) to reuse the drug again.

Taking synthetic cathinones can cause strong withdrawal symptoms such as depression, anxiety, tremors, difficulty falling asleep and paranoia.

Treatment

Benzodiazepines and antipsychotics are commonly used to treat withdrawal effects. Cognitive behavior therapy and motivation enhancement therapy are commonly used to control addictive behavior.

Disorders Due to Use of Hallucinogens

Most commonly abused hallucinogen, lysergic acid diethylamide (LSD) is a white odorless crystalline substance. It is a powerful, synthetic (man-made) drug belonging to the psychedelics group of drugs. When small doses are taken it can produce mild changes in perception, mood and thought. Larger doses may produce delusions, visual hallucinations and distortions of space and time. LSD presumably produces its effects by acting on 5 HT levels in the brain. A common pattern of LSD use is 'trip' (occasional use followed by a long period of abstinence).

Intoxication

It is characterized by perceptual changes occurring in clear consciousness. For example, depersonalization, derealization, illusions, synesthesias (colors are heard, sounds are felt), autonomic hyperactivity, marked anxiety, paranoid ideation and impairment of judgment.

Withdrawal Syndrome

Flashbacks (brief experiences of the hallucinogenic state)

Complications

Anxiety, depression, psychosis or visual hallucinosis

Treatment

Symptomatic treatment with antianxiety, antidepressant or antipsychotic medications

Disorders Due to Use of Nicotine

Nicotine is a plant alkaloid found in the tobacco plant. Present in cigarettes, cigar, e-cigarettes, liquid nicotine, nicotine gum, chewing tobacco, pipe tobacco and snuff, it provides little pleasure and energy. The main means of administration are smoking pipes/cigars, chewing, and also snorting fine powders. Nicotine addiction is one of the easiest addictions to fall into and the toughest addictions to get rid of. The effect can wear off fast and make the person to take more. An individual can abuse and get addicted to the nicotine in cigarettes just like other drugs. It is associated with significant morbidity and mortality worldwide.

Intoxication

Ingestion of liquid nicotine is the most common cause of nicotine intoxication. Salivation, nausea, vomiting, dehydration, headache, dizziness, tremors, anxiety, confusion, increased heart rate and elevated blood pressure.

Withdrawal Symptoms

Difficulty sleeping, dizziness, headache, increased weight gain, nausea, feeling uneasy, jittery, agitated or angry, depression.

Complications

Nicotine is a highly addictive chemical which can cause increased blood pressure, narrowing of arteries, contribute to hardening of the arterial wall and also a possible heart attack. It is one of the leading causes of preventable cancers.

Treatment

Nicotine replacement therapy includes nicotine patches, sprays, lozenges or gum. Medications which help to quit nicotine dependence are bupropion and varenicline. Psychotherapy and cognitive behavioral therapy can be very helpful in quitting nicotine.

Disorders Due to Use of Volatile Inhalants

Solvent abuse covers a range of gases or chemicals that evaporate at room temperature to form a vapor which can be inhaled. These nervous system depressants slow down the activity of central nervous system and affect the physical, mental and emotional responses. These are intentionally inhaled at high concentration. They alter the perception and sense of reality resulting in illusions, hallucinations and delusions. Users experience euphoria, dreamy high culminating in a short period of sleep. Some of the commonly used volatile solvents are petrol, aerosols, thinners, varnish remover and industrial solvents.

Intoxication

Inhalation of a volatile solvent leads to euphoria, excitement, belligerence, slurring of speech, apathy, impaired judgment and neurological signs.

Withdrawal Symptoms

Anxiety, depression

Complications

Irreversible damage to the liver and kidneys, peripheral neuropathy, perceptual disturbances and brain damage.

Treatment

Reassurance and diazepam for intoxication, haloperidol for psychotic symptoms.

General Nursing Interventions for a Patient with Acute Drug Intoxication

- ❖ Care for a substance abuse patient starts with an assessment to determine which substance he is abusing. Signs and symptoms vary with substance and dosage.
- ❖ During the acute phase of drug intoxication, care focuses on maintaining the patient's vital functions, ensuring his safety, and easing discomfort.
- ❖ During rehabilitation, caregivers help the patient to acknowledge his substance abuse problem and find alternative ways to cope with stress. Healthcare professionals can play an importance role in helping patients achieve recovery and stay drug-free.

❖ These general nursing interventions are appropriate for patients during and after acute intoxication with most types of psychoactive drugs.

During an Acute Episode

❖ Monitor patient's vital signs and urine output continuously; watch for complications of overdose and withdrawal such as cardiopulmonary arrest, seizures, and aspiration.

❖ Maintain a quiet, safe environment. Take appropriate measures to prevent suicide attempts and assaults in line with the facility policy; remove harmful objects from the room and use restraints only if you suspect the patient might harm himself or others.

❖ Approach the patient in a non-threatening way.

❖ Institute seizure precautions.

❖ Administer IV fluids to increase circulatory volume.

❖ Give medications as ordered; monitor and record their effectiveness.

During Drug Withdrawal

❖ Administer medications as ordered to reduce withdrawal symptoms; monitor and record their effectiveness.

❖ Maintain a quiet, safe environment as excessive noise might agitate the patient.

When the Acute Episode has Resolved

❖ Carefully monitor and promote adequate nutrition.

❖ Administer drugs carefully to prevent hoarding; check patient's mouth to ensure he has swallowed oral medication, and closely monitor visitors who might supply him with drugs.

❖ Refer the patient for rehabilitation as appropriate; give him a list of available resources.

❖ Encourage family members to seek help regardless of whether the abuser seeks it or not; suggest private therapy or community mental health clinics.

❖ Use the episode to develop personal self-awareness.

❖ Set limits when dealing with demanding, manipulative behavior.

Prevention of Substance Use Disorder

Prevention is an activity designed to avoid substance abuse and reduce its health and social consequences. The three levels of prevention are explained below:

Primary Prevention

It focuses on preventing initiation of substance abuse or delaying the age at which use begins. The interventions are as follows:

❖ Reduction of over prescribing by doctors (especially with benzodiazepines and other anxiolytic drugs).

❖ Identification and treatment of family members who may be contributing to the drug abuse.

❖ Introduction of social changes is likely to affect drinking patterns in the population as a whole. This is made possible by:
  ○ Putting up the price of alcohol and alcoholic beverages
  ○ Controlling or abolishing the advertising of alcoholic drinks
  ○ Controls on sales (by limiting hours or banning sales in supermarkets)
  ○ Restricting availability and lessening social deprivation (Governmental measures)

❖ Other approaches are to strengthen the individual's personal and social skills to increase self-esteem and resistance to peer pressure.

❖ Health education to college students and the youth about the dangers of drug abuse through curriculum and mass media. Such education should also include certain specific groups where a substance like alcohol may be culturally accepted. For instance, in certain tribal communities such as the Lambani group manufacture of arrack and its intake is considered normal. Some communities use it in the postnatal period as alcohol is believed to strengthen the pelvic muscles and also speed up retroversion of the uterus. Such attitudes should be addressed and corrected.

❖ An overall improvement in the socio-economic condition of the population.

Secondary Prevention

Secondary prevention interventions are aimed at individuals who are in the early stages of their substance abuse so as to prevent problematic substance use. It includes early detection and counseling. Secondary prevention interventions are as follows:

❖ Brief intervention in primary care (simple advice by a general practitioner plus an educational leaflet).

❖ Motivational interviewing which involves providing feedback to the patient on the personal risks that alcohol possesses together with a number of options for change.

❖ A full assessment including an appraisal of current medical, psychological and social problems. Assessment also includes ascertaining whether alcoholism is the primary or secondary problem. For example, a patient with diabetic neuropathy may be using alcohol to numb pain. Alcohol is also used by some to relieve asthmatic symptoms. In such instances, treatment of the medical problem can help to control alcoholism.

❖ Detoxification with benzodiazepines (diazepam, chlordiazepoxide).

Tertiary Prevention

Tertiary prevention aims at ending dependence and reducing complications associated with it so as to improve levels of functioning and health. Specific measures include:

❖ Alcohol deterrent therapy (disulfiram or antabuse).

❖ Other therapies include assertiveness training (to prevent yielding to peer pressure), teaching coping skills (some take drugs to combat stress), behavior counseling, supportive psychotherapy and individual psychotherapy.

❖ Agencies concerned with alcohol related problems: Alcoholics Anonymous (AA), Al-Anon, Al-Ateen, etc.

❖ Some practical issues related to relapse prevention are:

○ Motivation enhancement, including education about health consequences of alcohol use
○ Identifying high-risk situations and developing strategies to deal with them (craving management)
○ Drink refusal skills (assertiveness training)
○ Dealing with faulty cognitions
○ Handling negative mood states
○ Time management
○ Anger control
○ Financial management
○ Developing the work habit
○ Stress management
○ Sleep hygiene
○ Recreation and spirituality
○ Family counseling to reduce interpersonal conflicts which may otherwise trigger relapse

Rehabilitation

Rehabilitation is designed to help people recover from drug and alcohol addiction. The aim of rehabilitation is to enable individuals with substance use to leave the drug sub culture and develop new social contacts. The patients first engage in work and social activities in sheltered surroundings and then take greater responsibilities for themselves in conditions increasingly like those of everyday life. Continuing social support is usually required when the person makes the transition to normal work and living. Rehabilitation helps individuals to regain control over their life and reintegrate into the society.

CHILD AND ADOLESCENT PSYCHAITRIC DISORDERS

Child psychiatry is concerned with the assessment and treatment of children's emotional and behavioral problems. The child psychiatric nurse uses a wide range of treatment modalities including milieu therapy, behavior modification, cognitive behavior therapy, therapeutic play, group and family therapy and pharmacological agents.

Disorders of Intellectual Development (Mental Retardation/Mentally Challenged Individuals)

The term mental retardation is replaced with intellectual disability. Advocates for individuals with intellectual disability have rightfully asserted that the term "mental retardation" has negative connotations. The main reason to search for a new term is to find least stigmatizing terminology. While DSM-5 has replaced it with intellectual developmental disorder (IDD), ICD-11 has replaced it with disorders of intellectual development (DID).

Definition

According to ICD-11, disorders of intellectual development (DID) are a group of etiologically diverse conditions originating during developmental period characterized by significantly below average intellectual functioning and adaptive behavior that are approximately 2 or more standard deviations below the mean, based on appropriately normed, individually administered tests.

Intellectual disability (ID) is characterized by significant impairment in intelligence and adaptive behavior. Here intelligence includes the ability to learn, reason, problem solving and other skills. Adaptive behavior includes everyday social and life skills.

"Mental retardation/disorders or intellectual development refers to significantly sub-average general intellectual functioning resulting in or associated with concurrent impairments in adaptive behavior and manifested during the developmental period" *(American Association on Mental Deficiency, 1983).*

General intellectual functioning is defined as the result obtained by the administration of standardized general intelligence tests developed for the purpose, and adopted to the conditions of the region/country.

Significant subaverage is defined as an Intelligence Quotient (IQ) of 70 or below on standardized measures of intelligence. The upper limit is intended as a guideline and could be extended to 75 or more depending on the reliability of the intelligence test used.

Adaptive behavior is defined as the degree with which the individual meets the standards of personal independence and social responsibility expected of his age and cultural group. Expectations of adaptive behavior vary with chronological age. Deficits in adaptive behavior may be reflected in the following areas:

During Infancy and Childhood
- Sensory and motor skill development
- Communication skill (including speech and language)
- Self-help skills
- Socialization

During Childhood and Adolescence
- Application of basic academic skill to daily life activities
- Application of appropriate reasoning and judgment in the mastery of environment
- Social skills

During Late Adolescence
Vocational and social responsibilities and performance.

Developmental period is defined as the period of time between conception and the 18th birthday.

Epidemiology

According to Lakhan R et al. 2015 study, the overall intellectual disability in India stands at 10.5/1,000. Urban population has a slightly higher rate (11/1,000) than the rural population (10.8/1,000).

Etiology

In most of the cases the exact cause is unknown. The condition develops due to injury, disease or certain brain conditions (**Figure 5.25**).

1. Genetic Factors
- **Chromosomal abnormalities:**
  - Down's syndrome
  - Fragile X syndrome
  - Trisomy X syndrome

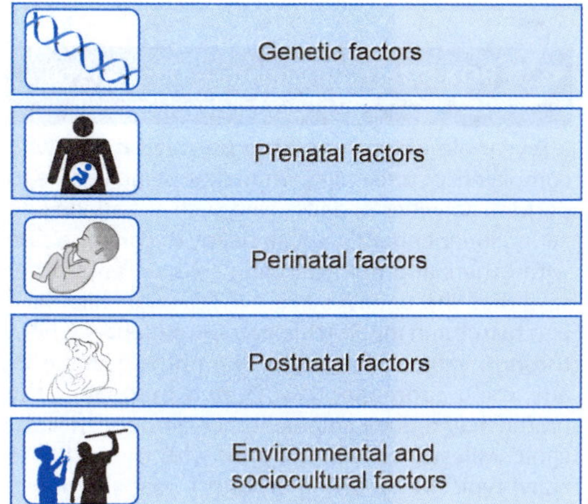

Figure 5.25: Etiology of intellectual disability

- ○ Turner's syndrome
- ○ Cat-cry syndrome
- ○ Prader-Willi syndrome
- ❖ **Metabolic disorders:**
  - ○ Phenylketonuria
  - ○ Wilson's disease
  - ○ Galactosemia
- ❖ **Cranial malformation:**
  - ○ Hydrocephaly
  - ○ Microcephaly
- ❖ **Gross diseases of brain:**
  - ○ Tuberous sclerosis
  - ○ Neurofibromatosis
  - ○ Epilepsy

2. Prenatal Factors

- ❖ **Infections:**
  - ○ Rubella
  - ○ Cytomegalovirus
  - ○ Syphilis
  - ○ Toxoplasmosis, herpes simplex
- ❖ **Endocrine disorders:**
  - ○ Hypothyroidism
  - ○ Hypoparathyroidism
  - ○ Diabetes mellitus
- ❖ **Physical damage and disorders:**
  - ○ Injury
  - ○ Hypoxia
  - ○ Radiation
  - ○ Hypertension
  - ○ Anemia
  - ○ Emphysema

- ❖ **Intoxication:**
  - ○ Lead
  - ○ Certain drugs
  - ○ Substance abuse
- ❖ **Placental dysfunction:**
  - ○ Toxemia of pregnancy
  - ○ Placenta previa
  - ○ Cord prolapse
  - ○ Nutritional growth retardation

3. Perinatal Factors

- ❖ Birth asphyxia
- ❖ Prolonged or difficult birth
- ❖ Prematurity (due to complications)
- ❖ Kernicterus
- ❖ Instrumental delivery (resulting in head injury, intraventricular hemorrhage)

4. Postnatal Factors

- ❖ **Infections:**
  - ○ Encephalitis
  - ○ Measles
  - ○ Meningitis
  - ○ Septicemia
- ❖ Accidents
- ❖ Lead poisoning

5. Environmental and Socio-cultural Factors

- ❖ Cultural deprivation
- ❖ Low socio-economic status
- ❖ Inadequate caretakers
- ❖ Child abuse

Classification

Intelligence quotient (IQ) is the ratio between Mental Age (MA) and Chronological Age (CA). While the chronological age is determined from the date of birth, mental age is determined by intelligence tests **(Box 5.37)**.

BOX 5.37: Classification of disorders of intellectual development based on intelligence quotient

Type	Intelligence quotient (IQ)
• Mild (educable)	50–70
• Moderate (trainable)	35–50
• Severe (dependent retarded)	20–35
• Profound (life support)	<20

Disorders of Intellectual Development Mild—6A00.0: Mild Retardation (IQ 50–70)

This is most common type of mental retardation accounting for 85–90% of all cases. These individuals have minimum retardation in sensory-motor areas.

Disorders of Intellectual Development Moderate—6A00.1: Moderate Retardation (IQ 35–50)

About 10% of mentally retarded fall under this group.

Disorders of Intellectual Development Severe—6A00.2: Severe Retardation (IQ 20–35)

Severe mental retardation is often recognized early in life with poor motor development and absent or markedly delayed speech and communication skills.

Disorders of Intellectual Development Profound—6A00.3: Profound Retardation (IQ below 20)

This group accounts for 1–2% of all mentally retarded. The achievement of developmental milestones is markedly delayed. They require constant nursing care and supervision. Associated physical disorders are common.

Behavioral Manifestations

Intelligence means ability to understand and interact with the world around us. There are many different signs and symptoms of intellectual disability that can exist in children and will vary depending upon specific type. These behavioral manifestations may first become apparent in infancy or in some cases may not be noticeable until child reaches school age **(Box 5.38)**. Some of the most common symptoms are presented in **Table 5.46**.

❖ Delay in milestone development such as neck holding, sitting, rolling over, crawling, walking, etc. Sometimes failure to achieve developmental milestones.

❖ Deficiencies in cognitive functioning such as inability to follow commands or directions, difficulties with reasoning, judging, critical thinking, distractable and difficulty in focusing.

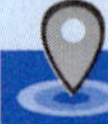

BOX 5.38: Case vignette—Disorders of intellectual development

A 9-year-old girl is brought to psychiatric OPD with complaints of screaming, irritability, being unable to perform activities of daily living such as bathing and eating independently, speak clearly or communicate with others and not attending school. Her mother says that she behaves like a 3-year-old child. Past psychiatric and medical history: The patient was born through vaginal delivery at 9 months gestational age, cried spontaneously. During pregnancy the mother had routine antenatal checkups from nearest clinic. Milestones were delayed with the ability to crawl typically occurring around 1 year and ability to walk independently occurring around 3 years. Family history was significant for one maternal uncle with developmental delay. There was no history of consanguinity. On examination the following were observed: high amount of salivation, normal vital signs, poor eye contact and display of repetitive behavior. Neurological examination (cranial nerves, motor, sensory and reflexes) was normal. The patient was diagnosed with severe mental retardation with significant behavioral disorder.

❖ Reduced ability to learn or meet academic demands
❖ Expressive or receptive language problems
❖ Psychomotor skill deficits
❖ Difficulty performing self-care activities
❖ Neurologic impairments
❖ Low self-esteem, depression and labile moods
❖ Irritability when frustrated or upset
❖ Acting-out behavior
❖ Lack of curiosity
❖ Children with severe intellectual disabilities may have additional health problems such as seizures, vision problems, hearing problems, etc.

Diagnosis

❖ History collection from parents and caretakers
❖ Physical examination
❖ Neurological examination
❖ Assessing milestones development
❖ Investigations:
   o Urine and blood examination for metabolic disorders

TABLE 5.46: Behavioral manifestations of intellectual disability in children

Type of intellectual disability/ behavioral manifestations	Mild intellectual disability (IQ: 50–70)	Moderate intellectual disability (IQ: 35–49)	Severe intellectual disability (IQ: 20–34)	Profound intellectual disability (IQ: <20)
Self-care ability	• Slower than normal in all areas • Can acquire daily living skills • The child may be able to live some-what independently with monitoring or assistance with life changes, challenges, or stressors (such as personal illness or the death of a loved one)	• Can participate in simple activities and self-care • The child requires close supervision and must be supervised when performing certain independent activities	• Significant delay in some areas • May be trained in simple self-care • The child requires complete supervision but may be able to perform simple hygiene skills such as brushing teeth and washing hands	• Significant delay in all areas • The child requires constant assistance and supervision • Not capable of self-care
Education level	• The child can achieve reading skills up to the level of primary school (grades 3 to 5) and master vocational training	• The child can achieve skills up to second class and may be trained in skills to participate in a workshop setting • Can learn elementary health and safety skills	• May learn a few simple skills • Can be taught daily routines and repetitive activities	• The child cannot benefit from academic training
Social skills	• The child can learn and use social skills in structured settings	• Can learn simple communication • The child has certain speech limitations and difficulty following expected social norms	• Little or no communication skills • The child has limited verbal skills and tends to communicate needs non-verbally or by acting them out	• The child has little speech development and lacks social skills
Psychomotor skills	• The child can develop average to good skills but may experience minor co-ordination problems	• The child may have difficulty with gross motor skills and limited vocational opportunities	• The child has poor psychomotor skills with limited ability to perform simple tasks even under direct supervision	• The child lacks both fine and gross motor skills

Contd...

Contd...

Type of intellectual disability/ behavioral manifestations	Mild intellectual disability (IQ: 50–70)	Moderate intellectual disability (IQ: 35–49)	Severe intellectual disability (IQ: 20–34)	Profound intellectual disability (IQ: <20)
Economic situation	• The child can per-form a job under close supervision and manage money with proper guidance	• The child may learn to handle a small amount of pocket money as well as how to make change	• The child may be taught how to use money and supervised while shopping	• The child must depend on others for money management

- ○ Culture for cytogenic and biochemical studies
- ○ Amniocentesis in infant chromosomal disorders
- ○ Chorionic villi sampling
- ○ Hearing and speech evaluation
- ○ EEG, especially if seizures are present
- ○ CT scan or MRI brain, for example, in tuberous sclerosis
- ○ Thyroid function tests when cretinism is suspected
- ○ Psychological tests like Stanford Binet Intelligence Scale and Wechsler Intelligence Scale for Children (WISC) for categorizing the child's level of disability
- ❖ Through psychological testing the mental age of the child is estimated. The Intelligence Quotient is then determined using the formula:

$$\frac{\text{Mental age (MA)}}{\text{Chronological age (CA)}} \times 100$$

Prognosis

As prognosis for children with mental retardation has dramatically improved, institutional care is no longer recommended. These children are mainstreamed whenever feasible mend are taught survival skills. A multidimensional orientation is used when working with these children, considering their physiological, cognitive, social and emotional development.

Treatment Modalities

- ❖ Behavior management
- ❖ Environmental supervision
- ❖ Monitoring child's developmental needs and problems
- ❖ Programs that maximize speech, language, cognitive, psychomotor, social, self-care, and occupational skills
- ❖ Ongoing evaluation for overlapping psychiatric disorders such as depression, bipolar disorder and attention-deficit hyperactivity disorder (ADHD)
- ❖ Family therapy to help parents develop coping skills and deal with guilt or anger
- ❖ Early intervention programs for children aged less than 3 years with mental retardation
  - ○ Provide day schools to train the child in basic skills such as bathing and feeding
  - ○ Vocational training

Prevention

Prevention of intellectual disability requires different methods depending on the cause. In this section prevention is explained under primary, secondary and tertiary level.

Primary Prevention

Focuses on measures taken at the early stage to decimate disability.

Measures at preconception

- ❖ Genetic counseling to determine risks of occurrence or recurrence of specific genetic or chromosomal disorders; parents can then make an informed decision as to the risks of having a retarded child.
- ❖ Immunization for maternal rubella.

❖ Blood tests for marriage licenses can identify the presence of venereal diseases.

❖ Adequate maternal nutrition can lay a sound metabolic foundation for later childbearing.

❖ Family planning in terms of size, appropriate spacing and age of parents can also affect a variety of specific causal agents.

During gestation

Two general approaches to prevention are associated with this period:

1. **Prenatal care:**
   ○ Adequate nutrition, fetal monitoring and protection from disease
   ○ Avoidance of teratogenic substances like exposure to radiation and consumption of alcohol and drugs
2. **Analysis of fetus for possible genetic disorders:** By amniocentesis, fetoscopy, fetal biopsy and ultrasound

At delivery

❖ Delivery conducted by expert doctors and staff especially in cases of high-risk pregnancy (e.g., maternal conditions of diabetes, hypertension, etc.).

❖ Apgar scoring done at 1 and 5 minutes after the birth of the child.

❖ Close monitoring of mother and child.

❖ Injection of gamma globulin which can prevent Rh-negative mothers from developing antibodies that might otherwise affect subsequent children.

Childhood

❖ Proper nutrition throughout the developmental period and particularly during the first 6 months after birth.

❖ Dietary restrictions for specific metabolic disorders until no longer needed.

❖ Avoidance of hazards in the child's environment to avert brain injury from causes such as lead poisoning, ingestion of chemicals or accidents.

Secondary Prevention

Secondary prevention focuses on early detection and treatment of preventable disorders.

❖ For example, phenylketonuria and hypothyroidism can be effectively treated at an early stage by dietary control or hormone replacement therapy.

❖ Early recognition of presence of mental retardation. A delay in diagnosis may cause unfortunate delay in rehabilitation.

❖ Psychiatric treatment for emotional and behavioral difficulties.

Tertiary Prevention

The focus at tertiary prevention is to promote recovery as well as to prevent further complications.

❖ This includes rehabilitation in vocational, physical and social areas according to the level of handicap. Rehabilitation is aimed at reducing disability and providing optimal functioning in a child with mental retardation.

Legal Aspects Concerning Persons with Mental Disabilities

❖ Mentally retarded are treated as persons with disabilities under Section 2 of the Persons with Disabilities (Equal Opportunities, Protection of Rights and Participation) Act, 1995 (PWD Act).

❖ The Rights of Persons with Disabilities (RPwD) Act 2016 has replaced the Person with Disabilities (PwD) Act 1995.

❖ Statutory provisions for the welfare of mentally retarded persons are included in PWD Act, 1995 and National Trust Act, 1999.

❖ Indian Railways and some State Governments have introduced schemes providing travel facility for persons with disability.

❖ The Income-Tax Act allows deduction in respect of maintenance including medical treatment of a dependent who is a person with disability which includes mental retardation and mental illness under Section 80DD.

Care and Rehabilitation

The main elements in comprehensive service for mentally retarded individuals and their families include:

- Early detection and early stimulation of mental handicaps.
- Regular assessment of the mentally retarded person's attainments and disabilities.
- Advice, support, and practical measures for families.
- Provision for education, training, occupation, or work appropriate for each handicapped person.
- Housing and social support to enable self-care.
- Medical, nursing, and other services for those who require them as outpatients, day patients, or inpatients.
- Psychiatric and psychological services.

Residential care: Parents should be supported in caring for their retarded children at home or if they are too heavy a burden for their parents, the child should be cared for in daycare centers, halfway homes, etc.

Specialist medical services: Retarded children and adults often have physical handicaps or epilepsy for which continuing medical care is needed.

Psychiatric services: Expert psychiatric care is an essential part of comprehensive community service for the mentally retarded.

Nursing Management

Determine child's strengths and abilities to develop a plan of care to enhance capabilities. Nursing management is explained under assessment, diagnosis, planning, implementation and evaluation.

Assessment

- Assessment of early infant behavior for cognitive disability among high-risk children should be closely done (for example, children born to elderly primiparas, birth trauma, etc.); Early infant behaviors that may indicate a cognitive disability include non-responsiveness to contact, poor eye contact during feeding, slow feeding, diminished spontaneous activity, decreased responsiveness to surroundings, decreased alertness to voice or movement and irritability.
- Documentation of daily living skills
- A careful family assessment for information on:
  - Family's response to the child
  - Presence of other members with impaired cognition in the family
  - Degree of independence encouraged at home
  - Stability of the family unit
- Psychological assessment—This is directed at the interaction between the individual and people who are closely involved in care, and determining the correct needs and wishes for the future. It should examine opportunities for learning new skills, making relationships, and achieving maximum choice about the way of life

Interventions

- The long-term goals for these children are highly individualized and are dependent on the level of mental retardation. Parents should be involved in establishing realistic goals for their child. Some of these goals can be:
  - The child dresses himself.
  - The child maintains continence of stool and urine.
  - The child demonstrates acceptable social behavior.
  - The adolescent participates in a structured work program.
- Monitor the child's developmental level and initiate supportive interventions such as speech, language or occupational skills as needed.
- Early intervention programs are essential to maximize children's potential development. This necessitates early recognition and referral. Nurses have an opportunity to evaluate children in the nursery, in the clinic during well-baby healthcare, in schools, and during acute management. The potential of each child will vary according to the degree of mental retardation. The key for success is that the child's strengths and potential abilities are emphasized rather than the deficits.

- ❖ The nurse can participate in programs that teach infant stimulation, activities of daily living and independent self-care skills.
- ❖ Teach the child adaptive skills such as eating, dressing, grooming and toileting. Encourage the child to perform tasks within their ability.
- ❖ Develop a daily schedule for the child and family.
- ❖ A successful technique in treatment of the mentally retarded is called operant conditioning. It focuses on changing or modifying the individual's response to the environment by reinforcing certain desirable patterns of behavior or eliminating undesirable patterns. Reward the child's accomplishments.
- ❖ In addition, learning social skills and adaptive behavior assists the child in building a positive self-image. For older children and adolescents, assistance is needed to prepare them for a productive work life.
- ❖ Maintain a consistent and supervised environment with adequate environmental stimulation.
- ❖ Prevent self-injury. Be prepared to intervene if self-injury occurs. Monitor the child for physical or emotional distress.
- ❖ Sexuality becomes a major concern as these children may form emotional attachment to those of the opposite sex and have normal sexual desires. However, their decision-making skills are limited. Teaching contraceptive methods are important to emphasize with both the child and family.
- ❖ In all instances it is important for the nurse to maintain a non-threatening approach. Very often, these children do not understand why physical assessment, therapeutic approaches and evaluative measures are needed. Proper explanation and relevant information should be given to the parents and their help enlisted in bringing out the best in the child. Close collaboration with all members of the team involved in child care is highly essential for a successful outcome. To a large extent the nurse is responsible for the emotional climate of the setting in which she is employed.

Prevention of Exploitation and Abuse of Persons with Mental Disabilities

- ❖ Persons with mental disabilities are one of the vulnerable groups likely to be exploited.
- ❖ Female persons with mental disabilities are the most vulnerable of the group. Therefore, the legal services institutions shall come to the assistance of these people in preventing their exploitation including sexual abuse and also for taking legal action against the abusers and exploiters.

Autism Spectrum Disorder

In ICD-11, autism spectrum disorder (ASD) is included in the category mental, behavioral or neurodevelopmental disorders (category 06).

The 11th edition of the International Classification of Diseases and Related Health Problems (ICD-11, 2018) notes that: "Autism spectrum disorder is characterized by persistent deficits in the ability to initiate and to sustain reciprocal social interaction and social communication, and by a range of restricted, repetitive, and inflexible patterns of behaviors and interests. The onset of disorder occurs during the developmental period. Deficits are sufficiently severe to cause impairment in personal, family, social, educational, occupational or other important areas of functioning.

Meaning

Autism spectrum disorder (ASD) is a neuro-developmental disorder often presenting in early childhood with restricted and repetitive behaviors, interests and activities and significant impairment in social communication.

Autism is a complex neurobehavioral disorder that includes impairments in social interaction, verbal and non-verbal communication combined with restricted and repetitive behavior. Parents usually notice

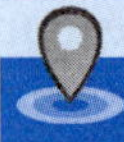

BOX 5.39: Characteristics of autistic disorder

- Inappropriate responses to environment
- Pronounced impairments in language, communication, and social interaction
- Repetitive interests and behaviors
- Disordered thinking
- Difficulty understanding feelings of others and world around him
- Repetitive, self-injurious, or other abnormal behaviors

signs in the first two years of their child's life **(Box 5.39)**.

Epidemiology

According Zeidan J et al. 2022 study on global prevalence of autism—a systematic review, it is estimated that worldwide about 1 in 100 children has autism. Male to female ratio is 4 or 5 : 1.

Etiology

There are many different factors involved in causation of ASD. A growing area of research focuses on interaction of genetic and environmental factors.

Genetic Factors

- ❖ The higher rate of autism in siblings of twins diagnosed with autism.
- ❖ For siblings of a person with autism, chances of having the condition are higher than for the general population.
- ❖ Having certain genetic conditions such as down syndrome or Fragile X syndrome or Rett syndrome.

Environmental Factors

- ❖ Advanced age of the mother at the time of conception.
- ❖ Prenatal exposure to pollutants and toxins such as pesticides, heavy metals, air pollution or nitrogen dioxide during fetal development.
- ❖ Maternal illness such as obesity, diabetes or immune system disorders.
- ❖ Any birth difficulty leading to periods of oxygen deprivation to the baby's brain.
- ❖ Having a very low birth weight.

Clinical Picture

The most obvious sign that a child has autism is its inability to interact socially (**Figure 5.26** and **Box 5.40**).

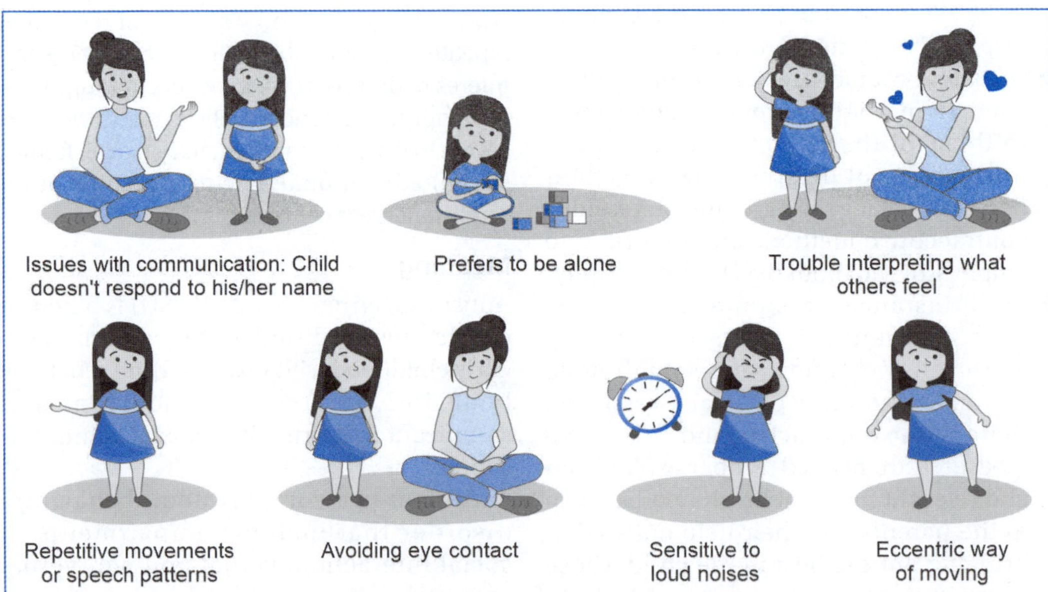

Figure 5.26: Signs of autism

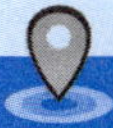

BOX 5.40: Case vignette—Autistic spectrum disorder

Arun, a 18-month-old male child came to psychiatric OPD with complaints of being unable to utter a single word, unresponsiveness to parent behavior, more tantrums, lack of eye-to-eye contact, dislike to be touched or kissed, not interactive with family members, no separation anxiety when left alone, less interested to play with toys. As an infant he was undemanding and placid.

On examination, motor development was found to be age appropriate. History stated that mother had induced labor at 37 weeks due to fetal distress. There was no family history suggestive of developmental delays. A comprehensive medical evaluation revealed normal MRI scan, EEG and other chromosomal analysis. Arun was diagnosed with autism spectrum disorder. Psychiatrist reassured the parents and encouraged them to visit a psychologist for behavioral problems and speech therapist for language development. Regular follow-up was also suggested.

At 24 months, motor skills were age appropriate, his language was delayed, it was noticed that he was resistant to changes in routine and had an unusual attachment to toys. His play skills were quite limited and he played with toys in idiosyncratic ways. He also has a repetitive rocking body, opens and closes drawers, has an intense fixed interest in a specific toy. Over the next two years, Arun was taken to various psychiatric hospitals and underwent several therapies after which he was enrolled in a special education program where he gradually began to speak.

Behavioral Characteristics

- Autistic aloofness (unresponsiveness to parent's smiling or cuddling affectionate behavior).
- Gaze avoidance or lack of eye-to-eye contact.
- Dislikes being touched or kissed.
- No separation anxiety on being left in an unfamiliar environment with strangers.
- No or abnormal social play. Failure to play with peers and unable to make friends.
- Failure to develop empathy.
- Marked lack of awareness of the existence or feelings of others.
- Anger or fear without apparent reason and absence of fear in the presence of danger.

Communication and Language

- Gross deficits and deviances in language development
- No mode of communication such as babbling, facial expression, gestures, mime, etc.
- Begin speaking late or do not speak by the age at which most children begin
- Absence of imaginative activity such as play acting of adult roles, fantasy characters of animals, lack of interest in imaginative stories
- Marked abnormality in the production of speech (volume, pitch, stress, rhythm, rate, etc.)
- Marked abnormalities in the form or content of speech including stereotyped or repetitive use of speech, use of "you" when "I" is meant, idiosyncratic use of phrases
- Marked impairment in the ability to initiate or sustain a conversation with others

Social Interaction

- No social interaction
- Inability to follow simple commands
- Prefer playing alone
- Indifferent and emotionless
- Do not mingle with parents, teachers and siblings

Activities

- Marked restricted, repertoire of activities and interests.
- Stereotyped body movements,,e.g., hand flicking or twisting, spinning, head banging, etc.
- Persistent preoccupation with parts of objects (for example, spinning wheels of toy cars) or attachment to unusual objects
- Marked distress over changes in trivial aspects of environment.
- Markedly restricted range of interests and a preoccupation with one narrow interest.

Other Features

- More than half of autistic children have moderate to profound mental retardation, while about 25% have mild mental retardation.

❖ Autistic children are resistant to transition and change.

❖ Over-responsive or under-responsive to sensory stimuli.

❖ May have a heightened pain threshold or an altered response to pain.

❖ Other behavioral problems like hyperkinesis, aggression, temper tantrums, self-injurious behavior, head banging, biting, scratching and hair pulling are common.

❖ **Idiot savant syndrome:** Inspite of a pervasive or abnormal development of functions, certain functions may remain normal, for example, calculating ability, prodigious remote memory, musical abilities, etc.

❖ Absence of hallucinations, delusions, loosening of associations as in schizophrenia.

❖ Kanner's "Autistic triad"—Kanner said autistic aloofness, speech and language disorder and obsessive desire for sameness constitute a triad characteristic of infantile autism.

Course and Prognosis

❖ Autistic disorder has a long course and guarded prognosis.

❖ Some people with autism can live independently while others have severe disabilities and require life-long care and support.

❖ About 10–20% autistic children begin to improve between 4 and 6 years of age and eventually attend an ordinary school and obtain work.

❖ About 10–20% can live at home but need to attend a special school or training center and cannot work.

❖ About 60% improve little and are unable to lead an independent life, mostly needing long-term residential care.

❖ Those who improve may continue to show language problem, emotional coldness and odd behavior.

❖ People with autism often have co-occurring conditions such as epilepsy, depression, anxiety, attention deficit hyperactivity, etc. The level of intellectual functioning among autistic people varies widely extending from profound impairment to superior levels.

Diagnosis

❖ No definitive diagnostic tool; usually diagnosed by age 3 after ruling out other disorders that resemble autism (neurologic disorders, hearing loss, speech problems, and mental retardation).

❖ The diagnostic evaluation is likely to include:
  ○ Medical examination
  ○ Neurological examination
  ○ Cognitive abilities assessment
  ○ Language abilities assessment
  ○ Observation of child behavior
  ○ Assessment of age-appropriate skills such as eating, dressing, toileting, etc.

❖ Autism identifying methods by an autism specialist:
  ○ Standardized rating scale to help evaluate the child's social behavior and language.
  ○ Tests for certain genetic and neurologic problems may be ordered.
  ○ Interviews with parents to seek information about the child's behavior and early development.

❖ Developmental screening to reveal behaviors suggestive of autism:
  ○ Failure to babble, coo, or gesture (point, wave, or grasp) by age of 12 months.
  ○ Failure to utter single words by age of 16 months and two-word phrases on his own by age of 24 months.
  ○ Loss of language or social skills at any age

❖ After evaluation and testing, diagnosis is based on clear evidence of poor or limited social relationships; underdeveloped communication skills; and repetitive behaviors, activities, and interests.

Treatment

There is no known cure for autism. However, with intensive therapy the child can learn certain skills and make conversation.

❖ **Pharmacotherapy** is a valuable treatment for associated symptoms like aggression, temper tantrums, self-injurious behavior, hyperactivity and stereotypic behavior. Some drugs that have been used are risperidone, serotonin specific reuptake inhibitors, clomipramine and lithium. Antiepileptic medication is used for generalized seizures.

- ❖ **Behavioral methods**: They are used to stop problematic behaviors and promote appropriate behaviors. Contingency management may control some of the abnormal behavior of autistic children. The term contingency management refers to a group of procedures based on the principle that, if any behavior persists, certain of its consequences are reinforcing it. If these consequences can be altered, the behavior will change. Parents are instructed and supervised by a clinical psychologist to often carry out this method at home.
- ❖ **Speech therapy and social skills training**: This training helps the child in communicating needs with words or gestures and express the needs to others.
- ❖ **Special schooling**: Most autistic children require special schooling while older adolescents may need vocational training.
- ❖ **Counseling and supportive therapy**: The family of an autistic child needs considerable help to cope with the child's behavior which is often distressing. Group-based parent training may be helpful to reduce distress among parents.
- ❖ **Home care** to assist with the child's physical or behavioral management at home; if the child's disruptive behavior persists, alternative residential placement may be necessary.
- ❖ **Others**: Development of a regular routine, positive reinforcements to teach self-care skills, speech therapy or sign language teaching, behavior techniques to encourage interpersonal interactions.

Nursing Management

Psychiatric nurses work as a team member of professionals helping children with autism. The nurse should be specialized in taking care of autistic children. The nurse's role is not restricted to hospital and clinics but extends to home environment.

Assessment

The following factors need to be considered in assessing an autistic child (Lord and Rutter, 1994):

- ❖ Cognitive level
- ❖ Language ability
- ❖ Communication skills, social skills, play, repetitive behavior and other abnormal behavior
- ❖ Stage of social development in relation to mental age and stage of language development
- ❖ Associated medical conditions
- ❖ Psychosocial factors

Interventions

- ❖ Work with the child on a one-to-one basis
- ❖ Protect the child when self-mutilative behavior occurs. Devices such as a helmet, padded mittens or arm cover may be used.
- ❖ Try to determine if self-mutilative behavior occurs in response to increasing anxiety and if so to what the anxiety may be attributed. Intervene with diversion or replacement activities as anxiety level starts to rise. These activities may provide needed feelings of security and substitute for self-mutilative behavior.
- ❖ Assign limited number of caregivers to the child. Ensure that warmth, acceptance and availability are conveyed.
- ❖ Provide child with familiar objects such as toys or a blanket. Support child's attempts to interact with others.
- ❖ Give positive reinforcement when eye contact is used to convey non-verbal expressions or when the child tries to speak. This can be done by giving something acceptable to the child which can either be a favorite food item or a toy.
- ❖ Gradually replace positive reinforcement with social reinforcement, for example, touching or hugging.
- ❖ Anticipate and fulfill the child's needs until communication can be established.
- ❖ Slowly encourage to express the needs verbally. Seek clarification and validation.

❖ Teach simple self-care skills by using behavior modification techniques.

❖ Language training plays a big part in teaching autistic children. At first, they have to learn the names of various objects by linking names to them. When teaching the word 'table' they must see and feel a real table and lots of different other tables. Otherwise, they may think that a table refers to only that particular object. Look at child's face and pronounce simple words. Ask the child to repeat the words. Show picture books and name the objects. Verbs like sitting, walking, running can be acted to show the child what these words mean.

❖ Autistic children have personal identity disturbance and need to be assisted to recognize separateness during self-care activities such as dressing and feeding. The child should be helped to name own body parts. This can be facilitated with the use of mirrors, drawings and pictures of himself. Encourage appropriate touching of and being touched by others.

❖ The role of the parent is crucial for any intervention with the autistic child; the parent generally acts as a co-therapist and plays an integral role in treatment. As the behavior of their autistic child is often very distressing, parental counseling begins with clarification of the diagnosis and an explanation of the characteristics of the disorder. To effectively participate in the treatment program the parents must have acknowledged the extent of their child's handicap and be able to work with him at the appropriate developmental level.

Prevention

❖ Genetic screening

❖ Refrain from using all addictive substances including alcohol, tobacco, etc.

❖ Avoid exposure to heavily polluted areas during pregnancy

❖ Exercise regularly

❖ Eat nutritious foods

❖ Early recognition and prompt treatment

Developmental Learning Disorder

The 11th edition of the International Classification of Diseases and Related Health Problems (ICD-11, 2018) notes that: Developmental learning disorder is characterized by significant and persistent difficulties in learning academic skills, which may include reading, writing or arithmetic. These individuals' performance in the affected academic skills is markedly below what would be expected for chronological age and general level of intellectual functioning and results in significant impairment in the individual's academic or occupational functioning. These disorders are not due to a disorder of intellectual development, sensory impairment, neurological or motor disorder.

Specific Areas of Learning Impairments

1. **Impairment in reading:** Specific reading disorders (dyslexia) should be clearly distinguished from general backwardness in scholastic achievement resulting from low intelligence or inadequate education. It is characterized by a slow acquisition of reading skills, slow reading speed, impaired comprehension, word omissions and distortions and letter reversals.

2. **Impairment in written expression (dysgraphia):** The main feature is significant impairment in writing skills such as spelling accuracy, grammar and punctuation accuracy, organization and cohesion of ideas in writing.

3. **Impairment in mathematics (dyscalculia):** Specific arithmetic disorder involves deficit in basic computational skills of addition, subtraction, multiplication and division.

Causes

❖ Family history

❖ Exposure to alcohol or drugs during antenatal period

❖ Emotional abuse of the child

❖ Head injury, neurological disorders

* Exposure to poisonous substances such as exposure to high levels of lead or other toxins

Symptoms of Learning Disorders

* Not being able to master skills in reading, spelling, writing or math at or near the expected age and grade levels.
* Trouble completing homework and assignments on time.
* Difficulty remembering what was just said or read.
* Difficulty in writing, drawing and under standing concepts.
* Children may feel frustrated that they cannot master a subject despite trying hard
* May feel helpless or withdraw.
* These disorders can also be present with emotional or behavioral disorders such as ADHD or anxiety or depression.

Treatment

* Special education services
* Individualized education program

Developmental Motor Co-ordination Disorder (Dyspraxia)

The 11th edition of the International Classification of Diseases and Related Health Problems (ICD-11, 2018) notes that: Developmental motor coordination disorder is characterized by a significant delay in the acquisition of gross and fine motor skills and impairment in the execution of coordinated motor skills that manifest in clumsiness, slowness or inaccuracy of motor performance.

Causes

Exact cause is unknown. It may be the result of delayed brain development, family history, mother taking alcohol or illegal drugs while pregnant. In some cases, this disorder is associated with attention deficit hyperactivity or disorders that cause intellectual disabilities.

Symptoms

* Impairment in fine and gross movement skills which include difficulty in maintaining balance, changing movement, learning new movements, predicting the outcome of their movements.
* Onset is in the early developmental period.
* During toddler period they are slow to learn to sit, walk and talk.
* During school age period they have an unsteady walk, difficulty going down stairs, dropping objects, frequent tripping, difficulty in performing school activities such as writing, coloring and using scissors.
* Motor skills difficulties are markedly below the individual's chronological age and level of intellectual functioning.
* These difficulties significantly interfere with activities of daily living and impact academic, vocational, leisure and play activities.
* They have difficulty adjusting movements and adapting to the demands of the environment.
* These children are physically inactive and may experience excessive weight gain.

Treatment

* Requires long-term physical therapy, occupational therapy and social skills training.
* Daily exercises
* **Training motor skills**: Breaking down difficult movements into smaller parts and practicing them regularly.

Attention-Deficit Hyperactivity Disorder

Attention-deficit hyperactivity disorder or ADHD or hyperkinetic disorder is a persistent pattern of inattention and/or hyperactivity more frequent and severe than is typical of children at a similar level of development. The syndrome was first described by Heinrich Hoff in 1854.

The 11th edition of the International Classification of Diseases and Related Health Problems (ICD-11, 2018) notes that: Attention-deficit hyperactivity disorder is characterized by a persistent pattern (at least 6 months) of inattention and or hyperactivity-impulsivity that has a direct negative impact on academic, occupational or social functioning.

Attention-deficit hyperactivity disorder is marked by an ongoing pattern of inattention and or hyperactivity-impulsivity that interferes with functioning or development.

Etiology

The exact cause of ADHD is unknown. Many studies suggest that genes play a larger role.

Genetic Factors

❖ There is greater concordance in monozygotic than in dizygotic twins.
❖ Siblings of hyperactive children have about twice the risk of having the disorder as does the general population.
❖ Biological parents of children with the disorder have a higher incidence of ADHD than do adoptive parents.

Non genetic Factors

❖ Being born prematurely before the 37th week of pregnancy
❖ Having low birthweight
❖ Smoking or alcohol or drug abuse during pregnancy
❖ Extreme stress during pregnancy

Clinical Features

Three main features of ADHD are (**Figure 5.27** and **Box 5.41**):

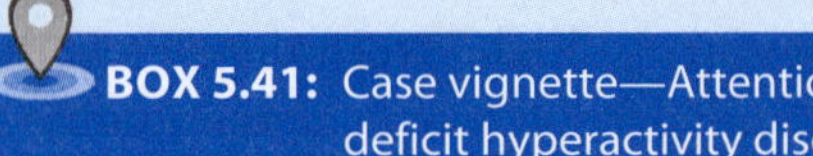

BOX 5.41: Case vignette—Attention-deficit hyperactivity disorder

Mourya is 10-year-old boy, fifth grader brought to psychiatric OPD with a history of problems at home and school. His mother reported about his school performance getting worse year on year. He has difficulties at home with following routines and remembering instructions. She has to repeat instructions over and over again. He has been exhibiting emotional and confrontational behavior, gets easily frustrated and is emotionally impulsive. There have been several incidents of hitting, crying outbursts and inappropriate behaviors.

Teachers reported that Mourya is restless and often requires reminders to help him stay on the task. He is described as constantly running around and presenting with difficulties in listening and following instructions. His approach to class work is very chaotic and is rarely able to focus on one task for over 2–3 minutes. He often blurts out answers and interrupts other students in the classroom. There have also been some difficulties in friendship groups with Mourya often getting involved in arguments during play. It is noticed that Mourya has become more and more disorganized over the past one year.

Mourya describes difficulties with focusing and sitting still in class, and sustaining attention at school. He recognizes this tendency in himself but says he cannot stop in spite of his best intentions. He has been struggling with his schoolwork and has fallen significantly behind in some subjects.

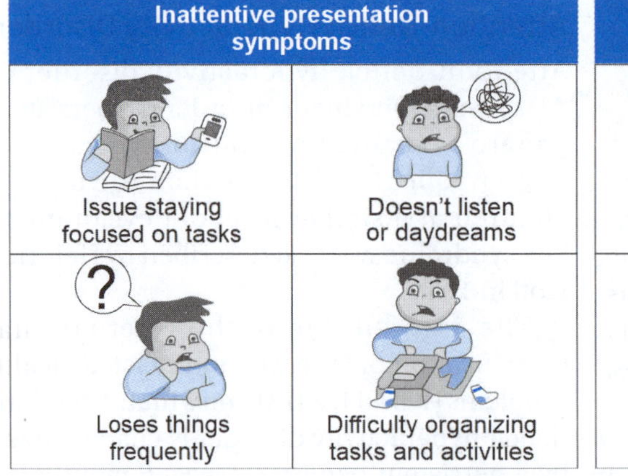

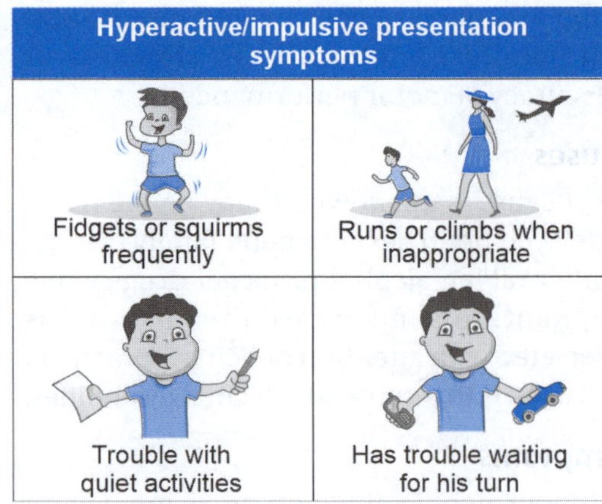

Figure 5.27: Symptoms of ADHD

1. **Inattention:** It refers to a person having difficulty in sustaining attention on task, sustaining focus and staying organized.
2. **Hyperactivity:** It refers to excessive motor activity and difficulties with remaining still. The person may seem to move about constantly including in situations when it is not appropriate or excessively fidgets, taps or talks.
3. **Impulsivity:** It means a person may act without thinking or have difficulty with self-control or act in response to immediate stimuli without consideration of the risks and consequences.

Inattention Symptoms

The symptoms can appear as early as between the ages of 3 and 6 and can continue through adolescence and adulthood. ADHD is more common in males than females, with females more likely to primarily have symptoms of inattention.

- General coordination deficit
- Have difficulty sustaining attention during play or tasks
- Not seem to listen when spoken to directly
- Easily distracted by unrelated thoughts or stimuli
- Have difficulty organizing task and activities, doing tasks in sequence, keeping materials and belongings in order, managing time and meeting deadlines
- Avoid tasks that require sustained mental effort such as homework
- Lose things necessary for tasks
- Be forgetful in daily activities
- Failure to finish tasks
- Memory and thinking deficits
- Specific learning disabilities
- Often lose things necessary for tasks or activities at school

Hyperactivity-impulsivity symptoms

- Sensitive to stimuli, easily upset by noise, light, temperature and other environmental changes.
- At times the reverse occurs and the children are flaccid and limp, sleep more and the growth and development are slow in the first month of life.
- More commonly active in crib, sleep little.
- Often fidgets with hands or feet or squirms in seat.
- Answers only the first two questions; often blurts out answers to questions before they have been completed.
- Unable to wait to be called on in school and may respond before everyone else.
- Has difficulty awaiting turn in games or group situations.
- Be constantly in motion or on the go or act as if driven by a motor.
- Talks excessively
- Explosive or irritable
- Emotionally labile and easily set off to laughter or tears.
- Mood is unpredictable
- Often engages in physically dangerous activities without considering possible consequences (e.g., runs into the street without looking both ways).
- In younger children with ADHD, hyper-activity-impulsivity is the most prominent of the symptoms. As the child reaches schooling the symptoms of inattention may become more prominent and cause the child to struggle academically.
- In adolescents' the symptoms more likely include feelings of restlessness or fidgeting but inattention and impulsivity may remain
- Inattention, restlessness and impulsivity tend to persist into adulthood.
- Children with ADHD may suffer with learning disabilities, anxiety disorders, conduct disorders, depression and substance abuse disorders.

Types

1. **ADHD:** Predominantly hyperactive-impulsive type
2. **ADHD:** Predominantly inattentive type
3. **ADHD:** Combined type

Diagnosis

- Most children with ADHD receive a diagnosis during elementary school years.
- Complete medical evaluation with emphasis on neurologic examination, hearing and vision.

❖ A psychiatric evaluation to assess intellectual ability, academic achievement and potential learning disorder problem.
❖ Detailed prenatal history and early developmental history.
❖ Direct observation, teacher's school report (often the most reliable), parent's report.

Treatment

Treatment includes a combination of psychological therapies and medications. In preschool-age and younger children the recommended first-line approach includes behavioral strategies in the form of parent management training and school intervention.

Medications

❖ **CNS/psychostimulants**: Dextroamphetamine, methylphenidate, pemoline are first line pharmacological treatments.
❖ **Alpha agonists**: Clonidine and serotonin specific reuptake inhibitors, atomoxetine are the other recommended drugs.

Psychological Therapies

❖ Behavior modification techniques
❖ Cognitive behavior therapy
❖ Social skills training
❖ Family education

Nursing Interventions

❖ Develop a trusting relationship with the child. Convey acceptance of the child separating from the unacceptable behavior.
❖ Ensure that patient has a safe environment. Remove objects from immediate area with which patient could injure self due to random hyperactive movements. Identify deliberate behaviors that could put the child at risk for injury. Institute consequences for repetition of such behavior. Provide supervision for potentially dangerous situations.
❖ Since there is non-compliance with task expectations provide an environment that is as free of distractions as possible.
❖ Ensure child's attention by calling his name and establishing eye contact before giving out instructions.

❖ Ask the patient to repeat instructions before starting a task.
❖ Establish goals that allow the patient to complete a part of the task with rewards at each step completion in the form of a break in physical activity.
❖ Provide assistance on a one-to-one basis beginning with simple concrete instructions.
❖ Gradually decrease the amount of assistance given to task performance while assuring the patient that assistance is still available if deemed necessary.
❖ Offer recognition for successful attempts and positive reinforcement for attempts made. Give immediate positive feedback for acceptable behavior.
❖ Provide quiet environment, self-contained classrooms and small group activities. Avoid over stimulating places such as cinema halls, bus stops and other crowded places.
❖ Help him learn how to take his turn, wait in line and follow rules.
❖ Assess parenting skill level considering intellectual, emotional and physical strengths and limitations. Be sensitive to their needs as there is often exhaustion of parental resources due to prolonged coping with a disruptive child.
❖ Provide information and materials related to the child's disorder and effective parenting techniques. Give instructional materials in written and verbal form with step-by-step explanations.
❖ Explain and demonstrate positive parenting techniques to parents or caregivers such as time-in for good behavior or being vigilant in identifying the child's behavior and responding positively to that behavior.
❖ Educate child and family on the use of psychostimulants and anticipated behavioral response.
❖ Coordinate overall treatment plan with schools, collateral personnel, the child and the family.

Conduct Disorders

Conduct disorders are characterized by a persistent and significant pattern of conduct in which the basic rights of others are violated or rules of society not followed. The onset occurs much before 18 years of age, usually even before puberty. The disorder is much more (about 5–10 times) common in boys **(Box 5.42)**.

Etiology

The etiology of conduct disorder is complex and results from an interaction between multiple biological and psychosocial factors.

> **BOX 5.42:** Characteristics of conduct disorder
>
> - Aggressive behavior is the hallmark
>   - Fights, bullies, intimidates, and assaults others physically or sexually
>   - Has poor relationships with peers and adults
>   - Violates other's rights and societal rules
> - A child with conduct disorder rarely performs at the level predicted by IQ or age, causing academic, social and developmental problems
>   - May perform poorly at school or work
>   - May be expelled from school and have problems with law
> - A child with conduct disorder is also at risk for sexually transmitted diseases, rape, teenage pregnancy, injuries, substance abuse, depression, suicidal thoughts, suicide attempts and suicide

Risk factors of conduct disorder are presented in **Figure 5.28**.

- ❖ **Genetic factors:** Studies with monozygotic and dizygotic twins as well as with non-twin siblings have revealed a significantly higher number of conduct disorders among those whose family members are affected with the disorder (Baum, 1989). Alcoholism and personality disorder in the father is reported to be strongly associated with conduct disorders.
- ❖ **Biochemical factors:** Various studies have reported a possible correlation between elevated plasma levels of testosterone and aggressive behaviors.
- ❖ **Organic factors:** Children with brain damage and epilepsy are more prone for developing conduct disorders.

Psychosocial Factors

- ❖ A home environment that lacks structure and adequate supervision with frequent marital conflicts between parents
- ❖ Parental rejection
- ❖ Inconsistent management with harsh discipline
- ❖ Frequent shifting of parental figures
- ❖ Large family size

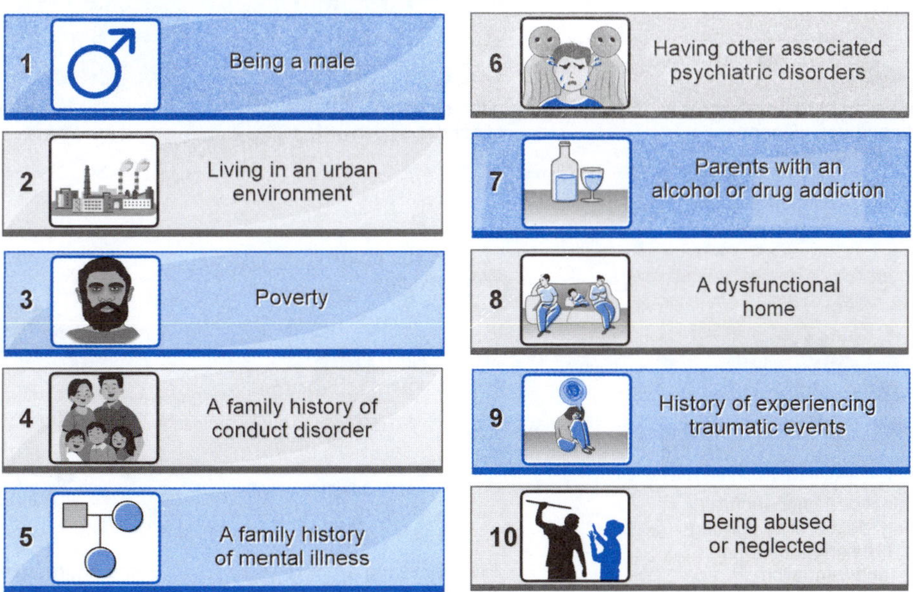

Figure 5.28: Risk factors for conduct disorder

❖ Absent father
❖ Parents with antisocial personality disorder or alcohol dependence
❖ Parental permissiveness
❖ Marital conflict and divorce in parents
❖ Associations with delinquent subgroups
❖ Inadequate/inappropriate communication patterns in the family
❖ Living in low socioeconomic conditions with overcrowding and unemployment

Clinical Features

❖ Fighting with family members and peers
❖ Frequent lying
❖ Stealing or robbery
❖ Running away from home and school
❖ Deliberate fire-setting
❖ Breaking someone else's house articles car, etc.
❖ Deliberately destroying other's property
❖ Cruelty towards other people and animals

❖ Physical violence like rape, assaultive behavior, use of weapons, etc.
❖ In addition to the typical symptoms of conduct disorder, secondary complications often develop like, drug abuse and dependence, unwanted pregnancies, syphilis, AIDS, criminal record, suicidal and homicidal behavior **(Figure 5.29).**

Diagnosis

❖ Complete psychiatric assessment to rule out psychiatric comorbidities like ADHD and mood disorders.
❖ Academic assessment with uncovering difficulties in learning and intellectual functioning.
❖ Neurological assessment to rule out head trauma and seizures.
❖ Assessment should be made in multiple settings with proper information from school authorities and feedback from parents and other caregivers.

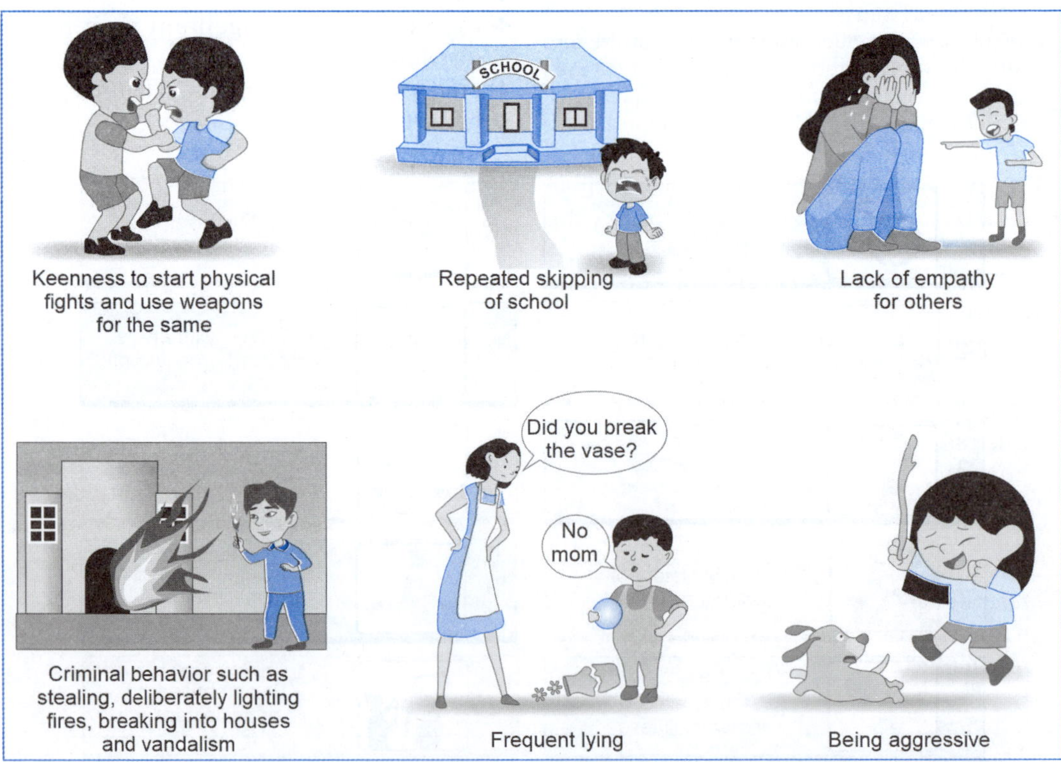

Figure 5.29: Clinical features of conduct disorder

❖ Laboratory investigations including drug screening to rule out comorbid medical illness or substance abuse disorders.

Treatment

The most common mode of management is placement in a corrective institution. Behavioral, educational and psychotherapeutic measures are employed for changing the behavior.

❖ Parent management training
❖ Anger management training
❖ Individual psychotherapy to resolve interpersonal conflicts and to teach assertive skills.
❖ Drug treatment may be indicated in the presence of epilepsy (anticonvulsants), hyperactivity (stimulant medication), impulse control disorder and episodic aggressive behavior (lithium, carbamazepine) and psychotic symptoms (antipsychotics).
❖ Therapeutic schools and Juvenile justice system if needed to provide structured rules and a means for monitoring and controlling the child's behavior.

Nursing Interventions

❖ The nurse should bear in mind that there is always the risk of violence in these children. She should therefore observe the child's behavior frequently during routine activities and interactions. She should be aware of behavior that indicates a rise in agitation.
❖ Redirect violent behavior with physical outlets for suppression of anger and frustration.
❖ Ensure that sufficient number of staff is available to indicate a show of strength if necessary. Administer tranquilizing medication as prescribed. Use of mechanical restraints or isolation should be used only if the situation cannot be controlled by less restrictive means.
❖ Explain to the patient the correlation between feelings of inadequacy and the need for acceptance from others and how these feelings provoke aggression or

defensive behavior such as blaming others for own faulty behavior. Practice more appropriate responses through role play.
❖ Set limits on manipulative behavior and identify its consequences. Administer the consequences in a matter-of-factly and non-threatening manner if such behavior occurs.
❖ Provide immediate positive feedback for acceptable behavior.
❖ Encourage the child to maintain a logbook and make daily entries of his behavior. The entry should consist of a brief statement of an incident when the patient was angry or disagreed with another person, what the patient thought about the incident afterwards (in his own words), what the patient thought about doing and what he actually did and the outcome. This provides an opportunity for the child to identify his predominant patterns of thinking and behaving in different situations and recognize new and acceptable ways of responding in situations which provoke such behaviors.
❖ Review the log with the patient before discharge. Provide feedback regarding improved behavioral responses and areas where continued work is needed. Encourage patient to continue the log after discharge.
❖ Provide social skills training by demonstrating the skills through modeling.
❖ Provide guidance and support to the parents.
❖ In parent training programs the nurse should emphasize that parents should reconnect with their children as positive, nurturing caregivers. However, management of difficult behavior is the key component of the program.
❖ Encourage parents to verbalize feelings of guilt and helplessness in dealing with the child. Involve siblings in family discussions and planning for more effective family interactions.
❖ Aggressive children often display problems across settings including the school. The nurse should therefore emphasize on close

collaboration between parents and school personnel likely to come into contact with the child (principal, assistant principal, guidance counselors, school psychologists, etc.). Children who see their parents and teachers working together find it easier to control their behavior both at home and school.

❖ **Truancy requires separate consideration**: Pressure should be brought upon the child to return to school and in case of need support of the family enlisted. At the same time an attempt should be made to resolve educational or other problems at school. During the whole process, it is essential to maintain good communication between the nurse, parents and teachers.

Elimination Disorders

Elimination disorders include the repeated voiding of urine into clothes or bed (enuresis) and the repeated passage of feces in inappropriate places (encopresis).

Non-organic Enuresis

It is a disorder characterized by involuntary voiding of urine by day and/or night which is abnormal in relation to the individual's mental age and which is not a consequence of a lack of bladder control due to any neurological disorder, epileptic attacks or any structural abnormality of urinary tract. Enuresis would not ordinarily be diagnosed in a child under the age of 5 years or with a mental age less than 4 years.

In most cases, enuresis is primary (the child has never attained bladder control). Sometimes it may be secondary (enuresis continuing after the child achieved continence for a certain period of time).

Factors Associated with Enuresis

❖ **Faulty training**: If toilet training is started too early and is especially coercive, it produces confusion and resentment rather than compliance. Also, if it is begun too late, loss of bladder control can result.

❖ **Emotional disturbances**: Emotional problems or conflicts can manifest in the form of disturbed bladder control. These conflicts may be due to such factors like dominating parents, harsh punishments and other problems in the family causing the child to feel neglected and isolated. As the children grow older they become sensitive about their habit of bed-wetting. They develop feelings of inferiority and a sense of being different from other children which aggravates the problem even further.

❖ Physical diseases and anatomic defects (e.g., congenital anomalies of the genitourinary tract, diseases involving the central nervous system) are relatively rare causes for enuresis.

Management

❖ Exclude any physical basis for enuresis by history, examination and if necessary, investigation of the renal tract.

❖ Explain to the child and parents about the maturational basis of the problem and the likelihood of spontaneous improvement.

❖ The child should be encouraged to keep a diary of the pattern of night time dryness/ wetness which can be done with a star chart. This consists of a record of dry nights with a star placed on the sheet for each dry night. The star chart system has three functions:
  ○ It provides an accurate record of the problem.
  ○ It tests motivation and cooperation of the child and the family.
  ○ It acts as a positive reinforcement for the desired behavior.

❖ Fluid restriction after 6 O'clock in the evening.

❖ Interrupting the child's sleep and emptying bladder in the toilet.

❖ **Bell and pad technique**: It is based on classical conditioning principle. A bell is attached to the napkin or panties and when the child passes urine the alarm goes off. The child has to then wake up, change his napkin, bed sheets, etc. Reinforcement is given for dry nights.

❖ **Medications**: Tricyclic antidepressants like imipramine or amitriptyline, 25–50 mg at night. Though mechanism of action is unknown the results have demonstrated their effectiveness.

❖ The parents should be instructed not to blame the child in any way. On no account should the child be embarrassed or humiliated which will only serve to aggravate the problem.

Non-organic Encopresis

It is the repeated voluntary or involuntary passage of feces, usually of normal or near normal consistency, in places not appropriate for that purpose in the individual's socio-cultural setting.

Management

❖ Family tensions regarding the symptoms must be reduced, while a non-punitive atmosphere is simultaneously created. Parental guidance and family therapy is often needed.

❖ Behavioral techniques, e.g., star charts, in which the child places a star on a chart for dry or continent nights.

❖ Individual psychotherapy to gain the co-operation and trust of the child.

Feeding or Eating Disorders

Feeding disorders involve behavioral disturbances that are not related to body weight and shape concerns such as eating of non-edible substances or voluntary regurgitation of foods.

Eating disorders involve abnormal eating behavior and preoccupation with food as well as prominent body weight and shape concerns. Feeding and eating disorders are anorexia nervosa and bulimia nervosa.

Anorexia Nervosa

Anorexia nervosa is characterized by behavioral and psychopathological symptoms and significant somatic signs. Majority are females and the onset is during adolescence.

Meaning

Anorexia nervosa is an eating disorder defined by restriction of energy intake relative to requirements leading to a significant low body weight. Patients have an intense fear of gaining weight and distorted body image with the inability to recognize the seriousness of their significant low body weight.

Anorexia nervosa is a psychiatric disease in which patients restrict their food intake relative to their energy requirements through eating less, exercising more, and/or purging food through laxatives and vomiting. Despite being severely underweight they do not recognize it and continue to have distorted body images.

Etiology

The exact cause of anorexia nervosa is not known.

a. **Biological factors**: Genetics and hormones might have an effect on the development of anorexia nervosa.

b. **Psychological factors:** A disturbance of body image, a struggle for control and a sense of identity are important factors in the causation of anorexia nervosa. Traits of low self-esteem and perfectionism are often found among individuals with anorexia nervosa.

c. **Environmental factors:** Unrealistic body images from media outlets like magazines and television can greatly influence young people and spark the desire to be thin. Influence of beauty contests, weight related concerns from family or peer environment also play an important role in causation of illness. Certain occupations demand a thin physique which may increase the risk of anorexia nervosa such as in sports, ballet or television and fashion industries.

Clinical Features

The most obvious sign of anorexia nervosa is being underweight. The core psycho-pathological feature is the dread of fatness, weight phobia and a drive for thinness. The clinical features can be classified into physical, psychological and behavioral signs (**Box 5.43** and **Figure 5.30**).

Physical Signs

❖ The body weight is 15% below the standard weight

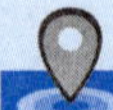

BOX 5.43: Case vignette—Anorexia nervosa

Mrs B, a 25-year-old female, married for 2 years, educated up to graduation, currently working in a private company as a receptionist, hailing from an upper social class, living with husband's family is referred by a gynecologist to tertiary mental healthcare facility with complaints of weight loss, recurrent episodes of vomiting since 1 year, amenorrhea since 6 months, inactive and decreased interest in sex.

Husband reports that after he casually remarked about her being slightly overweight she has reduced her food intake, began completely avoiding foods with high caloric value, gradual skipping of breakfast and lunch, and having minimal dinner. She also began to avoid eating in the presence of other family members. At times she would hide and eat or induce vomiting secretly.

Patient reported that she perceived herself as fat. She also experienced low self-esteem as she believed that she was not pretty and was not happy with her image. She eventually developed a morbid fear of looking fat and ugly, began eating less. She would use soap water enema and would occasionally use laxatives. Her weight dropped from 59 kg to 30 kg. Premorbid personality revealed an over concern about physical appearance inspired by skinny models.

On examination patient was found to be 30 kg in weight, height 5.4 ft and BMI 15.6. She looked emaciated, had dry and flaky skin, vitals were stable. Blood investigations which included full blood count, renal profile, liver function test, thyroid profile and serum calcium phosphate were within normal limits. Hemoglobin was 8 gm/dL. Tuberculosis, malabsorption syndrome and clinical depression were ruled out. Mrs B was diagnosed with anorexia nervosa.

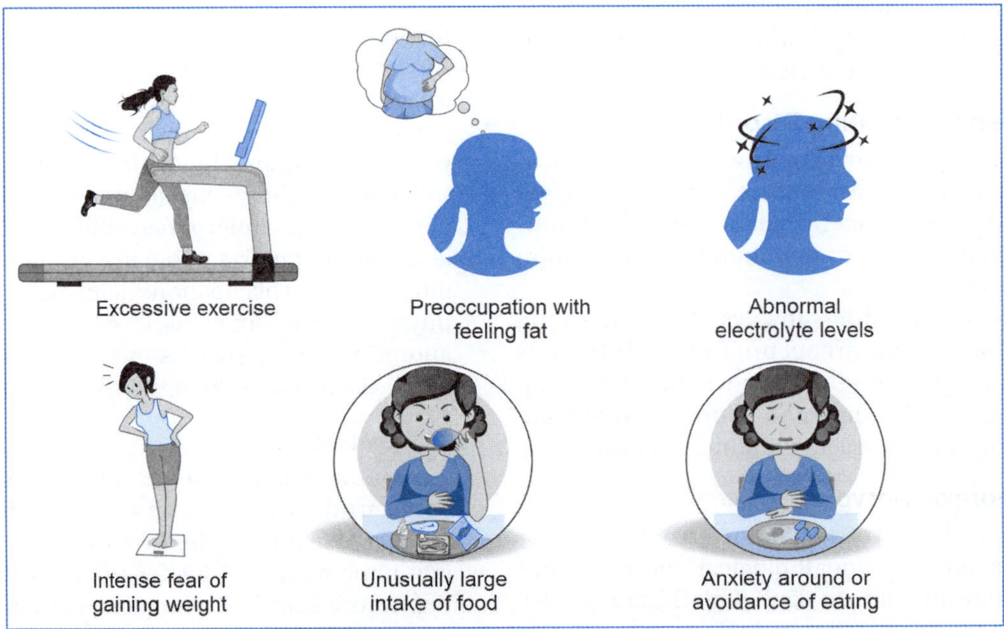

Figure 5.30: Clinical features of anorexia nervosa

- Amenorrhea
- Fainting or dizziness
- Poor sleep
- Looks pale, dry skin, sunken eyes, fine hair on the face and body
- Other signs and symptoms are secondary to starvation and include sensitivity to cold, delayed gastric emptying, constipation, low blood pressure, bradycardia, hypothermia and amenorrhea in females.
- Vomiting and abuse of laxatives may lead to a variety of electrolyte disturbances with the most serious being hypokalemia.
- Hormonal abnormalities also may be seen.

Psychological Signs

- Preoccupation with body size, distorted body image, description of herself as fat.
- There is an intense fear of becoming obese which does not reduce even if the person loses weight grossly and becomes very thin.
- There is a body image disturbance with the patient being unable to perceive the body size accurately.
- Being extremely dissatisfied with their body
- Depression and anxiety.
- Being anxious, perfectionism and having rigid thoughts about food.

Behavioral Signs

- The pursuit of thinness may take several forms. Patients generally eat little and set themselves daily calorie limits (often between 600 and 1000 calories). Some try to achieve weight loss by inducing vomiting, excessive exercise, misusing laxatives, appetite suppressants, enemas and diuretics.
- Counting calories and avoiding food.
- Self-harm, substance abuse or suicide attempts.

Complications

- Resulting from the malnutrition, dehydration and electrolyte imbalances caused by prolonged starvation, vomiting and laxative abuse.
- Increased susceptibility to infection
- Hypoalbuminemia

- Chronic inflammatory bowel disease (due to laxative abuse).
- Esophageal erosion, ulcers, tears, bleeding, gum erosion, dental caries (due to frequent vomiting).
- Amenorrhea
- Life-threatening cardiovascular complications.

Course and Prognosis

Anorexia nervosa often runs a fluctuating course with periods of exacerbations and partial remissions. Outcome is very variable.

Diagnosis

- Complete physical examination including laboratory tests to rule out endocrine, metabolic and central nervous system abnormalities; cancer; malabsorption syndrome and other disorders that cause physical wasting.
- Complete blood testing—hemoglobin levels, platelet count, cholesterol level, total protein, sodium, potassium, chloride, calcium and fasting blood glucose and serum amylase levels and blood urea nitrogen.
- ECG readings irregular
- Differential diagnosis to rule out other psychiatric disorders like substance abuse, anxiety disorder, body dysmorphic disorder, mood disorders, schizophrenia.

Treatment

Treatment is centered on nutritional rehabilitation and psychotherapy.

- In-patient treatment is required for existing psychiatric disorders, high risk for suicide, medically unstable, uncooperative, purging behavior.
- **Medications:** Antipsychotics (Olanzapine), appetite stimulants, antidepressants.
- Psychological therapies: Individual psychotherapy, behavioral therapy, cognitive behavior therapy and family therapy.

Nursing Interventions

- Maintain a strict intake and output chart
- Monitor status of skin and oral mucous membranes

❖ Encourage the patient to verbalize feelings of fear and anxiety related to achievement, family relationships and intense need for independence.

❖ Encourage the family to participate in education regarding connection between family process and patient's disorder.

❖ Avoid discussions that focus on food and weight.

❖ Short-term management is focused on ensuring weight gain and correcting nutritional deficiencies. Maintaining normal weight and preventing relapses are long-term goals to be achieved.

❖ Hospitalization is usually required. Successful treatment depends on good nursing care with clear aims and understanding on the part of the patient as well as the nurse.

❖ Eating must be supervised by the nurse and a balanced diet of at least 3,000 calories should be provided in 24 hours.

❖ In the early stages of treatment, it is best for the patient to remain in bed in a single room while the nurse maintains close observation. The goal should be to achieve a weight gain of 0.5–1 kg per week.

❖ Weight should be checked regularly. Monitor serum electrolyte levels and signs and symptoms like amenorrhea, constipation, hypoglycemia, hypotension, etc.

❖ Control vomiting by making the bathroom inaccessible for at least 2 hours after food.

❖ In extreme cases where the patient refuses to eat and comply with the treatment, gavage feedings may need to be instituted.

Bulimia Nervosa

Bulimia nervosa is characterized by episodes of binge-eating followed by feelings of guilt, humiliation, depression, and self-condemnation.

❖ A binge eating episode includes consuming abnormally large portions of food within a specific time period during which the individual experiences subjective loss of control over eating, i.e, eating more and being unable to stop.

❖ This binge eating is accompanied by use of compensatory measures to prevent weight gain (such as self-induced vomiting, diuretic or laxative use, dieting, fasting, strenuous exercises or a combination of these measures).

❖ There is a marked distress about the pattern of binge eating and inappropriate compensatory behavior.

❖ Significant impairment in personal, family, social, educational, occupational or other important areas of functioning.

Etiology

❖ More common in first-degree, biological relatives of people with bulimia.

❖ Possible role of altered serotonin levels in brain.

❖ Society's emphasis on appearance and thinness.

❖ Family disturbances or conflict

❖ Sexual abuse

❖ Learned maladaptive behavior

❖ Struggle for control or self-identity

Clinical Features

❖ Persistent sore throat, heartburn

❖ Callused or scarring on back of hands and knuckles.

❖ Tooth staining or discoloration, loss of dental enamel, and increased dental caries.

❖ History of eating amount of food larger than what most people would eat.

❖ Sense of lack of control during episodes of binge-eating.

❖ Thin, normal or slightly overweight appearance with history of frequent weight fluctuations.

❖ Abdominal and epigastric pain

❖ Amenorrhea

❖ Fluid and electrolyte imbalances

❖ Perfectionism

❖ Distorted body image

❖ Exaggerated sense of guilt

❖ Feelings of alienation

❖ Poor impulse control

❖ Low tolerance for frustration

❖ Peculiar eating habits or rituals

❖ Excessive exercise regimen

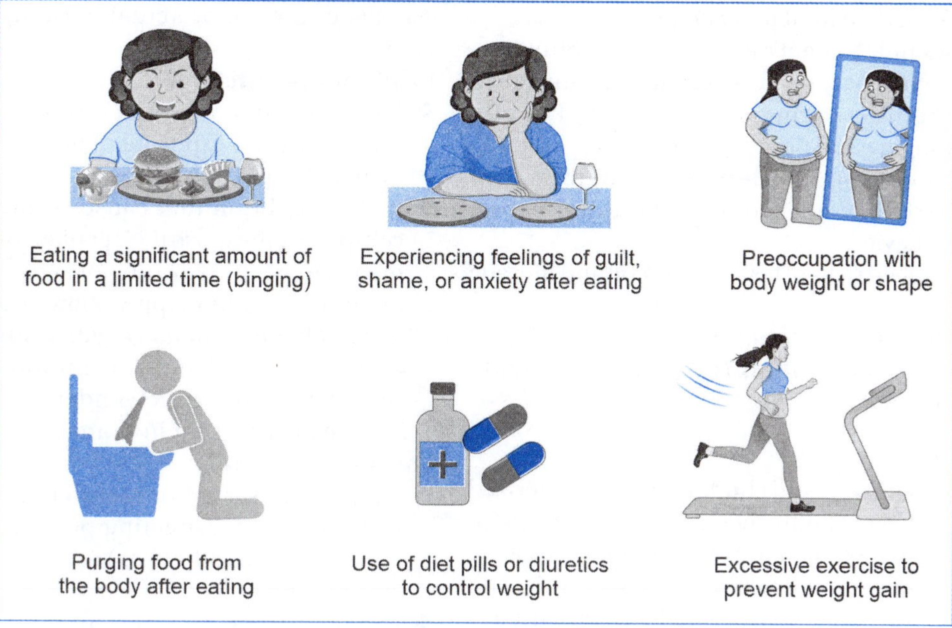

Figure 5.31: Clinical features of bulimia nervosa

❖ Withdrawal from friends and usual activities
❖ Frequent weighing (**Figure 5.31** and **Box 5.44**)

Complications

❖ Gastric rupture during periods of binge-eating
❖ Dental caries, erosion of tooth enamel, parotitis, and gum infections
❖ Dehydration or electrolyte imbalances

❖ Chronic, irregular bowel movements and constipation from laxative use
❖ Increased risk of suicide and psychoactive substance abuse

Diagnosis

❖ Medical evaluation to rule out upper gastrointestinal disorder
❖ Psychological evaluation and Beck Depression Inventory
❖ History
❖ Laboratory tests (serum electrolytes, blood glucose, baseline ECG)
❖ Confirmed, if ICD-10 criteria met

Treatment Modalities

❖ Psychotherapy
❖ TCAs or SSRIs
❖ Self-help groups
❖ Hospitalization

Nursing Interventions

❖ Engage patient in therapeutic alliance to obtain commitment to treatment.
❖ Establish contract with patient that specifies amount and type of food she must eat at each meal.

> **BOX 5.44:** Case vignette—Bulimia nervosa
>
> Ms A, a 20-year-old under graduate student visited psychiatric clinic with complaints of increased pulse rate, dizziness, difficulty in swallowing. On further questioning, Ms A said that she was more concerned about her weight, fear of becoming fat and had tried various measures to control her appetite. She has more craving for sweets and other high calorie foods. When such feelings occur she loses control and eats greedily at times. After such episodes of binge eating, Ms A induces vomiting to avoid weight gain. This induced vomiting relieves her guilt feelings due to overeating. Psychiatrist diagnosed it as a bulimia nervosa.

- ❖ Set a time limit for each meal
- ❖ Identify patient's elimination patterns
- ❖ Teach patient to maintain a journal to monitor high-risk situations that cue binging and purging behaviors
- ❖ Encourage patient to recognize and verbalize her feelings about her eating behavior
- ❖ Explain risks of laxative, emetic and diuretic abuse
- ❖ Provide assertiveness training
- ❖ Assess and monitor patient's suicide potential

Pica

Pica of infancy and childhood is characterized by eating non-nutritive substances (soil, paint chipping, paper, etc.). Treatment consists of common-sense precautions to keep the child away from abnormal items of diet. Pica usually diminishes as the child grows older.

SEXUAL DISORDERS

ICD-11 has redefined gender identity disorders by replacing transsexualism and gender identity disorder of children with 'gender incongruence of adolescence and adulthood' and 'gender incongruence of childhood' respectively. Gender incongruence has been moved out of the 'mental and behavioral disorders' chapter and into the new 'conditions related to sexual health' chapter.

In paraphilias, sexual arousal occurs persistently and significantly in response to objects which are not a part of normal sexual arousal.

The term paraphilia refers to a condition in which a persons' sexual arousal and gratification are based on fantasies about or engaging in sexual behavior that is considered atypical and extreme.

Paraphilias involve sexual excitement for atypical objects, situations and subjects, for example objects, children, dead bodies, animals, etc.

A paraphilic disorder is diagnosed when a paraphilia is causing significant distress or impairment to the individual in one or more aspects of his life or actual harm to self or others.

Exhibitionistic disorder

- ❖ It is a condition where a person is sexually aroused by the exposure of one's genitalia to an unsuspecting stranger.
- ❖ It is a condition that causes someone to compulsively expose their genitals or sexual organs to people who do not agree and are unknown and in inappropriate situations. This behavior elicits sexual stimulation and pleasure. Usually, exhibitionism is prevalent in the male gender but in rare cases can also occur in women.

Voyeuristic disorder

- ❖ This is a persistent or recurrent tendency to observe unsuspecting persons naked (usually of the other sex) and engaged in sexual activity.
- ❖ In voyeurism, the person gets sexual excitement and gratification from observing and watching the necked bodies of people often not aware of being observed and engaged in sexual activity.

Pedophilic disorder

- ❖ It is characterized by persistent or recurrent involvement of an adult in sexual activity with prepubertal children.
- ❖ It refers to recurrent sexual arousing fantasies, impulses or behaviors involving one or more prepubertal children.

Coercive sexual sadism disorder

- ❖ The person is sexually aroused by physical and psychological humiliation, suffering or injury of the sexual partner.
- ❖ In this disorder sexual excitement manifests itself in a recurring and intense way through desires, fantasies or behaviors in which the physical or psychological suffering of another person is deliberately and intentionally caused.

Frotteuristic disorder

- ❖ This is a persistent or recurrent involvement in the act of touching and rubbing against an unsuspecting, non-consenting person.
- ❖ It is characterized by intense and recurrent sexual excitement manifested through fantasies, desires and real behaviors related

to touching or rubbing against a non-consenting person.

Treatment

- ❖ Behavior therapy
- ❖ Supportive psychotherapy
- ❖ Drug therapy: Antipsychotics have been used for severe aggression associated with paraphilias

Nursing Interventions

- ❖ Assess patient's sexual history and previous level of satisfaction in sexual relationships; also assess patient's perception of the problem.
- ❖ Note cultural, social, ethnic, racial and religious factors that may contribute to conflicts regarding variant sexual practices.
- ❖ Assess for any medications which might be affecting libido.
- ❖ Provide information regarding sexuality and sexual functioning, correct any misconceptions if necessary. Teach patient that sexuality is a normal human response and that it involves complex inter-relationships among one's self-concept, body image, family and cultural influences.
- ❖ Both the patient and his/her partner may need additional assistance if problems in sexual relationship are severe or remain unresolved.
- ❖ Refer for additional counseling or sex therapy if required.
- ❖ Assist therapist as necessary in plan of behavior modification to help decrease variant behavior.
- ❖ In all cases, an accepting and non-judgmental attitude on the part of the nurse is highly essential for successful resolution of these problems as these are highly sensitive issues and may be causing significant distress to the patient.

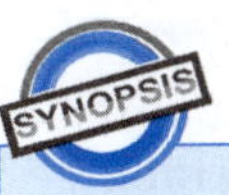

- ❖ The World Health Organization reports that psychiatric disorders are the leading cause of disability globally.
- ❖ Many factors are responsible for the causation of mental illness. These factors may predispose an individual to mental illness, precipitate or perpetuate the mental illness.
- ❖ Predisposing factors are risk factors that determine an individual's susceptibility to mental illness.
- ❖ Precipitating factors are events that occur shortly before the onset of a disorder and appear to have induced it.
- ❖ Perpetuating factors are factors in the patient, family, community or larger systems that are responsible for aggravating or prolonging the disease already existing in an individual rather than subsiding it.
- ❖ Mental illnesses are caused by a combination of biological, physiological, environmental, psychological and social factors.
- ❖ Psychopathology is the scientific study of mental disorders including efforts to understand their genetic, biological, psychological and social causes; effective classification schemes; course across all stages of development; manifestations and treatment.
- ❖ The common signs and symptoms of mental illnesses are alterations of personality and behavior, alteration of biological function, disorders of consciousness, disorders of attention and concentration, disorders of orientation, volitional disturbances, disorders of motor activity, disorders of perception, disorders of mood.

- ❖ At present there are two major classifications in psychiatry namely ICD-11 (2022) and DSM-5TR (2022). In both forms of classification mental disorders are grouped by their symptoms in categories that compose the classification.
- ❖ Personality disorders result when personality traits become abnormal, i.e., become inflexible and maladaptive and cause significant social or occupational impairment or significant subjective distress.
- ❖ Personality disorders may occur due to a combination of genetic, biological, social, psychological, developmental and environmental factors.
- ❖ Four core features of personality disorders are distorted thinking, problematic emotional responses, over or under regulated impulse control and interpersonal difficulties.
- ❖ Organic mental disorders are behavioral or psychological disorders associated with transient or permanent brain dysfunction.
- ❖ Delirium is an acute organic mental disorder characterized by disturbance of attention, orientation and awareness that develops within a short period of time.
- ❖ Some of the common causes of delirium are drug interactions, dehydration, hospitalization and surgery, illness or infections.
- ❖ The clinical features are impairment of consciousness, impairment of attention, perceptual disturbances, disturbance of cognition, psychomotor disturbance, disturbance of the sleep wake cycle, emotional disturbance and other symptoms.
- ❖ Dementia is an acquired global impairment of intellect, memory and personality but without impairment of consciousness. It is a general term used to describe brain disorders that primarily affect person's memory and behavior.
- ❖ Common signs and symptoms of dementia are personality changes, memory impairment, thought impairment, cognitive impairment, affective impairment, perceptual impairment, behavioral impairment.
- ❖ Schizophrenia is a chronic, severe mental disorder that affects the way a person thinks, acts, expresses emotions, perceives reality and relates to others.
- ❖ The exact cause of schizophrenia is unknown. Several studies suggest that multiple factors are responsible for causation of schizophrenia. It is characterized by positive symptoms, negative symptoms and cognitive symptoms.
- ❖ Mood disorders or affect disorders are described by marked disruptions in emotions, severe lows called depression or highs called mania.
- ❖ Acute mania is referring to a syndrome in which the central features are mood change (which may be towards elation or irritability), over-activity and self-important ideas.
- ❖ The cause for manic episode is a combination of neurochemical, genetic, psychological and environmental factors.
- ❖ Depressive episode is characterized by low or depressed mood, loss of interest in most activities, tiredness, changes in appetite, feelings of worthlessness and recurrent thoughts of death.
- ❖ There are several factors that contribute to cause of depressive disorder. These are neurochemical imbalances, hormonal abnormalities, psychosocial factors and other factors.
- ❖ Neurotic disorder (neurosis) is a less severe form of psychiatric disorder where patients show either excessive or prolonged emotional reaction to any given stress. The neuroses term is no longer used in the current scientific literature.

❖ Normal anxiety becomes pathological when it causes significant subject distress and impairment in the normal functioning of the individual.

❖ Generalized anxiety disorders are those in which anxiety is unrealistic, excessive and persistent, present all the time and not restricted to certain situations or exposure to certain objects.

❖ The central feature is the occurrence of panic attacks, i.e., sudden attacks of anxiety in which physical symptoms predominate and are accompanied by fear of a serious consequence such as a heart attack.

❖ In phobic anxiety disorders, the individual experiences intermittent anxiety which arises in particular circumstances, i.e., in response to the phobic object or situation.

❖ Obsessive-compulsive disorder (OCD) is a chronic mental health condition that involves obsessions (uncontrollable and recurring thoughts), compulsions (repetitive behaviors) or both.

❖ The cause for OCD is multifactorial. It involves genetic factors, biochemicals, regression to the pre-oedipal phase and stimulus to anxiety.

❖ Patients are present with multiple obsessions and compulsions. These include obsession thoughts, images, ruminations, doubts and impulses.

❖ PTSD is characterized by re-experiencing the traumatic event, avoidance of thoughts and memories of the event/events and hyper vigilance state.

❖ Dissociative disorders involve experiencing a loss of connection between thoughts, memories, feelings, behavior and identity.

❖ Somatoform disorder or somatic symptoms disorder or somatization is a form of mental illness characterized by repeated presentation with physical symptoms which do not have any physical basis, and a persistent request for investigations and treatment despite repeated assurance by the treating doctors.

❖ Substance use disorder (SUD) is a complex condition in which there is uncontrolled use of substance despite harmful consequences.

❖ Commonly abused substances are alcohol, opioids, cannabinoids, cocaine, amphetamines, hallucinogens, sedatives and hypnotics, inhalants, nicotine and ketamine.

❖ Substance use disorders are caused by multiple factors. These include genetic vulnerability, biochemical factors, deficiency of endomorphins, withdrawal and reinforcing effects of drugs, stimuli and settings associated with drug use, individual personality characteristics, social factors, easy availability of drugs, psychiatric disorders.

❖ Child psychiatry is concerned with the assessment and treatment of children's emotional and behavioral problems.

❖ Intellectual disability (ID) is characterized by significant impairment in intelligence and adaptive behavior. Various types of disorders of intellectual development are mild, moderate, severe and profound.

❖ Some of the most common symptoms are delay in milestone development, deficiencies in cognitive functioning, reduced ability to learn, psychomotor skill deficits, difficulty to perform self-care activities.

❖ Autism spectrum disorder is characterized by persistent deficits in the ability to initiate and sustain reciprocal social interaction and social communication, and by a range of restricted, repetitive and inflexible patterns of behaviors and interests.

❖ Attention-deficit hyperactivity disorder is marked by an ongoing pattern of inattention and or hyperactivity-impulsivity that interferes with functioning or development.

❖ Conduct disorders are characterized by a persistent and significant pattern of conduct in which the basic rights of others are violated or rules of society not followed.

❖ Elimination disorders include the repeated voiding of urine into clothes or bed (enuresis) and the repeated passage of feces in inappropriate places (encopresis).

❖ Eating disorders involve abnormal eating behavior and preoccupation with food as well as prominent body weight and shape concerns.

❖ Anorexia nervosa is an eating disorder defined by restriction of energy intake relative to requirements leading to a significant low body weight.

❖ Bulimia nervosa is characterized by episodes of binge-eating followed by feelings of guilt, humiliation, depression, and self-condemnation.

❖ The term paraphilia refers to a condition in which a persons' sexual arousal and gratification are based on fantasies about or engaging in sexual behavior that is considered atypical and extreme.

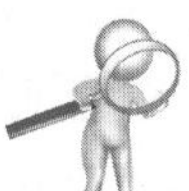

REVIEW QUESTIONS

Long Essays

1. Describe in detail the etiological factors for psychiatric disorders.
2. Explain common signs and symptoms of mental illness.
3. What is dementia? List various causes for Alzheimer's disease. Describe nursing management for dementia patient.
4. What is the meaning of schizophrenia? Explain etiological factors and clinical characteristics for schizophrenia. Write a note on nursing management for positive symptoms of a person with schizophrenia.
5. Define mania. List etiological factors related to manic episode. Describe nursing management for an acute manic state patient.
6. Explain causes of depression. Describe nursing management for a severe depression patient.
7. What is obsessive compulsive disorder? Describe nursing management for obsessive compulsive disorder.
8. Describe role of a nurse in the prevention of intellectual disability.
9. Define autism spectrum disorder. List characteristics of autistic disorder. Explain nursing intervention for ASD.
10. Describe etiological factors and clinical features of ADHD. Explain nursing interventions for ADHD.
11. Define conduct disorder. List core symptoms of conduct disorder. Explain nursing management of a child with conduct disorder.
12. What is the meaning of anorexia nervosa? List etiological factors and clinical manifestations. Enlist nursing interventions.

Short Essays

1. List various personality disorders and explain general nursing interventions for personality disorder patients.
2. Nursing interventions for delusions.
3. Nursing interventions for suicidal behavior of a patient.

4. Describe signs and symptoms of depression.
5. Describe nursing management for generalized anxiety disorders.
6. Describe nursing interventions for somatoform disorder.
7. Enumerate nursing interventions for acute intoxication of alcohol.
8. Explain role of a nurse in prevention of substance abuse.
9. Describe complications of bulimia nervosa.
10. Explain clinical features of anorexia nervosa.

Short Answers

1. List paraphilic disorders
2. List the symptoms of mania
3. List the signs and symptoms of delirium tremens
4. List the signs and symptoms of anxiety
5. List complications of alcohol abuse
6. List some of the commonly abused substances
7. Core symptoms of ADHD

Give the Meaning of the Following

Addiction	Conversion	Euphoria	Phobia
Akinesia	Delirium	Euphoria	Projection
Alogia	Delusion	Flight of ideas	Schizophrenia
Amnesia	Dementia	Hallucinations	Stupor
Anorexia nervosa	Depression	Insight	Sundown
Apathy	Echolalia	Mania	Thought block
Autism	Echo praxia	Mutism	Thought insertion
Bulimia nervosa	Encopresis	Neologism	Thought withdrawal
Compulsions	Enuresis	Obsessions	

Fill in the Blanks

1. Lack of awareness of correct time, place and person is called __________.
2. Frequent washing of hands, checking repeatedly are symptoms of __________.
3. Delirium and dementia are classified as __________ disorders.
4. Repetition or echoing by the patient of the words of the examiner is called as __________.
5. Deliberate self-harm is also known as __________.
6. First rank symptoms of schizophrenia were described by __________.
7. __________ is a major self-help organization for the treatment of alcohol use disorder.
8. Misinterpretation of external stimuli is termed as __________.
9. Repeated thinking of contamination of dirt or germs is known as __________.
10. False filling of memory is called __________.
11. An irrational fear resulting in desire to avoid the fearful object or situation is __________.

State the Following Statements are True or False

1. Compulsion is repetitive unwanted urge to perform an act.
2. Mania is a state of excess cheerfulness and increased activity.
3. Palpitations are not the symptoms of anxiety.
4. Delusions of grandiose is usually seen in depression.
5. Children with autism can be orally communicative and crossing social boundaries.
6. Aversion therapy is given for client with alcohol dependence syndrome.
7. Psychoeducation is one of the important approaches in psychiatric rehabilitation.
8. Flight of ideas is found in mania.
9. Mild mental retardation relates to an IQ between 50 to 70.
10. Blank and flat affect is seen in mania.
11. Altered perception is called delusion.
12. Coining of new word is called neologism.

13. Suicide is considered as a psychiatric emergency.
14. False perception of smell is known as gustatory hallucination.
15. Opioids are examples of narcotic drugs.
16. Delirium tremens occurs during alcohol withdrawal.
17. Flight of ideas is seen in mental retardation.
18. Loss of insight occurs in anxiety neurosis.
19. IQ of a normal person ranges between 15–70.

Multiple Choice Questions

1. **Apathy means:**
   a. Absence of affect
   b. Absence of mind
   c. Absence of speech
   d. Absence of pain

2. **Hallucinations are:**
   a. Perceptual abnormalities
   b. Mood abnormalities
   c. Thought abnormalities
   d. Cognitive abnormalities

3. **Which of the options best represents neologism?**
   a. Coining new words
   b. Making abrupt stops in the flow of conversation
   c. Providing excessive details
   d. Talking excessively while frequently shifting from one idea to another

4. **Which of the following best suits a patient exhibiting flight of ideas?**
   a. Coin new words
   b. Make abrupt stops in the flow of conversation
   c. Provide excessive details
   d. Talk excessively while frequently shifting from one idea to another

5. **A delusion in which the patient believes that others, oneself or the world do not exist:**
   a. Persecutory delusion
   b. Nihilistic delusion
   c. Bizarre delusion
   d. Secondary delusion

6. **False perception of taste is termed as:**
   a. Gustatory hallucination
   b. Tactile hallucination
   c. Somatic hallucination
   d. Olfactory hallucination

7. **Which of the following factors causes abnormal behavior in mentally ill patients?**
   a. Higher education
   b. Unemployment
   c. Black magic
   d. Changes in neurochemicals

8. **In which of the following personality disorders are mistrust and suspiciousness the main clinical features?**
   a. Paranoid personality disorder
   b. Antisocial personality disorder
   c. Anxious personality disorder
   d. Histrionic personality disorder

9. **Which of the following is a characteristic of antisocial personality disorder?**
   a. Argumentative
   b. Loss of cognitive function
   c. Violates social norms
   d. Not capable of carrying on regular activities

10. **Sexual arousal with the help of a non-living object is called:**
    a. Fetishism
    b. Transvestism
    c. Exhibitionism
    d. Fortteurism

11. **A condition in which the person seeks sexual excitement by giving pain to the partner is termed as:**
    a. Masochism
    b. Fetishism
    c. Sadism
    d. Transvestism

12. **Following are all organic brain disorders, *except:***
    a. Amnestic disorder
    b. Dementia
    c. Delirium
    d. Mental retardation

13. **An acquired global impairment of intellect, memory and personality without impairment of consciousness is:**
    a. Delirium
    b. Dementia
    c. Amnestic syndrome
    d. Parkinson's disease

14. **Which of the following is the most common cause of dementia?**
    a. Alzheimer's disease
    b. Addison's disease
    c. Multi-infarct dementia
    d. Lead poisoning

15. **A 75-year-old patient is diagnosed with Alzheimer's dementia and confabulates. The nurse understands that this patient:**
    a. Fills in memory gaps with false description of events
    b. Rationalizes his behavior
    c. Denies confusion using jokes
    d. Pretends to be someone else

16. **Which of the following will the nurse use when communicating with a patient who has cognitive impairment?**
    a. Provide detailed explanation with examples
    b. Use gestures instead of words
    c. Use short words and simple sentences
    d. Use stimulating words and sentences to capture the patient attention

17. **Sundowner syndrome means:**
    a. Restlessness and confusion worsening in the evenings
    b. Unconsciousness filling of memory gaps
    c. Attempts to compensate for defects
    d. Stereotyped behavior and activities

18. **Which of the following is an acute organic psychiatric disorder?**
    a. Dementia
    b. Delirium
    c. Amnestic disorder
    d. Organic mood disorder

19. **Which of the following nursing interventions is most appropriate to reduce accidents among dementia patients?**
    a. Do not allow the patient to walk in the house
    b. Remove sharp items from patient environment
    c. Provide well fitted shoes with straps
    d. Provide help to walk at all times

20. **Which of the following interventions will improve orientation among dementia patients?**
    a. Use calendar with larger writings
    b. Clock with large dial
    c. Provide newspapers with current events
    d. All of the above

21. **A 65-year-old male patient has been admitted to the psychiatric unit with symptoms of fatigue, inability to concentrate, inability to complete everyday tasks and preferring to sleep all the day, one of the most important intervention for this patient is:**
    a. Encourage him to perform regular activities
    b. Explain causes of fatigue
    c. Encourage him to join in ward activities
    d. Develop a structured routine for him to follow

22. **Which of the following is a negative symptom of schizophrenia?**
    a. Delusions
    b. Apathy
    c. Hallucinations
    d. Thought disturbances

23. Which of the following is a positive symptom of schizophrenia?
a. Delusions
b. Apathy
c. Ambivalence
d. Avolition

24. Which information is the most essential in the initial teaching session for the family of a young adult recently diagnosed with schizophrenia?
a. Symptoms of this disease are due to imbalance in the brain
b. Genetic history is an important factor related to the development of schizophrenia
c. Schizophrenia is a serious disease affecting every aspect of a person's functioning
d. Distressing symptoms of this disorder respond to treatment with medications

25. Mr D is a 32-year-old male diagnosed with chronic schizophrenia. You find him sitting in the corner of the ward with hands crossed over the chest, face down, totally unaware of people around him, emotionally unresponsive of any happenings in the ward. He tries to cover himself when approached by staff members and is not willing to participate in daily activities of the ward. Which is the best method to make the patient interact with others and continue the same?
a. Observe the patient closely and verbally praise him when he talks to others.
b. Praise him with a token even for a little interaction which can later be utilized in favorable situations.
c. Praise him with tokens when he talks properly to others which can later be utilized in favorable situations.
d. Encourage him to talk to others.

26. A female patient who is actively hallucinating approaches the nurse and states; I am hearing voices that are saying bad things about me. The nurse should:
a. Simply state, "I do not hear the voices."
b. Suggest the patient to join other patients playing cards
c. Encourage the patient to not listen to what the voices are saying
d. State, "The staff understands that you are frightened and will stay with you while the voices are speaking."

27. During his assessment interview, a schizophrenic patient tells the nurse, "My life partner is unfaithful and having an extramarital affair". The nurse documents that the patient is experiencing:
a. Delusion of persecution
b. Delusion of jealousy
c. Delusion of grandiosity
d. Illogical thinking

28. A patient is refusing to take food. He says the food is poisoned. Which of the following is the most appropriate nursing intervention?
a. Assure the patient that the food is not poisoned
b. Assure the patient by tasting the patient's food
c. Explain the patient that it is a symptom of disease
d. Allow the patient to take packed foods, fruits, eggs, etc.

29. Which of the following statements of a patient would require immediate attention of the nurse?
a. I am getting thoughts of hurting myself, they are scary to me
b. I am not getting sleep
c. I want to consume alcohol
d. I want to be free from all these medicines

30. Which of the following nursing interventions is most appropriate for a patient talking and laughing to self?

a. Explain to the patient that such behavior is inappropriate
b. Ignore the patient behavior
c. Divert the patient by engaging him in one or other activities
d. Isolate the patient in another room

31. Which of the following nursing intervention/s is most appropriate for a patient exhibiting agitation and violent behavior?
a. Maintain low level of stimuli in the environment
b. Frequent observation of behavior
c. Remove all dangerous objects from patient's environment
d. All of the above

32. Following are the clinical features of mania, *except:*
a. Elation of mood
b. Disorientation
c. Increased psychomotor activity
d. Self-important ideas

33. Grandiose delusions occur in which of the following disorder?
a. Manic disorder
b. Obsessive compulsive disorder
c. Phobic disorder
d. Anxiety disorder

34. The drug of choice for mood disorder is:
a. Haloperidol
b. Imipramine
c. Lithium
d. Chlorpromazine

35. A patient with mania says, "we can, pan, scan, ran, plan.." the nurse identifies this as:
a. Clang association
b. Echolalia
c. Word salad
d. Neologism

36. A patient is on Lithium drug for 10 days. On the 10th day his serum lithium level is 1.0 mEq/L. The nurse knows that this value indicates:
a. Atoxic level
b. Laboratory error
c. A therapeutic blood level of the drug
d. Unusual response of the drug

37. A patient has been taking Lithium carbonate for his hypomania. While taking this drug which mineral would you recommend in adequate quantities?
a. Sodium
b. Iron
c. Iodine
d. Calcium

38. All of the following nursing interventions are most appropriate for a patient with violent behavior, *except:*
a. Recognize that violent behavior is a part of manic episode
b. Set limits for his behavior
c. Ignore patient behavior
d. Provide safe environment

39. Which of the following foods are recommended for manic patients?
a. Finger foods
b. Liquid foods
c. Semi-solid foods
d. Favorite foods

40. Depression is characterized by all, *except:*
a. Psychomotor retardation
b. Loosening of association
c. Inability to experience pleasure in any activity
d. Pervasive sadness

41. Triad symptoms of depression include:
a. Suicidal ideas, hopelessness, decreased appetite
b. Pervasive sadness, anhedonia, decreased psychomotor activity
c. Worthlessness, disturbed sleep, delusions
d. Monotonous voice, preoccupations, poor memory

42. **Worthlessness, hopelessness and help-lessness are characteristic features of:**
    a. Paranoid schizophrenia
    b. Depression
    c. Mania
    d. Obsessive compulsive disorder

43. **Which patient among the following requires nurse's immediate attention?**
    a. A patient who is refusing to attend group meetings
    b. A patient with rapid and irrelevant speech
    c. A patient who has been sleeping for only 2 hours in the night
    d. A patient who is expressing suicidal ideation

44. **Which of the following would be a priority intervention for a patient who attempted suicide previously?**
    a. Ask the patient frankly if he/she has a thought of, or has plans of committing suicide
    b. Avoid bringing up the subject of suicide in case you induce ideas of self-harm in the patient
    c. Involve the patient actively in unit activities so that he/she will not think of suicide
    d. Explain the consequences of suicidal attempts to the patient

45. **A patient was hospitalized following a suicide attempt after losing his job. One week later, a sudden apparent improvement is observed in the patient. The nurse understands that the most probable reason is that the patient:**
    a. Has gotten some information about a new job
    b. Has established supportive relationship with the personnel
    c. Has been relieved of a stressful work environment
    d. May be committed to suicide and has a workable plan

46. **Characteristic features of neurotic disorder include all the following, *expect:***
    a. Having insight
    b. Subjective distress
    c. Reasonably preserved behavior
    d. Delusions and hallucinations

47. **State of uneasiness arising out of anticipation of danger is termed as:**
    a. Anxiety
    b. Phobia
    c. Obsessions
    d. Compulsions

48. **Social phobia refers to an:**
    a. Irrational fear of a specific object
    b. Irrational fear of performing activities in the presence of others
    c. Irrational fear of being in places away from the home setting
    d. Irrational fear of society

49. **Which of the following is an example of simple phobia?**
    a. Fear of public places
    b. Fear of insects
    c. Fear of performing activities
    d. Avoidance of public places

50. **Irrational fear of being in places away from home setting is termed as:**
    a. Agoraphobia
    b. Acrophobia
    c. Algophobia
    d. Claustrophobia

51. **Following are the symptoms of anxiety, *except:***
    a. Palpitations
    b. Gastric discomfort
    c. Frequency of urination
    d. Bradycardia

52. **A patient has sudden attacks of anxiety predominated by physical symptoms accompanied by fear of serious consequence such as a heart attack. This is a characteristic of which disorder?**

a. Panic disorder
b. Phobia disorder
c. Generalized anxiety disorder
d. Obsessive compulsive disorder

53. **Which of the following behavior modification technique is useful in the treatment of phobias?**
a. Token economy
b. Modeling
c. Desensitization therapy
d. Positive reinforcement

54. **Following are all characteristics of obsessional thoughts in OCD, *except:***
a. Arising of unwanted thoughts
b. Feeling of subjective compulsions
c. Experiencing subjective distress
d. Experiencing powerlessness

55. **Signs and symptoms of OCD include all, *except*:**
a. Obsessive thoughts
b. Compulsive acts
c. Lack of concentration and task completion
d. Ordered flight of ideas

56. **Which of the following medications can be used to treat patients with anxiety disorders?**
a. Haloperidol
b. Alprazolam
c. Clozapine
d. Resperidone

57. **Recurrent, intrusive, senseless ideas, thoughts, and images that are ego-dystonic and involuntary are termed as:**
a. Obsessions
b. Compulsions
c. Hypochondriasis
d. Obtrusiveness

58. **Which of the following nursing interventions is most appropriate for a patient with compulsive acts?**
a. Recognize that this behavior is a part of OCD
b. Set limits for his compulsive acts
c. Ignore patient behavior
d. Provide positive reinforcement for non-ritualistic behavior

59. **Three months after a traumatic experience Ms Z is re-experiencing images of stressful events, insomnia and depression. She is likely to be suffering from:**
a. Acute stress reaction
b. Post-traumatic stress disorder
c. Adjustment disorder
d. Somatic disorder

60. **All the following features characterize a hysterical fit, *except*:**
a. Movements are irregular and bizarre
b. Incontinence of urine does not occur
c. Tongue bite is absent
d. It usually occurs in the absence of people and unsafe places

61. **A sudden unexpected travel away from home/work place with assumption of new identity and inability to recall the past is called:**
a. Dissociative identity disorder
b. Dissociative amnesia
c. Dissociative fugue
d. Trance and possession disorder

62. **All the following features characterize a hypochondriasis, *except*:**
a. Persistent preoccupation with a fear of having serious diseases
b. Repeated health care visits
c. Unconvinced by repeated investigations
d. Physical symptoms are managed by denial defense mechanism

63. **A condition wherein the individuals have excessive worry or belief that they are suffering from a physical illness despite lack of medical evidence is typical of:**
a. Generalized anxiety disorder
b. Hypochondriasis
c. Somatoform disorder
d. Dissociative disorder

64. **The best nursing intervention for a patient with hypochondriasis is to:**
    a. Collect detailed history to rule out physical disorder
    b. Instruct the patient to take prescribed medications
    c. Assist the patient to focus on his/her abilities and strengths
    d. Explain side effects of medication

65. **Drug dependence means:**
    a. Physiological and psychological dependence on drugs
    b. Maladaptive pattern of substance use
    c. Experiencing psychotic symptoms
    d. Developing complications

66. **Delirium tremens usually starts how many days after the last drink of alcohol?**
    a. 2–5 days
    b. 1–2 days
    c. 6–8 days
    d. 8–10 days

67. **Which of the following drug is a deterrent agent in the treatment of alcohol dependence syndrome?**
    a. Acamprosate
    b. Naltrexone
    c. Disulfiram
    d. Buproprion

68. **Detoxification means:**
    a. Alcohol-induced disorder
    b. Treatment for alcohol withdrawal symptoms
    c. Treatment for alcohol complications
    d. Removal of toxins from body

69. **Which of the following nursing interventions is most appropriate for a patient during acute intoxication?**
    a. Decrease in environmental stimuli
    b. Educate on ill effects of alcoholism
    c. Educate family members on how to control alcohol behavior
    d. Encourage the use of positive coping skills

70. **For a nurse who wants to give health education to an alcoholic patient, which of the following will be most appropriate?**
    a. Group discussion
    b. Individual discussion
    c. Demonstration
    d. Role play

71. **Drug/s of choice in the management of alcohol withdrawal is/are:**
    a. Antidepressants
    b. Benzodiazepines
    c. Disulfiram
    d. Acamprosate

72. **Which of the following is the most common complication of alcoholism?**
    a. Fever
    b. Liver disorders
    c. Skeletal problems
    d. Skin lesions

73. **Which of the following chromosomal abnormalities cause intellectual disability?**
    a. Down's syndrome
    b. Toxemia of pregnancy
    c. Kernicterus
    d. Septicemia during infancy

74. **A child with an IQ score 30 would be categorized under which of the degrees of intellectual disability?**
    a. Mild   b. Moderate
    c. Severe   d. Profound

75. **Following are all primary preventive measures of MR, *except*:**
    a. Genetic counseling
    b. Immunization for maternal rubella
    c. Proper nutrition throughout the developmental period
    d. Reduction of disability by rehabilitation

76. **Following are all core features of anorexia nervosa disorder,** *except:*
    a. Fear of becoming obese
    b. Body image disturbance
    c. Excess body weight
    d. Drive for thinness

77. **Following are all characteristics of childhood autism,** *except:*
    a. Unresponsiveness to parent's affection
    b. Gross deficits in language development
    c. Stereotype body movements
    d. Attention deficit and hyperactivity

78. **Autism mainly involves:**
    a. Over activity and inattention
    b. Poor eating skills
    c. Poor intelligence
    d. Poor communication

79. **Which of the following measures is a priority for the parents of an autistic child who engages in head banging?**
    a. Stimulant administration
    b. Home safety measures
    c. Face-to-face communication
    d. Regular routines

80. **Which of the following nursing interventions is most appropriate to develop language skills among autistic children?**
    a. Teach the names of objects by linking them with the actual object
    b. Assign limited number of care givers
    c. Provide child with familiar toys
    d. Encourage child to talk

81. **Which of the following characteristics is the nurse most likely to observe in ADHD children?**
    a. More attentive, less focused, impulsive
    b. Sensitive to stimuli, more attentive and focused
    c. More attentive, hyperactive, unable to wait
    d. Less attentive, hyperactive, impulsive

82. **Following are all conduct disorders,** *except:*
    a. Aggressive behavior
    b. Violating others rights
    c. Poor performance in school
    d. Poor communication skills

83. **Following are all core features of bulimia nervosa,** *except:*
    a. Binge eating
    b. Use of diuretics or laxatives
    c. Dieting or fasting
    d. Fear of thinness

84. **An elimination disorder in which the child suffers from incontinence of urine during sleep is termed as:**
    a. Enuresis
    b. Encopresis
    c. Dyspareunia
    d. Pseudocyesis

85. **Craving and eating of non-food substances such as paint and clay is termed as:**
    a. Binge eating
    b. Verbigeration
    c. Polyphagia
    d. Pica

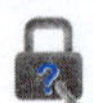 **ANSWER KEY**

Fill in the Blanks

1. Disorientation	2. Obsessive compulsive disorder	3. Organic psychiatry	4. Echolalia	5. Suicide	6. Kurt Schneider	7. Alcohol anonymous
8. Illusion	9. Obsession	10. Confabulation	11. Phobia			

State the Following Statements are True or False

1. True	2. True	3. False	4. False	5. False	6. True	7. True
8. True	9. True	10. False	11. False	12. True	13. True	14. False
15. True	16. True	17. False	18. False	19. False		

Multiple Choice Questions

1. a	2. a	3. a	4. d	5. b	6. a	7. d
8. a	9. c	10. a	11. c	12. d	13. b	14. a
15. a	16. c	17. a	18. b	19. c	20. d	21. d
22. b	23. a	24. d	25. b	26. d	27. b	28. d
29. a	30. c	31. d	32. b	33. a	34. c	35. a
36. c	37. a	38. d	39. a	40. b	41. b	42. b
43. d	44. a	45. d	46. d	47. a	48. b	49. b
50. a	51. d	52. a	53. c	54. d	55. d	56. b
57. a	58. d	59. b	60. d	61. c	62. d	63. b
64. c	65. a	66. a	67. c	68. b	69. a	70. d
71. b	72. b	73. a	74. c	75. d	76. c	77. d
78. d	79. b	80. a	81. d	82. d	83. d	84. a
85. d						

Bio-Psycho and Social Therapies

Patients suffering from physical illnesses are given specific treatment because the causes are specific and the signs and symptoms are also specific. In a psychiatric setting, the cause may not be so specific and most patients are given more than one treatment. These treatment methods vary from patient to patient. Some patients refuse treatment and may not co-operate with doctors and nurses. Some do not realize that they are ill and may actively resist all forms of treatment.

The nurse has an extremely important role to play in the treatment of the mentally ill. She is the one who has closer contact with the patient than any other member of the hospital team. She also has a greater opportunity to get to know him and report on his improvement.

PHYSICAL THERAPIES

Physical therapies are treatment approaches that use physiologic or physical interventions to effect behavioral change. The most commonly used physical therapies are: psychopharmacology, electroconvulsive therapy, ketamine therapy, light therapy, repetitive transcranial magnetic stimulation.

Psychopharmacology

Psychopharmacology is the study of medications used to treat psychiatric disorders. It discusses many psychoactive medications that alter synaptic transmission in the brain in certain and specific ways. Medications that affect cognitive function, emotion and behavior are called psychotropic medications. They have significant effect on higher mental functions. Psychopharmacological agents are first line treatment for almost all psychiatric ailments nowadays. The nurse plays a pivotal role in medication administration and patient education. It is also important for the nurse to be aware of the potential side effects and interactions of these drugs. Assisting the patient to understand the importance of taking psychotropic medications as prescribed and the issues surrounding medication adherence is an important skill for the mental health nurse. It is important for the nurse to understand the terms used in drug therapy.

- ❖ **Efficacy** refers to the maximal therapeutic effect that a drug can achieve.
- ❖ **Potency** describes the amount of drug needed to achieve that maximum effect; low potency drugs require higher dosages

to achieve efficacy, whereas high potency drugs achieve efficacy at lower dosages.

❖ **Half-life** is the time it takes for half of the drug to be removed from the bloodstream. Drugs with a shorter half-life may need to be given once a day.

❖ Drugs that activate receptors are termed **agonist,** and those that block are termed **antagonists.**

Core Concept (Neurotransmitters)

❖ Neurotransmitters are endogenous chemicals that enable communication between neurons.

❖ These are the chemical messengers that travel from one brain cell to another and are synthesized by enzymes from certain dietary amino acids or precursors.

❖ These are stored in the axon terminals of the presynaptic neuron. An electrical impulse through the neuron stimulates the release of the neurotransmitter into the synaptic cleft which in turn determines whether another electrical impulse is generated.

❖ Neurotransmitters help relay messages from one part of the brain to another and between the brain and the rest of the body, primarily through synaptic transmission.

❖ Signals sent by neurotransmitters are responsible for the vast majority of brain and motor functions such as memory, planning, heart rate, respiration, digestion, hormonal responses, movement and others.

❖ Many different diseases involve increased or decreased levels of neurotransmitters in the brain such as anxiety, depression, schizophrenia, Parkinson's disease, drug addiction, etc.

❖ Neurotransmitters are synthesized and stored in the presynaptic neuron.

❖ An action potential in the presynaptic neuron causes an influx of Ca^{2+} into the neuron.

❖ The influx of Ca^{2+} causes the neurotransmitter to be released into the synapse.

❖ The neurotransmitters bind to neurotransmitter receptors that are located on the membrane of the postsynaptic cell.

❖ Receptors are molecules situated on the cell membrane that are binding sites for neurotransmitters. The synapse separates the two neurons (pre- and postsynaptic cells). These neurotransmitters are stored in the vesicles waiting to be released into the synapse **(Figure 6.1)**.

❖ After neurotransmission, they are either reabsorbed (reuptake) and stored by the presynaptic cell for later use or metabolized (broken down) by enzymes such as monoamine oxidase (MAO) and cholinesterase (ChE).

❖ During neurotransmission, the chemical neurotransmitter released from a storage vesicle in the presynaptic cell crosses the synapse and is recognized by the receptor on the postsynaptic cell membrane termed as binding.

❖ Depending on the type of neurotransmitter they have either an excitatory effect or an inhibitory effect on the postsynaptic cell.

❖ An excitatory effect causes depolarization of the postsynaptic cell; an inhibitory effect causes hyperpolarization making the postsynaptic cell less active.

❖ After release and binding, the neurotransmitter is either degraded by an enzyme or brought back by the transport molecules to the presynaptic neuron, a reuptake process.

❖ Drugs affect neurotransmission in several ways **(Figure 6.2)**:
  - *Release:* Many neurotransmitters are released into the synapse from the storage vesicles in presynaptic cell.
  - *Blockade:* Neurotransmitters are prevented from binding to the postsynaptic receptors.
  - *Receptor sensitivity changes:* Receptor becomes more or less responsive to the neurotransmitter.
  - *Blocked reuptake:* As the presynaptic cell does not reabsorb the neurotransmitter it is retained in the synapse and therefore enhances or prolongs the action.
  - *Interference with storage vesicles:* Either released more or less.

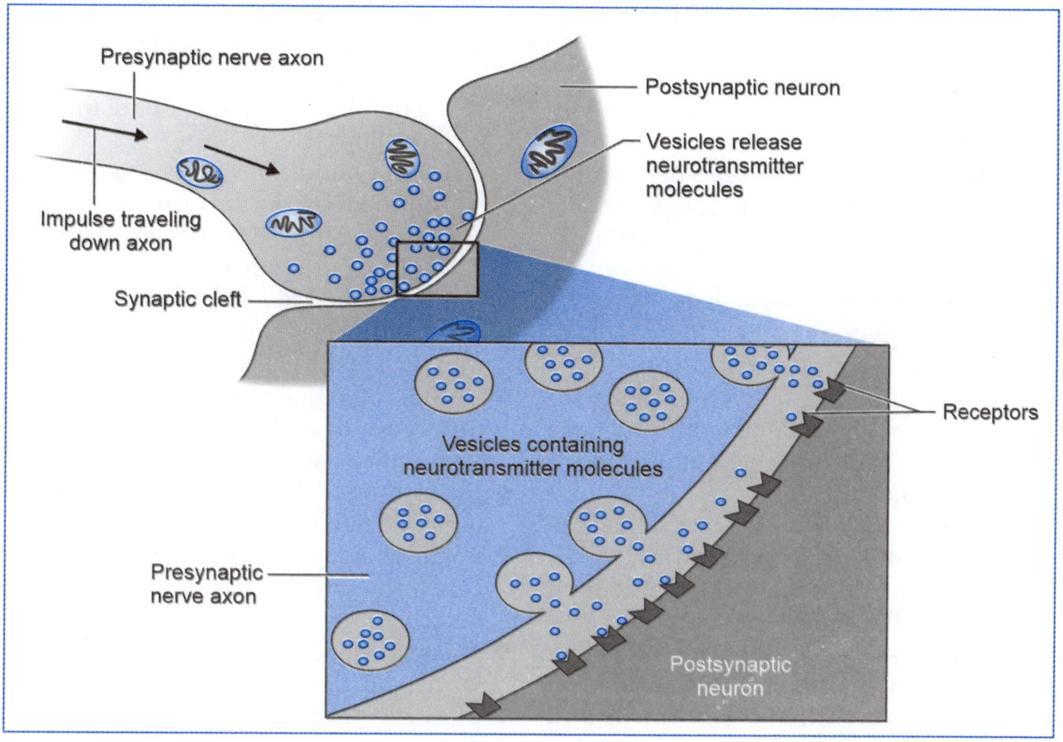

Figure 6.1: Synapse

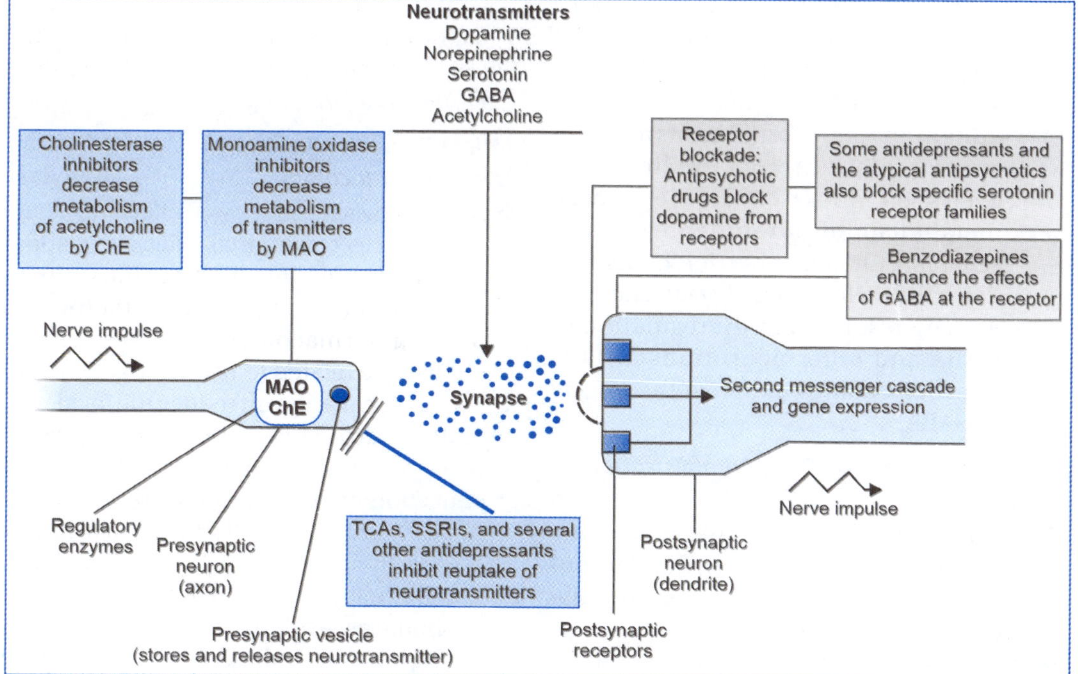

Figure 6.2: Neurotransmission and drug effects at the synapse

- ○ *Precursor chain interference:* The process that 'makes' the neurotransmitter either synthesized more or less.
- ❖ **Psychotropic drugs alter synaptic activity by:**
  - ○ Modifying the reuptake of a neurotransmitter into the presynaptic neuron.
  - ○ Activating or inhibiting postsynaptic receptors.
  - ○ Inhibition of enzyme activity.
- ❖ **Biological theories suggest that:**
  - ○ Many of the psychiatric disorders are caused by dysregulation (imbalance) in the complex process of brain structures communicating with each other through neurotransmission.
  - ○ Psychosis involves excessive dopamine and serotonin dysregulation. Antipsychotic drugs block dopamine from the receptor site.
  - ○ Mood disorders result from disruption of normal patterns of neurotransmission of norepinephrine, serotonin and other transmitters. Antidepressants block the reuptake of norepinephrine or serotonin and regulate the areas of the brain that manufacture these chemicals. Some antidepressants and atypical antipsychotics block specific subtypes of serotonin receptors thereby enhancing serotonin transmission at serotonin receptors implicated in depression. MAOIs slow down enzymatic metabolism of norepinephrine and serotonin. Cholinesterase inhibitors slow down the metabolism of acetylcholine.
  - ○ Anxiety results from dysregulation of GABA and other neurotransmitters. Benzodiazepines enhance the effects of GABA.

General Guidelines on Drug Administration in Psychiatry

- ❖ The nurse should not administer any drug unless there is a written order. Do not hesitate to consult the doctor when in doubt about any medication.
- ❖ All medications given must be charted on the patient's case record sheet.

- ❖ **While administering medication:**
  - ○ Always address the patient by name and make certain of his/her identification.
  - ○ Do not leave the patient until the drug is swallowed.
  - ○ Do not permit the patient to go to the bathroom to take the medication.
  - ○ Do not allow one patient to carry medicine to another.
- ❖ If it is required to leave the patient to get water, do not leave the medicine tray within the reach of the patient.
- ❖ Do not force oral medication because of the danger of aspiration. This is especially important in stuporous patients.
- ❖ Check drugs daily for any change in color, odor and number.
- ❖ Bottles should be tightly closed and labeled. Labels should be written legibly and in bold lettering.
- ❖ Make sure that an adequate supply of drugs is on hand, but do not overstock.
- ❖ Make sure no patient has access to the drug cupboard.
- ❖ Drug cupboards should always be kept locked when not in use. Never allow a patient or worker to clean the drug cupboard. The drug cupboard keys should not be given to patients. *(See Appendices 21 and 25 for Drug Book Format and Drug Guide)*

Patient Education Related to Psychopharmacology

- ❖ Nurses assess for drug side effects, evaluate desired effects, and make decisions about prn (pro re neta) medication. Thus, nurses must understand general principles of psychopharmacology and have specific knowledge related to psychotropic drugs.
- ❖ Teaching patients can reduce the incidence of side effects while improving compliance with the drug regimen. Specific areas of education include the following:
  - ○ *Discussion of side effects:* Side effects can directly affect the patient's willingness to adhere to the drug regimen. The nurse should always inquire about the patient's response to a drug, both therapeutic responses and adverse responses.

○ *Discussion of safety issues*: Because some drugs such as tricyclic antidepressants have a narrow therapeutic index, thoughts of self-harm must be discussed. Discussion should also include abruptly discontinued effects. Many psychotropic drugs cause sedation or drowsiness. Discussions concerning use of hazardous machinery, driving must be reviewed.

○ *Drug interactions*: Patients and families must be taught to discuss the effects of the addition of over-the-counter drugs, alcohol and illegal drugs to currently prescribed drugs.

○ *Instructions for older adult patients:* Because older individuals have a different pharmacokinetic profile than younger adults, special instructions concerning side effects and drug-drug interactions should be explained.

○ *Instructions for pregnant or breastfeeding patients:* As pregnant or breastfeeding patients have special risks associated with psychotropic drug therapy, special instructions should be tailored for these individuals. Teaching patients about their medications enables them to not only be mature participants in their own care but also decreases undesirable side effects. Furthermore, effective teaching can reduce noncompliance **(Box 6.1)**.

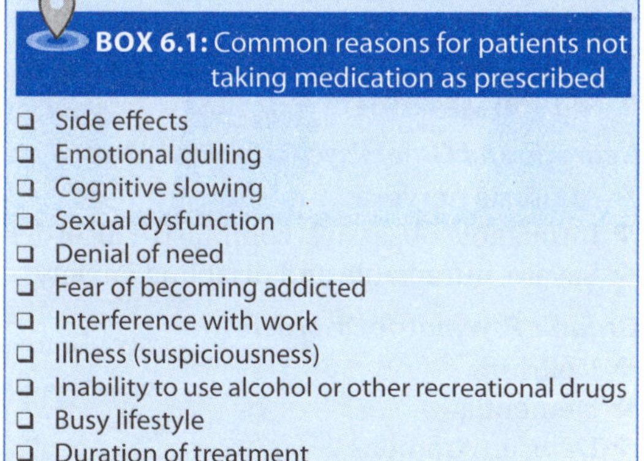

Classification of Psychotropic Drugs

Psychotropic drugs can traditionally be classified based on clinical indication as under **(Figure 6.3)**:

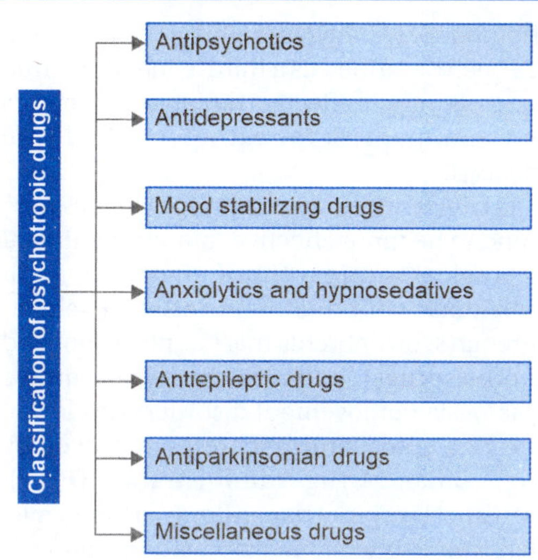

Figure 6.3: Classification of psychotropic drugs

ANTIPSYCHOTICS

Antipsychotics are psychotropic drugs that are used for the treatment of psychotic symptoms. These medications cannot 'cure' the illness but can take away many of the symptoms or make them milder, help patients to lead a more normal and fulfilling life by alleviating psychotic symptoms. In some cases they can shorten the course of an episode of the illness as well. Antipsychotic drugs are also known as neuroleptics, major tranquilizers, anti-schizophrenic drugs or D2-receptor blockers.

Classification

The first antipsychotic medications were introduced in the 1950s with the invention of phenothiazines. Also known as typical antipsychotics or conventional antipsychotics, these first-generation antipsychotics are dopamine receptor antagonists. These often have unpleasant side effects such as muscle stiffness, tremor, and abnormal movements thereby leading the researchers to continue their search for better drugs.

The 1990s saw the development of second-generation antipsychotics. Also known as atypical antipsychotics, these are serotonin-dopamine antagonists. Due to fewer side-effects than the older drugs they are now being used as first-line treatment. More recently, aripiprazole (Abilify) an atypical antipsychotic has been described as a third-generation drug due to its unique effect on dopamine receptors and minimal risk for extrapyramidal side effects (EPS).

In clinical trials, atypical antipsychotics were found to be more effective than conventional or "typical" antipsychotic medications in individuals with treatment-resistant schizophrenia (schizophrenia that has not responded to other drugs), and also the risk of tardive dyskinesia (a movement disorder) was lower. The 12 atypical antipsychotics approved by the Food and Drug Administration (FDA), 2016 are clozapine, risperidone, aripiprazole, olanzapine, quetiapine, ziprasidone, amisulpride, paliperidone, asenapine, lurasidone, iloperidone, cariprazine and brexpiprazole. Though each of these has a unique side effect profile, these medications are in general better tolerated than the earlier drugs.

Antipsychotics are classified based on pharmacological mechanism of dopamine D2 receptor antagonism which is linked to clinical efficacy. Classification of antipsychotics is presented in **Table 6.1**.

Pharmacokinetics

Antipsychotics when administered orally are absorbed variably from the gastrointestinal tract due to uneven blood levels. They are highly bound to plasma as well as tissue proteins. Brain concentrations are significantly higher than plasma concentrations. They are metabolized in the liver, and excreted mainly through the kidneys. The elimination half-life varies from 10 to 24 hours.

Most of the antipsychotics tend to have a therapeutic window. If the blood level is below this window, the drug is ineffective. If the blood level is higher than the upper limit of the window, it results in toxicity or the drug is again ineffective.

Mechanism of Action

Typical antipsychotics work by inhibiting dopaminergic neurotransmission. These drugs block D2 receptors in the mesolimbic and mesofrontal systems (concerned with emotional reactions). They also have noradrenergic, cholinergic and histaminergic blocking action. Sedation is caused by alpha-adrenergic blockade. Antidopaminergic actions on basal ganglia are responsible for causing EPS **(Figure 6.4)**.

Atypical antipsychotics work by blocking D2 dopamine receptors as well as serotonin receptor antagonist action such as anti-serotonergic (5-hydroxytryptamine or 5-HT), antiadrenergic and antihistaminergic actions. These are therefore called serotonin-dopamine antagonists.

Indications

The main indicators for antipsychotic drugs are management of schizophrenia, mania and depression with psychotic symptoms, behavioral problems in childhood disorders, eating and organic psychiatric disorders.

Psychiatric Disorders

❖ Schizophrenia
❖ Schizoaffective disorders
❖ Paranoid disorders

Mood Disorders

❖ Acute mania
❖ Major depression with psychotic symptoms
❖ Severe agitation

Childhood Psychiatric Disorders

❖ Attention-deficit hyperactivity disorder
❖ Autism
❖ Enuresis
❖ Conduct disorder

Neurotic and Other Psychiatric Disorders

❖ Anorexia nervosa
❖ Intractable obsessive-compulsive disorder
❖ Severe, intractable and disabling anxiety

Organic Psychiatric Disorders

❖ Delirium
❖ Dementia
❖ Delirium tremens
❖ Drug-induced psychosis

Medical Disorders

❖ Huntington's chorea
❖ Intractable hiccough
❖ Nausea and vomiting

TABLE 6.1: Classification of antipsychotics

Category		Subclass	Common drugs (Generic name)	Trade names	Oral dose mg/day	Parental dose mg/day
Typical antipsychotics	Dopamine antagonist	Phenothiazines	Chlorpromazine	Thorazine, Largactil	300–1500 mg	50–100 IM only
			Triflupromazine	Vesprin, Siquil	100–400 mg	30–60 IM only
			Thioridazine	Mellaril, Thioril	300–800 mg	—
			Trifluoperazine	Espazine	15–60 mg	1–5 IM
			Fluphenazine Decanoate	Prolinate	—	25–50 IM every 1–3 weeks
		Thioxanthenes	Flupenthixol	Depixol, Fluanxol	3–40 mg	
		Butyrophenones	Haloperidol	Haldol, Serenace	5–100 mg	5–20 IM
		Diphenylbutyl Piperidines	Pimozide	Orap	4–20 mg	—
			Penfluridol	Flumap	20–60 mg/weekly	
		Indolic derivatives	Molindone	Moban	50–225 mg	
		Dibenzoxazepines	Loxapine	Loxitane	25–100 mg	
Atypical antipsychotics	Dopamine and serotonin antagonist	—	Clozapine	Clozaril, Sizopin, Denzapine	50–450 mg	Zyprexa Relprevv is a long-acting injectable (LAI) (Olanzapine) 10 mg, 2–4 weeks
			Risperidone	Risperdal, Sizodon, Sizomax	2–10 mg	
			Olanzapine	Zyprexa, Olanz	10–20 mg	
			Quetiapine	Seroquel, Qutan	150–750 mg	
			Ziprasidone	Geodon	20–80 mg	
			Amisulpride (Noval)	Solian	50–300 mg	
	Partial dopamine antagonist	—	Aripiprazole (Noval)	Abilify, Aristada	05–30 mg	Aripiprazole lauroxil is a long-acting intramuscular injection administered 4–6 weeks

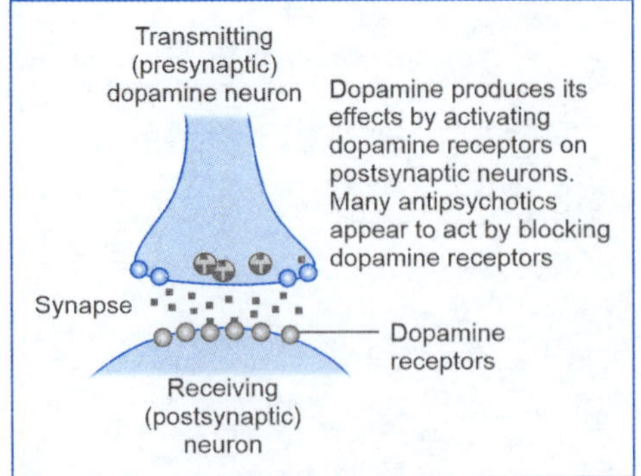

Figure 6.4: Dopamine neurotransmission and drug effects at the synapse

❖ Tic disorder
❖ Eclampsia
❖ Heat stroke
❖ Severe pain in malignancy
❖ Tetanus

Contraindications

Contraindicated Situations for First-generation Antipsychotics

❖ History of severe allergy
❖ Use of central nervous system depressants like barbiturates, benzodiazepines, opioids
❖ Severe cardiac, renal and liver disorders
❖ Poorly controlled seizures
❖ Narrow-angle glaucoma
❖ Prostatic hypertrophy
❖ Parkinson's disease

Contraindicated Situations for Atypical Antipsychotics

❖ History of severe allergy.
❖ Elderly patients diagnosed with dementia.
❖ Caution in the presence of a prolactinoma.
❖ Glaucoma, liver disease, cardiac arrhythmias, severe cardiac disorders, severe neutropenia or bone marrow depression.

Antipsychotics should be avoided during first trimester pregnancy. For women taking antipsychotics and considering breastfeeding, alternative treatments may be typically advised due to drug accumulation in breast milk.

Adverse Effects of Antipsychotic Drugs

The most common side-effects of conventional antipsychotic medication include anticholinergic effects, photosensitivity and extrapyramidal side-effects **(Figure 6.5)**.

Extrapyramidal Symptoms (EPS)

Antipsychotics cause four main extrapyramidal symptoms **(Figure 6.6)**. These occur due to blockade of D2 receptors in the midbrain region of the brainstem. Conventional antipsychotic drugs cause a greater incidence of EPS than do atypical antipsychotic drugs.

❖ **Neuroleptic-induced parkinsonism (Pseudoparkinsonism):** Symptoms include rigidity in the arms and shoulders, tremors in the hands and arms, bradykinesia, stooped posture, drooling, akinesia, masked facies and shuffling gait. The disorder can be reversible and treated with anticholinergic agents.

❖ **Acute dystonia:** Dystonic reactions are spastic contractions of the muscles resulting from a slow sustained muscular spasm that led to an involuntary movement. Dystonia can involve the neck, jaw, tongue and the entire body (opisthotonos). There is also the involvement of eyes leading to upward lateral movement of the eye known as oculogyric crisis. Dystonia can be prevented

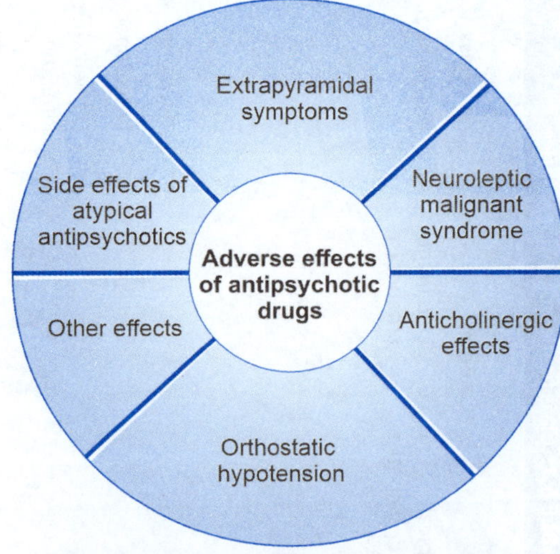

Figure 6.5: Adverse effects of antipsychotic drugs

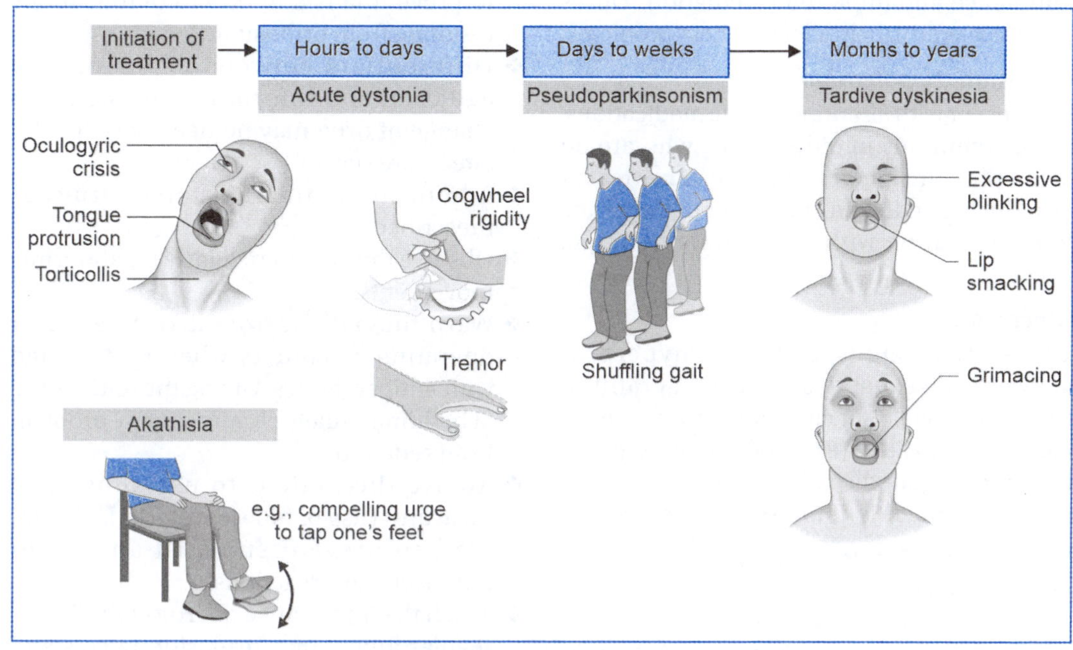

Figure 6.6: Extrapyramidal symptoms

by anticholinergic, antihistaminergic, dopamine agonists, beta-adrenergic antagonists, benzodiazepines, etc. These reactions are uncomfortable and can be life-threatening if left untreated.

❖ **Akathisia:** Akathisia is a subjective feeling of inner restlessness which is evident from the inability to remain still. It is associated with psychomotor restlessness with the individual experiencing an intense sensation of unease usually involving the lower extremities. Akathisia can be treated with low doses of beta blockers such as propranolol and also with benzodiazepines.

❖ **Tardive dyskinesia:** It is a delayed adverse effect of antipsychotics which may not be reversible even if the medication is discontinued. It consists of abnormal, irregular choreoathetoid movements of the muscles of the head, limbs and trunk. It is characterized by chewing, sucking, grimacing and perioral movements.

Neuroleptic Malignant Syndrome

It is a rare but serious disorder occurring in a small minority of patients taking neuroleptics, especially high-potency compounds. The onset is often in the first 10 days of treatment. The clinical picture includes rapid onset (usually over 24–72 hours) of severe motor, mental and autonomic disorders, the most prominent motor symptom being generalized muscular hypertonicity. Stiffness of the muscles in the throat and chest may cause dysphasia and dyspnea. Mental symptoms include akinetic mutism, stupor or impaired consciousness. Hyperpyrexia develops with evidence of autonomic disturbances in the form of unstable blood pressure, tachycardia, excessive sweating, salivation, and urinary incontinence. Creatine phosphokinase (CPK) in the blood may rise to very high levels; also the white cell count may increase. Secondary features may include pneumonia, thromboembolism, cardiovascular collapse, and renal failure. The syndrome lasts for one to two weeks after stopping the drug. *(Refer Chapter 8—Page No. 283 for Management of Neuroleptic Malignant Syndrome)*

Anticholinergic Effects

Dry mouth, constipation, cycloplegia, mydriasis, urinary retention, blurred vision, impotence and impaired ejaculation. Doses can be lowered to help alleviate these problems.

Orthostatic Hypotension

It can occur with all antipsychotic medications, more commonly in older adults who are on blood pressure medications. It can be treated by reducing or dividing the doses or switching to a medication with lesser antiadrenergic effect.

Other Effects

These are seizures, sedation, hyperprolactinemia, sexual dysfunction, agranulocytosis (especially for clozapine), sialorrhea or increased salivation (especially for clozapine), weight gain, jaundice, dermatological effects (contact dermatitis, photosensitive reaction).

Common Side Effects with Atypical Antipsychotics

Hormonal side effects such as weight gain, diabetes mellitus; other side effects such as QTc prolongation, hypertension, abnormal cholesterol and triglycerides, extrapyramidal side effects, myocarditis, agranulocytosis, cataract, and sexual side effects. In females there may be abnormal menstrual cycles and infertility. Some drugs cause a high increase in prolactin levels.

Nurse's Responsibility for a Patient Receiving Antipsychotics

❖ To manage extrapyramidal symptoms either alter the dosage or discontinue the drug or change to a different antipsychotic.

❖ Instruct the patient to take sips of water frequently to relieve dryness of mouth. Frequent mouth washes, use of chewing gum, applying glycerin on the lips can also be helpful.

❖ Include a high-fiber diet, ensure increased fluid intake and laxatives to reduce constipation.

❖ Advise the patient to get up from the bed or chair very slowly. Patient should sit on the edge of the bed for one full minute dangling his feet before actually standing up. Check BP before and after medication is administered. It is an important measure

to prevent falls and other complications resulting from orthostatic hypotension.

❖ Differentiate between akathisia and agitation and inform the physician. A change of drug may be necessary if side-effects are severe.

❖ Administer antiparkinsonian drugs as prescribed.

❖ Observe the patient regularly for abnormal movements.

❖ Warn the patient from driving a car or operating machinery when first treated with antipsychotics. Giving the entire dose at bedtime usually eliminates any problem from sedation.

❖ Advise the patient to use sunscreen measures (use of full sleeves, dark glasses, etc.) to prevent sunburn and other photosensitive reactions.

❖ Teach the importance of drug compliance, regular follow-ups, drug side-effects and reporting if too severe. Give reassurance and reduce unfounded fears and anxieties.

❖ A patient receiving clozapine is at risk for developing agranulocytosis. Monitor TC, DC essentially in the first few weeks of treatment. Stop the drug if WBC count drops to less than $3,000/mm^3$ of blood. The patient should also be told to report if sore throat or fever develops which might indicate infection.

❖ Take all seizure precautions as clozapine reduces seizure threshold. The dose should be regulated carefully and patient put on anticonvulsants such as eptoin.

❖ Instruct the patient to report any fever, muscle rigidity, diaphoresis, tachycardia, etc.

❖ Assess vital signs regularly including temperature.

❖ For hormonal side effects assess for history of diabetes, evaluate blood sugar levels, teach the importance of diet and exercise.

❖ **Additional patient teaching:**
   ○ Smoking increases the metabolism of antipsychotics. Hence patient is encouraged to discuss it with the treating doctor.
   ○ Must be advised not to consume alcohol while on antipsychotics treatment.

○ Should not take any other prescribed or OTC medicines without the approval of the treating physician.

○ Patient must report immediately to the physician if any pregnancy occurs, is suspected or planned as safe use of antipsychotics during pregnancy has not been established yet.

(See Appendix 25 for Drug Guide)

ANTIDEPRESSANTS

Antidepressants are drugs used for treatment of depressive illness. These are also called mood elevators or thymoleptics. It is believed that during depressive episode there is a functional deficiency of dopamine (DA), serotonin (5-HT), norepinephrine (NE) and acetylcholine (ACh) neurotransmitters or hyposensitive receptors. Antidepressant medications increase the amount of available neurotransmitters by inhibiting neuro-transmitter reuptake or monoamine oxidase (MAO) or blocking certain receptors.

Classification

There are several types of antidepressants. For classification and details see **Table 6.2**.

Indications

Antidepressants are one of the most frequently prescribed medications for following conditions **(Figure 6.7):**

Depression
❖ Depressive episode
❖ Dysthymia
❖ Reactive depression
❖ Secondary depression
❖ Abnormal grief reaction

Childhood Psychiatric Disorders
❖ Enuresis
❖ Separation anxiety disorder
❖ Somnambulism
❖ School phobia
❖ Night terrors

Other Psychiatric Disorders
❖ Panic attack

TABLE 6.2: Classification of antidepressants

Class	Mechanism of action	Examples of drugs	Trade names	Oral dosage (mg/day)
Tricyclic antidepressants (TCAs)	Inhibit reuptake of serotonin (5-HT) and norepinephrine (NE); block NE, ACh and histamine receptors	Imipramine	Antidep	75–300
		Amitriptyline	Tryptomer	75–300
		Clomipramine	Anafranil	75–300
		Dothiepin	Prothiaden	75–300
		Mianserin	Depnon	30–120
Selective serotonin reuptake inhibitors (SSRIs)	Inhibit reuptake of serotonin (5-HT)	Fluoxetine	Fludac	10–80
		Sertraline	Serenata	50–200
		Fluvoxamine	Faverin	50–100
Selective serotonin and norepinephrine re-uptake inhibitors (SNRI)	Potent inhibitors of serotonin and norepinephrine reuptake	Venlafaxine	Effexor	25–100
		Levomilnacipran	Fetzima	20–120
Atypical antidepressants (noradrenaline and dopamine reuptake inhibitors)	Inhibit the reuptake of both dopamine and norepinephrine	Bupropion Mitazapine Nefazodone Vortioxetine	Survector	100–400
Monoamine oxidase inhibitors (MAOIs)	Increase NE and 5-HT by inhibiting the enzyme that degrades them (MAO-A)	Trazodone	Trazalon	150–600
		Isocarboxazid	Marplan	10–30

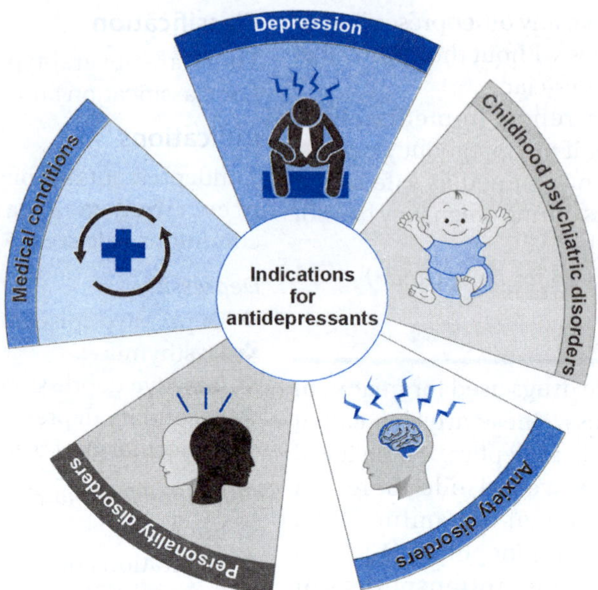

Figure 6.7: Indications for antidepressants

❖ Generalized anxiety disorder
❖ Agoraphobia, social phobia
❖ OCD with or without depression
❖ Eating disorder
❖ Borderline personality disorder
❖ Post-traumatic stress disorder
❖ Depersonalization syndrome

Medical Disorders
❖ Chronic pain
❖ Migraine
❖ Peptic ulcer disease

Contraindications

❖ History of seizures
❖ Person with cardiac disease and liver dysfunction.
❖ Avoid use in older people and children
❖ Use cautiously during pregnancy and lactation period.

Pharmacokinetics

Antidepressants are highly lipophilic and protein-bound. The half-life is long and usually more than 24 hours. It is predominantly metabolized in the liver. These drugs do not cause any dependence, tolerance, addiction or withdrawal.

Mechanism of Action

Though the exact mechanism is unknown, the predominant action is to increase catecholamine levels in the brain. TCAs are also called mono amine reuptake inhibitors (MARIs). The main mode of action is by blocking the reuptake of norepinephrine (NE) and/or serotonin (5-HT) at the nerve terminals thus increasing the NE and 5-HT levels at the receptor site.

MAOIs act on MAO (monoamine oxidase) which is responsible for the degradation of catecholamines after reuptake. The final effect is the same, a functional increase in the NE and 5-HT levels at the receptor site. The increase in brain amine levels is probably responsible for the antidepressant action. It takes about 5–10 days for MAOIs and 2–3 weeks for TCAs to bring down depressive symptoms. When a patient does not respond even after a trial period of 4–6 weeks, a different antidepressant is tried. SSRIs act by inhibiting the re-uptake of serotonin and increasing its levels at the receptor site **(Figure 6.8)**.

Side Effects

Each type of antidepressant has different possible side effects which may vary from

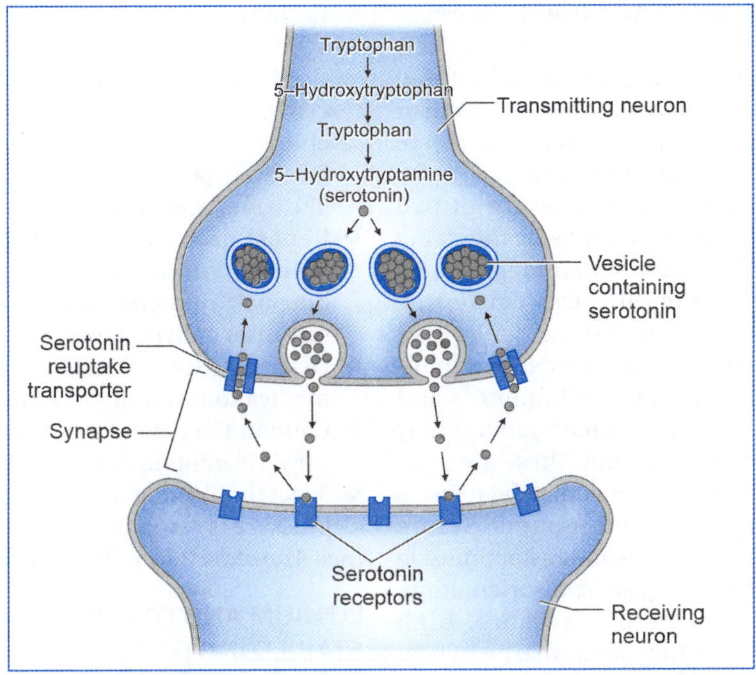

Figure 6.8: Serotonin neurotransmission and drug effects at the synapse

person to person. Selective serotonin reuptake inhibitors are the most commonly prescribed class of antidepressants because of fewer side effects than other types of antidepressants. The common side effects of antidepressants are presented in **Figure 6.9**.

❖ **Autonomic side effects:** Dry mouth, constipation, cycloplegia, mydriasis, urinary retention, orthostatic hypotension, impotence, impaired ejaculation, delirium and aggravation of glaucoma.

❖ **CNS effects:** Sedation, tremor and other extrapyramidal symptoms, withdrawal syndrome, seizures, jitteriness syndrome, precipitation of mania.

❖ **Cardiac side effects:** Tachycardia, ECG changes, arrhythmias, direct myocardial depression, quinidine-like action (decreased conduction time).

❖ **Allergic side effects:** Agranulocytosis, cholestatic jaundice, skin rashes, systemic vasculitis.

❖ **Metabolic and endocrine side effects:** Weight gain.

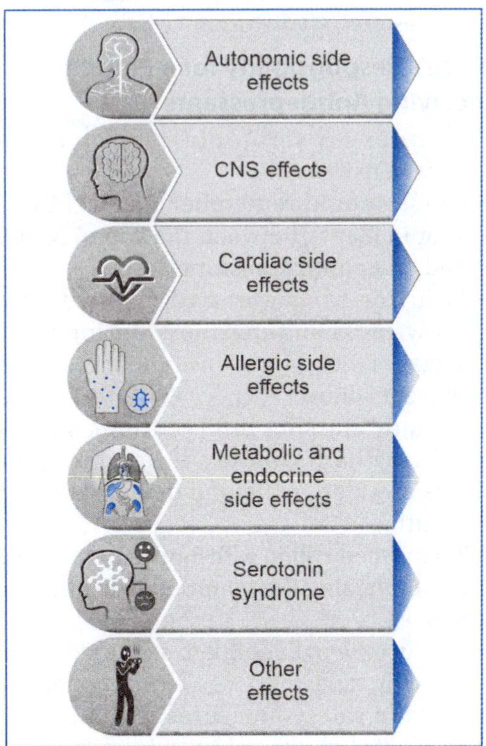

Figure 6.9: Side effects of antidepressants

❖ **Special effects of MAOI drugs:** Hypertensive crisis (occipital headache, neck stiffness, nausea or vomiting, sweating, dilated pupils, photophobia, shortness of breath or confusion and severe hypertension), severe hepatic necrosis, hyperpyrexia.

❖ **Serotonin syndrome:** The use of two high dose serotonin drugs at the same time or MAOI and other antidepressants administered together can cause this syndrome. High doses of drugs like monoamine oxidase inhibitors, serotonin-norepinephrine reuptake inhibitors and selective serotonin reuptake inhibitors may also cause this syndrome. These are mild or severe. Mild symptoms may be nausea, vomiting, diarrhea and tremors. Severe symptoms may include confusion, muscle twitching, muscle spasms, disorientation, delirium, high blood pressure, high temperature, seizures, abnormal heart beat which can be fatal.

❖ **Other effects:** Blurred vision, weight gain, sexual dysfunction, hyponatremia, elevated cholesterol, GI disturbances.

Nurse's Responsibility for a Patient Receiving Antidepressants

❖ Monitor for serotonin syndrome and hypertensive crisis.

❖ Nurse should remember that 7–14 days should elapse between the use of MAOIs and other antidepressants.

❖ Monitor for signs and symptoms of drowsiness and dizziness during initial stages of therapy and institute measures to prevent falling.

❖ General nursing interventions such as offering hard candies, ice and frequent sips of water are helpful in alleviating dry mouth.

❖ Taking medication with food may be helpful in minimizing the common side effects of nausea.

❖ Instruct the patient not to stop medication abruptly, taper the dose when discontinued.

❖ Provide safety measures. For example, adequate lighting, raised side, rails, etc., to prevent injuries.

❖ Patients on MAOIs should be warned against the danger of ingesting tyramine-rich foods which can result in hypertensive crisis. Some of these foods are beef liver, chicken liver, fermented sausages, dried fish, overripe fruits, chocolate and beverages like wine, beer and coffee.

❖ Report promptly if occipital headache, nausea, vomiting, chest pain or other unusual symptoms occur; these can herald the onset of hypertensive crisis.

❖ Instruct the patient not to take any medication without prescription.

❖ Caution the patient to change his position slowly to minimize orthostatic hypotension.

❖ Strict monitoring of vitals especially blood pressure is essential.

(See Appendix 25 for Drug Guide)

LITHIUM AND OTHER MOOD STABILIZING DRUGS

Mood stabilizers are used for the management and treatment of bipolar affective disorders (having disturbance in mood including mania and depression). The clinical effects of mood stabilizing medications are reducing acute (severe) symptoms of mania or depression to a more manageable level, stabilizing mood swings, preventing symptoms relapse and re-hospitalizations. Some of the commonly used mood stabilizers are:

❖ Lithium

❖ Carbamazepine

❖ Sodium valproate

Lithium was discovered by FJ Cade in 1949. The clinical properties of carbamazepine and valproic acid were discovered in the 1970s and 1980s.

Lithium

Lithium is an element with atomic number 3 and atomic weight 7. It was the first mood stabilizer and the first-line treatment option in the treatment of mania. It is available in brand names as Carbolith, Eskalith, Lithonate, Lithotabs, etc.

Indications

❖ Acute mania

❖ Prophylaxis for bipolar and unipolar mood disorder
❖ Schizoaffective disorder
❖ Cyclothymia
❖ Major depressive disorder as an adjunct therapy
❖ **Other disorders**
  ○ Premenstrual dysphoric disorder
  ○ Bulimia nervosa
  ○ Borderline personality disorder
  ○ Episodes of binge drinking
  ○ Trichotillomania (trich)
  ○ Cluster headaches

Pharmacokinetics

❖ Lithium is readily absorbed with peak plasma levels occurring 2–4 hours after a single oral dose of lithium carbonate.
❖ Lithium is distributed rapidly in liver and kidney and more slowly in muscle, brain and bone. Steady state levels are achieved in about 7 days.
❖ Elimination is predominantly via kidneys. In the body lithium substitutes for sodium, calcium, potassium and magnesium. Lithium is reabsorbed in the proximal tubules and is influenced by sodium balance. Depletion of sodium can precipitate lithium toxicity.
❖ About 95% of lithium excretion is through the kidneys and the rest through sweat and feces. It is widely known to affect thyroid function most commonly resulting in hypothyroidism and goiter. Because of its narrow therapeutic index and quickly becoming fatal, initial and ongoing health assessment and laboratory monitoring is required.

Mechanism of Action

Specific action of lithium though unclear, probable mechanisms of action can be an impact on the neurotransmitters such as serotonin, norepinephrine, glutamate, GABA and dopamine. It has been suggested that lithium may correct an ion exchange abnormality in the neuron, normalize synaptic neurotransmission of norepinephrine, serotonin, dopamine and acetylcholine and regulate second-messenger systems during neurotransmission.

Dosage

Lithium is administered orally in tablet form, capsules or liquid. The tablet is available in a controlled release 450 mg tablet or a slow-release formulation in a 300 mg tablet. Capsules are available in 150 mg, 300 mg and 600 mg strength. Liquid formulation is available as 8 mEq/5 mL strength. The dosage usually starts at 300 mg twice or three times a day.

Treatment starts after serial lithium estimation with a loading dose of 600 mg or 900 mg of lithium per day. A single night time dose may be a considered to minimize side effects in stabilized patients. Lower doses and lower serum levels of lithium are preferred in elderly patients.

Blood Lithium Levels

Serum lithium levels are to be monitored 12 hours after the last dose. Monitoring should be done every 1 to 2 weeks until reaching the desired therapeutic levels. Then check lithium levels every 2 to 3 months.

❖ Therapeutic levels = 0.8–1.2 mEq/L (for treatment of acute mania)
❖ Prophylactic levels = 0.6–1.2 mEq/L (for prevention of relapse in bipolar disorder/chronic therapy)
❖ Toxic lithium levels >2.0 mEq/L

Side Effects

Lithium can cause several adverse effects which are dose-related. Notable side-effects are as follows **(Box 6.2):**

❖ **Neurological:** Fine hand tremors, motor hyperactivity, muscular weakness, cogwheel rigidity, confusion, memory problems, seizures, neurotoxicity (delirium, abnormal involuntary movements, seizures, coma).
❖ **Renal:** Polydipsia, polyuria, tubular enlargement, nephrotic syndrome.
❖ **Cardiovascular:** Bradycardia, flattened or inverted T waves, heart block and sick sinus syndrome.
❖ **Gastrointestinal:** Nausea, vomiting, diarrhea, abdominal pain and metallic taste.
❖ **Endocrine:** Euthyroid goiter or hypothyroid goiter and weight gain.

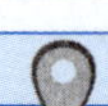

> **BOX 6.2:** Side effects of lithium
>
> ❑ Neurological effects
> ❑ Renal effects
> ❑ Cardiovascular effects
> ❑ Gastrointestinal effects
> ❑ Endocrine effects
> ❑ Hematological effects
> ❑ Dermatological effects
> ❑ Pregnancy and lactation effects
> ❑ Lithium toxicity

❖ **Hematologic:** Leukocytosis and aplastic anemia.

❖ **Dermatological:** Acne, skin rash and exacerbation of psoriasis.

❖ **Side-effects during pregnancy and lactation:** Teratogenic possibility, increased incidence of Ebstein's anomaly (distortion and downward displacement of tricuspid valve in right ventricle) when taken in first trimester. Secreted in milk, can cause toxicity in infant.

❖ **Lithium toxicity:** Lithium has a very narrow therapeutic index. Drug levels above 2 mEq/L are toxic which is very close to its therapeutic range. Common causes for an increase in lithium levels are reduced sodium intake, diuretic therapy, low renal function, fluid and electrolyte loss, sweating, diarrhea, dehydration, fever, vomiting, medical illness, over dose, etc. **(Box 6.3)**.

Management of Lithium Toxicity

❖ Lithium toxicity has no antidote.
❖ Discontinue the drug immediately.

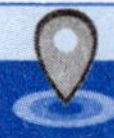

> **BOX 6.3:** Signs and symptoms of lithium toxicity
>
> ❑ Lithium toxicity can cause interstitial nephritis, arrhythmia, sick sinus syndrome, hypotension, T wave abnormalities and bradycardia.
> ❑ Prodrome of intoxication (lithium level ≥2.0 mEq/L) symptoms include anorexia, nausea, vomiting, diarrhea, deep tendon reflexes, ataxia, tinnitus, vertigo, weakness, drowsiness.
> ❑ Lithium intoxication (lithium level ≥2.5 mEq/L) symptoms include fever, decreased urine output, decreased blood pressure, irregular pulse, ECG changes, impaired consciousness, seizures, coma and death.

❖ Give hydration with normal saline which will enhance lithium excretion.

❖ For significant short-term ingestions, residual gastric content should be removed by induction of emesis, gastric lavage and adsorption with activated charcoal.

❖ If possible, instruct the patient to ingest fluids.

❖ Avoid all diuretics.

❖ Assess serum lithium levels, serum electrolytes, renal functions, ECG as soon as possible.

❖ Maintain fluid and electrolyte balance.

❖ In a patient with serious manifestations of lithium toxicity, hemodialysis should be initiated.

Contraindications of Lithium Use

❖ Pregnancy, breastfeeding
❖ Children below 12 years
❖ Cardiac, renal, thyroid or neurological dysfunctions
❖ Presence of blood dyscrasias
❖ During first trimester of pregnancy and lactation
❖ Severe dehydration
❖ History of seizures

Nurse's Responsibilities for a Patient Receiving Lithium

Every patient on lithium needs close monitoring. The psychiatrist generally prescribes lithium, but drug levels are monitored by the nurse.

The pre-lithium work up: A complete physical history, ECG, blood studies (TC, DC, FBS, BUN, creatinine, electrolytes) and urine examination (routine and microscopic), fasting blood sugar level must be carried out. It is important to assess renal function as renal side effects are common and the drug can be dangerous in an individual with compromised kidney function. Thyroid function should also be assessed as the drug is known to depress the thyroid gland.

Precautions to achieve therapeutic effect and prevent lithium toxicity

❖ Use of sustained-release capsules or dividing doses.

❖ Ensure adequate dietary sodium and fluid intake (2–3 liters per day).

❖ Replace fluid and electrolyte lost during exercise or gastrointestinal illness.

❖ Monitor signs and symptoms of lithium side effects and toxicity.

❖ Lithium must be taken on a regular basis preferably at the same time daily. If a patient misses the dose and fewer than 2 hours have elapsed, the missed dose can be taken right away; however, if longer than 2 hours have elapsed, the dose should be skipped and the next dose taken as scheduled; never double up on doses.

❖ When lithium therapy is initiated, mild side-effects such as fine hand tremors, increased thirst and urination, nausea, anorexia, etc. may develop. Most of them are transient and do not represent lithium toxicity.

❖ Serious side effects of lithium that necessitate its discontinuance include vomiting, extreme hand tremors, sedation, muscle weakness and vertigo. The psychiatrist should be notified immediately if any of these effects occur.

❖ Since polyuria can lead to dehydration with the risk of lithium intoxication, patients should be advised to drink enough water to compensate for the fluid loss.

❖ Various situations may require an adjustment in the amount of lithium administered to a patient such as the addition of a new medicine to the patient's drug regimen, a new diet or an illness with fever or excessive sweating. In this connection, people involved in heavy outdoor labor are prone to excessive sodium loss through sweating. They must be advised to consume large quantities of water with salt to prevent lithium toxicity due to decreased sodium levels. If severe vomiting or gastroenteritis develops, the patient should be told to report immediately to the doctor. These conditions have a high potential for causing lithium toxicity by lowering serum sodium levels.

❖ Frequent serum lithium level evaluation is important. Blood for determination of lithium levels should be drawn in the morning approximately 12 hours after the last dose was taken.

❖ Patient should be told about the importance of regular follow-up. Blood sample should be taken every six months for estimation of electrolytes, urea, creatinine, full blood count, and thyroid function test.

Carbamazepine

Carbamazepine is an anticonvulsant drug used as a mood stabilizer. It is available in the market under different trade names like Tegretol, Mazetol, Zeptol and Zen Retard.

Indications

❖ Seizures—complex partial seizures, generalized tonic clonic seizures, seizures due to alcohol withdrawal.

❖ Psychiatric disorders—bipolar disorder, resistant schizophrenia, acute depression, impulse control disorder, aggression, psychosis with epilepsy, schizoaffective disorders, alcohol withdrawal, and cocaine withdrawal syndrome.

❖ Paroxysmal pain syndromes—trigeminal neuralgia, restless leg syndrome and phantom limb pain.

Contraindications

❖ Hypersensitivity to carbamazepine or TCAs
❖ History of bone marrow depression
❖ Pregnancy and lactation
❖ Concomitant use of MAOIs
❖ Use cautiously with history of adverse hematologic reaction to any drug
❖ Glaucoma
❖ History of cardiac, hepatic or renal damage

Dosage

It is available as conventional 100 mg or 200 mg tablets, extended-release tablets of 100/200/300/400 mg, suspensions and solutions. The initial dose of 200 mg twice daily in adults and 100 mg twice daily in children aged under 12 is slowly increased to minimum effect level. The average daily dose of 600–1800 mg orally is administered in divided doses. Therapeutic blood levels are 6–12 µg/mL with toxic blood levels being more than 15 µg/mL.

Mechanism of Action

Its mood stabilizing mechanism is not clearly established. Its anticonvulsant action may be by decreasing the abnormal and excessive activity of the nerve cells in the brain.

Side Effects

Drowsiness, confusion, headache, ataxia, hypertension, arrhythmias, skin rashes, Steven-Johnson syndrome, nausea, vomiting, diarrhea, dry mouth, abdominal pain, jaundice, hepatitis, oliguria, leukopenia, thrombocytopenia, bone marrow depression leading to aplastic anemia.

Nurse's Responsibilities

- ❖ Since the drug may cause dizziness and drowsiness advise the patient to avoid driving and other activities requiring alertness.
- ❖ Advise patient not to consume alcohol when he is on the drug.
- ❖ Emphasize the importance of regular follow-up visits and periodic examination of blood count and monitoring of cardiac, renal, hepatic and bone marrow functions.
- ❖ Administer drug with food to prevent GI upset.
- ❖ Advise patient not to discontinue drug abruptly or change dosage except on the advice of physician.
- ❖ Counsel women who wish to become pregnant; advise the use of barrier contraceptives.

Sodium Valproate

Sodium valproate is an anticonvulsant drug used as a mood stabilizer. It is also known by the trade names Encorate Chrono, Valparin, Epilex, Epival, Epilim and Depakote.

Indications

- ❖ Acute mania, prophylactic treatment of bipolar I disorder, rapid cycling bipolar disorder
- ❖ Schizoaffective disorder
- ❖ Seizures
- ❖ Other disorders like bulimia nervosa, obsessive-compulsive disorder, agitation and post-traumatic stress disorder (PTSD)

Contraindications

Hypersensitivity to valproic acid, hepatic disease, use cautiously with children below 2 years, pregnancy and lactation.

Mechanism of Action

The drug acts on gamma-aminobutyric acid (GABA), an inhibitory amino acid neurotransmitter. GABA receptor activation serves to reduce neuronal excitability.

Dosage

The usual dose is 15 mg/kg/day with a maximum of 60 mg/kg/day orally.

Side Effects

Nausea, vomiting, diarrhea, sedation, dry or sore mouth or swollen gums, tremors, feeling tired or sleepy, headache, weight gain, loss of hair, thrombocytopenia, platelet dysfunction, irregular periods.

Nurse's Responsibilities

- ❖ Assess for hypersensitivity to valproic acid, hepatic dysfunction, pregnancy and lactation.
- ❖ Advise the patient to take the drug immediately after food to reduce GI irritation.
- ❖ Advise regular follow-up and periodic examination of blood count, hepatic function and thyroid function. Therapeutic serum level of valproic acid is 50–100 µg/mL.
- ❖ Discontinue drug at any sign of pancreatitis.
- ❖ Advise patient not to discontinue drug abruptly.
- ❖ Avoid alcohol and sleep inducing and over-the-counter drugs.

ANXIOLYTICS (ANTIANXIETY DRUGS) AND HYPNOSEDATIVES

Also called minor tranquilizers, most of them belong to the benzodiazepine group of drugs.

Classification

1. **Barbiturates:** For example, phenobarbital, pentobarbital, secobarbital and thiopentone.
2. **Non-barbiturate non-benzodiazepine antianxiety agents:** For example, Meprobamate glutethimide, ethanol, diphenhydramine and methaqualon.

3. **Benzodiazepines:** Presently benzodiazepines are the drugs of first choice in the treatment of anxiety and insomnia.
   - *Very short-acting*: For example, Triazolam, Midazolam
   - *Short-acting*: For example, Oxazepam (Serepax), Lorazepam (Ativan, Trapex, Larpose), Alprazolam (Restyl, Trika, Alzolam, Quiet, Anxit)
   - *Long-acting*: For example, Chlordiazepoxide (Librium), Diazepam (Valium, Calmpose), Clonazepam (Lonazep), Flurazepam (Nindral), Nitrazepam (Dormin).

Indications for Benzodiazepines

- Anxiety disorders
- Insomnia
- Depression
- Panic disorder and social phobia
- Obsessive-compulsive disorder
- Post-traumatic stress disorder
- Bipolar I disorder
- Other psychiatric indications include alcohol withdrawal, substance-induced and psychotic agitation

Contraindications

- Hypersensitivity to any antianxiety drugs
- Should not be taken in combination with other CNS depressants
- Pregnancy, lactation
- Narrow angle glaucoma
- Shock and coma
- Caution in elderly, debilitated clients
- Hepatic or renal dysfunction
- Caution in individuals with history of drug abuse and depressed or suicidal patients

Dosage (mg/day)

- **Alprazolam:** 0.5–6 mg PO
- **Oxazepam:** 15–120 mg PO
- **Lorazepam:** 2–6 mg PO/IV/IM
- **Diazepam:** 2–10 mg PO/IM/ slow IV
- **Clonazepam:** 0.5–20 mg PO/IM
- **Chlordiazepoxide:** 15–100 mg PO; 50–100 mg slow IV
- **Nitrazepam:** 5–20 mg PO

Mechanism of Action

Benzodiazepines bind to specific sites on the GABA receptors and increase the GABA level. Since GABA is an inhibitory neurotransmitter, it has a calming effect on the central nervous system thereby reducing anxiety.

Side Effects

Nausea, vomiting, weakness, vertigo, blurring of vision, body aches, epigastric pain, diarrhea, impotence, sedation, increased reaction time, ataxia, dry mouth, retrograde amnesia, impairment of driving skills, dependence and withdrawal symptoms (as a result the drug should be withdrawn slowly).

Symptoms of toxicity: Euphoria, slurred speech, disorientation, unsteady gait and impaired judgement. Symptoms of overdose: Respiratory depression, cold and clammy skin, hypotension, weak and rapid pulse, dilated pupils and coma.

Nurse's Responsibility in the Administration of Benzodiazepines

- Administer with food to minimize gastric irritation.
- Advise the patient to take medication exactly as directed. Abrupt withdrawal may cause insomnia, irritability and sometimes even seizures.
- Explain about adverse effects and advise him to avoid activities that require alertness.
- Caution the patient to avoid alcohol or any other CNS depressants along with benzodiazepines. Also instruct him not to take any over-the-counter (OTC) medications.
- If IM administration is preferred give deep IM.
- For IV administration do not mix with any other drug. Give slow IV as respiratory or cardiac arrest can occur; monitor vital signs during IV administration. Prevent extravasation as it might cause phlebitis and venous thrombosis.
- Regular use of these drugs often leads to "drug tolerance."

❖ Assess for symptoms of toxicity and overdose. These must be reported immediately to the physician.

(See Appendix 25 for Drug Guide)

ANTIPARKINSONIAN AGENTS

In clinical practice anticholinergic drugs, amantadine and antihistamines have their primary use as treatments for medication-induced movement disorders particularly neuroleptic-induced parkinsonism, acute dystonia and medication-induced tremor. The commonly used antiparkinsonian agents are: Anticholinergics (Examples: Trihexyphenidyl, Benztropine, Biperiden); Dopaminergic Agents (Examples: Bromocriptine, Carbidopa/Levodopa); Monoamine oxidase type B inhibitors (Example: Selegiline).

Trihexyphenidyl (Artane, Trihexane, Trihexy, Pacitane)

Indications

❖ Drug-induced parkinsonism
❖ Adjunct in the management of Parkinsonism

Mechanism of Action

It acts by increasing the release of dopamine from presynaptic vesicles, blocking the reuptake of dopamine into presynaptic nerve terminals or by exerting anagonist effect on postsynaptic dopamine receptors. Trihexyphenidyl reaches peak plasma concentrations in 2–3 hours after oral administration with duration of action up to 12 hours.

Dosage

1–2 mg/day orally initially, maximum dose up to 15 mg/day in divided doses.

Side Effects

Dizziness, nervousness, drowsiness, weakness, headache, confusion, blurred vision, mydriasis, tachycardia, orthostatic hypotension, dry mouth, nausea, constipation, vomiting, urinary retention and decreased sweating.

Nurse's Responsibilities

❖ Assess parkinsonian and extrapyramidal symptoms. Medication should be tapered gradually.
❖ Caution patient to change the position slowly to minimize orthostatic hypotension.
❖ Instruct the patient about frequent rinsing of mouth and good oral hygiene.
❖ Caution the patient that this medication reduces perspiration and overheating may occur during hot weather.

MISCELLANEOUS DRUGS

These include drugs used in deaddiction, child psychiatry, eating disorders, stimulants, vitamins, calcium channel blockers, etc.

Drugs Used in Deaddiction

Commonly used drugs are antabuse and anticraving drugs.

Disulfiram (antabuse drug): It is an important drug in this class and is used to ensure abstinence in the treatment of alcohol dependence. Its main effect is to produce a rapid and violently unpleasant reaction in a person who ingests even a small amount of alcohol while taking disulfiram.

Anticraving drugs: Through detoxification process withdrawal symptoms of a particular type of drug or chemical are managed as the toxins from the drug are removed from the body. Removal of the drug from the body is accompanied by physical, psychological and emotional cravings. A number of stimuli can put off a craving response within the brain. Anticraving drugs seem to work by blocking the receptors associated with cues that setoff relapse. Several different addictions (alcoholism, opiate addiction, nicotine addiction and cocaine addiction) are being treated with use of anticraving medications after detoxification. These drugs are used to help prevent relapse both during the detox phase and in early recovery phase. Commonly used anticraving drugs are Naltrexone, Naloxone, Subutex, Topiramate, Baclofen, Acamprosate, Methadone, Neurontin, etc. *(Refer Chapter 5—Page No. 251 for detailed description on disulfiram and anticraving drugs)*

Drugs Used in Child Psychiatry

Commonly used medications in child psychiatry are clonidine and methylphenidate.

Clonidine

Clonidine is an imidazoline derivative used as an antihypertensive agent.

Indications

- Attention deficit hyperactivity
- Control of withdrawal symptoms from opioids
- Tourette's disorder
- Control of aggressive or hyperactive behavior in children
- Autism
- Highly irritable, impulsive and aggressive children

Mechanism of action

- Alpha 2 adrenergic receptor agonist.
- The agonist effects of clonidine on presynaptic alpha 2 adrenergic receptors result in a decrease in the amount of neurotransmitter released from the presynaptic nerve terminals. This decrease serves generally to reset the sympathetic tone at a lower level and reduce arousal.

Dosage

Usual starting dosage is 0.1 mg orally twice a day; the dosage can be raised by 0.3 mg a day to an appropriate level.

Side effects

Dry mouth, dryness of eyes, fatigue, irritability, sedation, dizziness, nausea, vomiting, hypotension and constipation.

Nurse's responsibility

Monitor BP. The drug should be withheld if the patient becomes hypotensive. Advise frequent mouth rinses and good oral hygiene for dry mouth.

Methylphenidate (Ritalin)

Methylphenidate, dextroamphetamine and pemoline are sympathomimetics.

Indications

- Attention-deficit hyperactivity disorder
- Narcolepsy
- Depressive disorders
- Obesity

Mechanism of action

Sympathomimetics cause the stimulation of alpha and beta-adrenergic receptors directly as agonists and indirectly by stimulating the release of dopamine and norepinephrine from presynaptic terminals. Dextroamphetamine and methylphenidate are also inhibitors of catecholamine reuptake especially dopamine reuptake and inhibitors of monoamine oxidase. The net result of these activities is believed to be the stimulation of several brain regions.

Dosage

Starting dose is 5–10 mg/day orally, maximum daily dose is 80 mg/day.

Side effects

Anorexia or dyspepsia, weight loss, slowed growth, dizziness, insomnia or nightmares, dysphoric mood, tics and psychosis.

Nurse's responsibilities

- Assess mental status for change in mood, level of activity, degree of stimulation and aggressiveness.
- Ensure patient is protected from injury.
- Keep stimuli low and environment as quiet as possible to discourage over stimulation.
- To treat anorexia, administer the medication immediately after meals.
- Weigh the patient regularly (at least weekly) during hospitalization and at home while on therapy with CNS stimulants due to the potential for anorexia/weight loss and temporary interruptions of growth and development.
- To prevent insomnia, administer last dose at least 6 hours before bedtime.
- In children with behavioral disorders, a drug 'holiday' should be attempted periodically under the direction of the physician to determine effectiveness of the medication and the need for continuation.
- Ensure that parents are aware of the delayed effects of ritalin. They should be asked not to discontinue the drug for lack of immediate results as the therapeutic response may not be seen for 2–4 weeks.

- ❖ Inform parents that OTC (over-the-counter) medications should be avoided while the child is on stimulant medication. Some OTC medications particularly cold and hay fever preparations contain certain sympathomimetic agents that could compound the effects of the stimulant and create drug interactions that may be toxic to the child.
- ❖ Ensure parents are aware that the drug should not be withdrawn abruptly. Withdrawal should be gradual and under the direction of the physician.

ELECTROCONVULSIVE THERAPY

Electroconvulsive therapy (ECT) is a type of somatic treatment, first introduced by Bini and Cerletti in April 1938. From 1980 onwards ECT is being considered as a unique psychiatric treatment. In this form of treatment, a seizure is artificially induced in an anesthetized patient by passing an electric current through electrode applied to the patient's head. It involves applying a brief electrical pulse to the scalp after the patients are administered muscle relaxants and general anesthesia.

Parameters of Electrical Current Applied

ECT uses an electrical current to cause a seizure which is when a burst of electrical activity happens in the brain causing affected brain cells to fire rapidly. This causes electrical and chemical changes. Presently, ECT uses constant current (0.8 or 0.9 Ampere) administered in brief pulses (typically with a pulse width of 0.25–1.5 ms) in varying frequencies and stimulus train durations (typically up to 8 s).

Type of Seizure Produced

- ❖ ECT stimulation induces a typical generalized tonic-clonic seizures.
- ❖ Seizures from ECT typically last between 30 and 90 seconds.

Mechanism of Action

Though the exact mechanism of action is not known, the ECT however affects multiple central nervous system components including hormones, neuropeptides, neurotropic factors and neurotransmitters. The induction of a bilateral generalized seizures is required for effects of ECT.

Types of ECT

Direct ECT: In this, ECT is given in the absence of anesthesia and muscular relaxation. This is not a commonly used method now. Use of direct or unmodified ECT is prohibited under 'The Mental Health Care Act 2017'.

Modified ECT: Here ECT is modified by drug-induced muscular relaxation and general anesthesia.

Frequency and Total Number of ECT

Frequency: Two or three times per week or as indicated.

Total number: A course of ECT for depression consists of 6 to 12 sessions. Patients with schizophrenia require more treatment sessions.

Once the patient achieves remission of symptoms, the ECT course can be terminated. If a patient does not show noticeable improvement within 6 sessions, change of technique may be considered.

Application of Electrodes

There are three different ways that electrodes can be applied **(Figure 6.10)**:

1. **Unilateral ECT (ULECT):** In this, both electrodes are placed on the non-dominant side (usually right side) of the head to minimize cognitive deficits.
2. **Bilateral/bitemporal ECT (BTECT):** Electrodes are placed on the fronto-temporal sites on each side.
3. **Bifrontal ECT (BFECT):** Electrodes are placed 5 cm vertically above the outer canthus of each eye along an imaginary vertical line perpendicular to a line connecting the pupils.

Indications

ECT is indicated in patients with following conditions **(Figure 6.11)**:

1. **Major depression**: With suicidal risk; stupor; poor intake of food and fluids; melancholia with psychotic features;

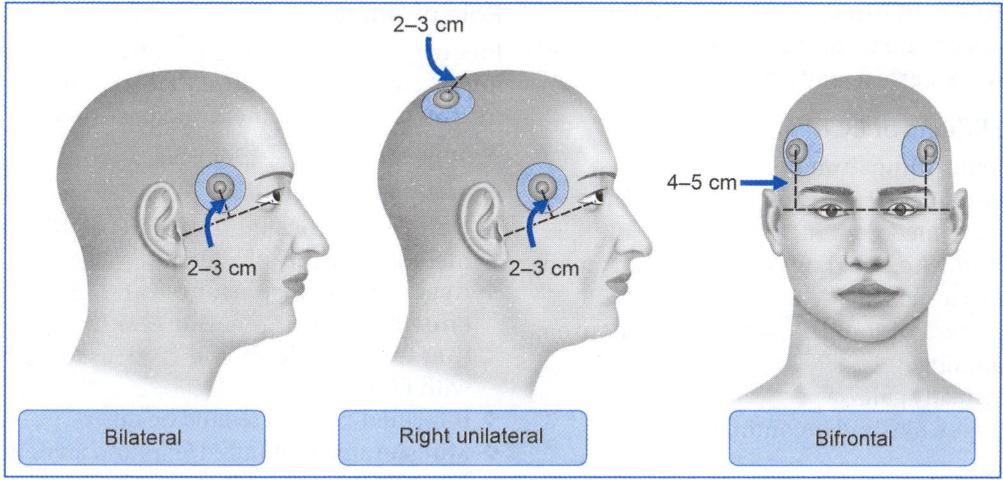

Figure 6.10: Application of ECT electrodes

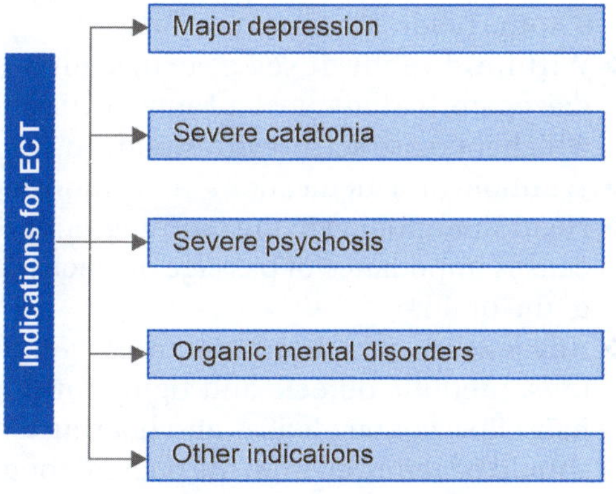

Figure 6.11: Indications for ECT

unsatisfactory response to drugs or where drugs are contraindicated or have serious side effects.

2. **Severe catatonia (functional):** With stupor; poor intake of food and fluids; unsatisfactory response to drug therapy, or when drugs are contraindicated or have serious side effects.

3. **Severe psychosis (schizophrenia or mania):** With risk of suicide, homicide or danger of physical assault; depressive features; unsatisfactory response to drug therapy or when drugs are contraindicated or have serious side effects.

4. **Organic mental disorders:**
   - Organic mood disorders
   - Organic psychosis

5. **Other indications:** ECT is preferred over antidepressant therapy in some cases such as patients with cardiac disease; when tricyclics are contraindicated because of the potential for dysrhythmias and congestive heart failure; and for pregnant women in whom antidepressants place the fetus at risk for congenital defects. It may have a safer profile than antidepressants or antipsychotics in debilitated elderly and breastfeeding patients. It is also recommended for patients who have exhibited a favorable response to ECT previously.

Contraindications

A. Absolute: Raised ICP (intracranial pressure)
B. Relative:
   - Cerebral aneurysm
   - Cerebral hemorrhage
   - Brain tumor
   - Acute myocardial infarction
   - Congestive heart failure
   - Pneumonia or aortic aneurysm
   - Retinal detachment
   - High-risk pregnancies

Complications of ECT

Life-threatening complications of ECT are rare. ECT does not cause any brain damage. Fractures can sometimes occur in elderly patients with osteoporosis. In patients with a history of heart disease, dysrhythmias and respiratory arrest may occur.

Side Effects of ECT

- Memory impairment
- Drowsiness, confusion and restlessness
- Poor concentration, anxiety
- Headache, weakness/fatigue, backache, muscle aches
- Dryness of mouth, palpitations, nausea, vomiting
- Unsteady gait
- Tongue bite and incontinence

ECT Team

It is typically administered by a team of trained medical professionals that includes a psychiatrist, anesthesiologist, trained nurses and aides.

Treatment Facilities and Equipment

There should be a suite of three rooms:
1. A pleasant, comfortable waiting room (pre-ECT room).
2. ECT room equipped with ECT machine and accessories **(Table 6.3)**.
3. A well-equipped recovery room

TABLE 6.3: List of drugs and equipment in ECT station	
List of drugs in ECT station	**List of equipment in ECT station**
• IV fluids • Thiopentone • Succinylcholine • Atropine • Diazepam • Beta blockers • Vasodilators • Antiarrhythmic drugs • Ketamine • Bronchodilators • Antiemetics • Analgesics (According to American Psychiatric Association, 2005)	• Mouth gags • Resuscitation apparatus • Infusion sets • Intravenous fluids • Oxygen masks • Airways • Curved tongue depressors • Endotracheal tubes • Suction catheters • Electrode gel • Electrode pads and leads • ECT devise • Disposable gloves • Biometric waste bins • Immediate access to defibrillator

Role of Nurse

Electroconvulsive therapy is treated like a minor surgical procedure that requires pre-treatment, intra treatment and post-treatment nursing care.

Pre-treatment Evaluation

- Detailed medical and psychiatric history including history of allergies.
- Assessment of patients' and family's knowledge of indications, side-effects, therapeutic effects and risks associated with ECT.
- Informed consent should be taken.
- Mitigate any unfounded fears and anxieties regarding the procedure.
- Assess baseline vital signs.
- Patient should avoid food intake for at least 6 hours before treatment.
- Withhold night doses of drugs such as diazepam, barbiturates and anticonvulsants which increase seizure threshold.
- Withhold oral medications in the morning.
- Head shampooing in the morning since oil causes impedance of passage of electricity to the brain.
- Any jewelry, prosthesis, dentures, contact lens, metallic objects and tight clothing, hair clips, contact lenses and hearing aids should be removed from the patient's body.
- Hair should be dry and clean (damp hair and presence of cream may lead to short circuiting of the current over scalp).
- Empty bladder and bowel just before ECT.
- Administration of 0.6 mg atropine IM or SC 30 minutes before ECT or IV just before ECT.

Intraprocedure Care

- Place the patient comfortably on the ECT table in supine position.
- Stay with the patient to allay anxiety and fear.
- Assist in administering the anesthetic agent (thiopental sodium 3–5 mg/kg body weight) and muscle relaxant (0.5–1 mg/kg body weight of succinylcholine).
- Since the muscle relaxant paralyzes all muscles including respiratory muscles, patent airway should be ensured and ventilatory support started.

- ❖ Mouth gag should be inserted to prevent possible tongue bite.
- ❖ The place(s)of electrode placement should be cleaned with normal saline or 25% bicarbonate solution, or a conducting gel applied.
- ❖ Monitor voltage, intensity and duration of electrical stimulus given.
- ❖ Monitor seizure activity using cuff method.
- ❖ 100% oxygen should be provided.
- ❖ During seizure monitor vital signs, ECG, oxygen saturation, EEG, etc.
- ❖ Record the findings and medicines given in the patient's chart.

Post-procedure Care

- ❖ Monitor vital signs.
- ❖ Continue oxygenation till spontaneous respiration starts.
- ❖ Assess for postictal confusion and restless-ness.
- ❖ Take safety precautions to prevent injury (side-lying position and suctioning to prevent aspiration of secretions, use of side rails to prevent falls).
- ❖ If there is severe postictal confusion and restlessness, IV diazepam may be adminis-tered.
- ❖ Reorient the patient after recovery and stay with him until fully oriented.
- ❖ Close monitoring of cognitive deficits.
- ❖ Documentary findings as relevant in the patient's record.

  (See Appendix 14 for ECT History Collection Format)

REPETITIVE TRANSCRANIAL MAGNETIC STIMULATION (rTMS)

It is a noninvasive brain stimulation therapy which uses electromagnetic pulses to stimulate nerve cells through the production of the high or low intensity magnetic field. rTMS refers to applying recurring TMS pulses to a specific region of the brain.

Mechanism of Action

TMS is a medical device which applies electrical pulses to the brain using a magnetic coil held over the head. An electric current is delivered to the coil by a stimulator and the current flowing through the loops in the coil generates a magnetic field. This magnetic field goes through the head to the brain where it produces an electric stimulation to the brain. Through TMS a series of short magnetic pulses are directed to the brain to stimulate nerve cells. The magnetic pulses stimulate areas of neurons and change the functioning of the brain circuits involved.

Indications

- ❖ Treatment resistant depression
- ❖ Obsessive compulsive disorder
- ❖ Post-traumatic stress disorder
- ❖ Generalized anxiety disorder
- ❖ Bipolar disorder
- ❖ Movement disorders

Contraindications

- ❖ Patient with seizures
- ❖ Substance use
- ❖ Person with metal or implanted medical devices such as pacemakers, cochlear implants for hearing, aneurysm clips, etc.
- ❖ Psychosis
- ❖ Brain tumor
- ❖ Traumatic brain injury
- ❖ Stroke
- ❖ Frequent headaches

Side Effects

- ❖ Headache
- ❖ Tingling, spasms or twitching of facial muscles
- ❖ Light-headedness
- ❖ Seizures
- ❖ Hearing loss if ears are not protected during the procedure

Care Before Procedure

- ❖ Obtain informed consent
- ❖ Evaluate for contraindications
- ❖ Remove all metals, jewelry or anything that would be sensitive to a magnet
- ❖ Cover ears with earplugs as rTMS makes a loud noise

Care During Procedure

- ❖ Make the patient to sit in a comfortable reclining chair.

❖ Technician will take measurements to find the best place to put the electromagnetic coil that will deliver the magnetic pulses.

❖ Technician positions the electromagnetic coil on the head and moves the coil around the head.

❖ The patient feels and hears rapid tapping on the scalp. The pattern may be few seconds of tapping followed by a pause.

❖ Depending on the type of stimulation pattern used, the procedure will last for 5–20 minutes. The course is approximately 4–6 weeks.

❖ The patient remains awake during the procedure and will be sitting comfortably in a recliner throughout the session.

After Care

❖ Patient can return to normal daily activities immediately following the procedure.

❖ Patient may have headache for a short time.

KETAMINE THERAPY

Ketamine is a noncompetitive *N*-methyl-D-aspartate (NMDA) receptor antagonist that has traditionally been used for the induction and maintenance of anesthesia. Ketamine infusion therapy involves the administration of a single infusion or a series of infusions for the management of major depressive disorder, post-traumatic stress disorder, acute suicidality or chronic pain.

Mechanism of Action

❖ Ketamine infusion therapy has been shown to have antidepressant properties.

❖ Ketamine targets the brain's NMDA receptors. It binds to these receptors and increases the level of glutamate.

❖ Glutamate activates AMPA receptors. The activation allows the neurons to communicate better along the new pathways. This process enhances cognition, mood and thought patterns.

❖ Ketamine can also affect depression by reducing inflammatory signals. These signals have a connection to several mood disorders.

Dose

❖ Usual starting dose is 0.5 mg/kg with an increase up to 1.0 mg/kg depending on the response.

❖ Frequency: Twice per week for 4–5 weeks with taper.

❖ Most patients could receive 3–6 infusions.

Considerations

❖ Intravenous ketamine therapy should not be considered for the initial treatment of psychiatric disorders or chronic pain management.

❖ It should only be considered after failure of standard treatment such as no improvement after administration of antidepressants, different medication combinations and or ECT or transcranial magnetic stimulation, no sustained change in response to psychological therapies such as cognitive behavioral therapy or individual therapy.

Indications

❖ Adults with moderate to severe depression.

❖ Adults experiencing acute suicidality.

❖ Adults experiencing post-traumatic stress disorder.

❖ Individuals diagnosed with bipolar disorder.

❖ Individuals diagnosed with personality disorders.

❖ Individuals suffering with chronic pain.

Contraindications

❖ Active substance abuse

❖ History of psychosis

❖ History of increased intracranial pressure

❖ Pregnancy

❖ Uncontrolled hypertension

❖ Acute or unstable cardiovascular disease

❖ Previous negative response to ketamine

Side Effects

Nausea, high blood pressure, some patients may experience perceptual disturbances, there could also be dissociation or out of body experiences.

Equipment

❖ Infusion room

❖ Recovery area
❖ IV infusion equipment
❖ BP apparatus
❖ Oxygen administration equipment
❖ Emergency medications
❖ Clinical assessment tools to assess level of depression, anxiety, etc.

Procedure

❖ The patient should not eat or drink before the therapy.
❖ Trained nurse will start the IV connection.
❖ Slow infusion with over 40 minutes.

Risks

❖ Ketamine may have addictive properties.
❖ The patient must only receive it under the supervision of medical staff.

Role of a Nurse Before Ketamine Therapy

❖ Provide education to patient and caregiver.
❖ **Obtain informed consent:** It includes risks, benefits, potential side effects as well as alternative therapies and the risks and potential side effects.
❖ Comprehensive diagnostic assessment is got done to rule out diagnosis of current and past substance use and psychotic disorders.
❖ A baseline urine toxicology screen is recommended to ensure the accuracy of the reported substance use and medication record.
❖ Collect detailed and thorough history of previous antidepressant treatment to confirm adequate trial.
❖ Review current medications and allergies including histories of opiate and benzodiazepine use.
❖ Obtain baseline symptom severity to assess clinical improvement with treatment at a later stage.
❖ Obtain physician consultation for general medical clearance, specialty medical clearance—cardiac, neurological, ophthalmological, urologic as necessary based on history.
❖ Pre-procedure labs—Ensure liver function test and creatinine levels are got done.

❖ Establish process for infusion and medication orders.
❖ Evaluate contraindications to ketamine.
❖ Ketamine procedure may take 90–120 minutes.

Role of a Nurse During Treatment

❖ Ketamine is administered intravenously.
❖ Keep low stimuli environment when ketamine is administered.
❖ During procedure monitor the following—vital signs, blood pressure, level of consciousness, signs and symptoms of ketamine toxicity, dissociative effects.
❖ During administration the nurse monitors the patient and side effects. Common side effects include sedation, dissociation, dizziness, nausea, vertigo, anxiety, increased blood pressure and changes in reaction time and motor skills.
❖ After the procedure normal diet and medications may resume.

Role of a Nurse After Treatment

❖ The nurse monitors cognitive and physical functioning until the patient gets back to baseline. These include limb movement, vital signs, pupillary response, etc.
❖ Patients are not released to ward/unit until they are at baseline or no longer feeling the effects of ketamine. These are stable vital signs, alert and absence of dissociative effects.
❖ Assess depression and anxiety level 24 hours after administration of ketamine to assess progress.

Follow-up

❖ Patient should be monitored closely using a rating scale to assess clinical change to better re-evaluate the risk to benefit ratio of continued treatment.
❖ Assessments of cognitive function, urinary discomfort and substance use should be considered if repeated administrations are provided.
❖ Considering the known potential for abuse of ketamine, clinicians should be vigilant

about assessing the potential for patients to develop ketamine use disorder.

❖ The number and frequency of treatments should be limited to the minimum necessary to achieve clinical response.

PSYCHOLOGICAL THERAPIES

Psychological therapies refer to a variety of treatments that aim to help an individual to identify and manage disturbed thoughts, emotions and behavior. There are several types of therapies that are used to deal with psychological problems. Most of these therapies are conducted by a psychologist or a psychiatrist. Though the nurses may or may not be actively involved in the therapy, to provide continuity in patient care they must understand the basic principles of various therapies. Commonly used therapies are psychotherapy, behavioral therapy and cognitive behavior therapy.

Psychotherapy

Psychotherapy is referred to as a systemic treatment primarily employing verbal communication as the means of treatment aimed at relieving the patient's symptoms and helping him to understand and modify his conduct so as to lead a well-adjusted life. Various types of psychotherapies are presented in **Table 6.4**.

Psychoanalytic Therapy

Psychoanalysis was first developed by Sigmund Freud at the end of the 19th century. The most important indication for psychoanalytical therapy is the presence of long-standing mental conflicts which may be unconscious but produce symptoms. In psychoanalysis focus is on the cause of the problem, which is buried somewhere in the unconscious. The therapist tries to take the patient into the past in an effort to determine where the problem began. The aim of the therapy is to bring all repressed material to conscious awareness so that the patient can work towards a healthy resolution of his problems which are causing the symptoms.

TABLE 6.4: Types of psychotherapy

Dimension	Types
Depending on the number of patients taking part	◆ Individual psychotherapy ◆ Group psychotherapy
Depending on the duration of treatment	◆ Long-term psychotherapy ◆ Short-term psychotherapy
Depending on the depth of exploration	◆ Supportive psychotherapy ◆ Deep psychotherapy
Depending on the amount of responsibility given to the patient	◆ Directive ◆ Non-directive
Depending on the nature of the group	◆ Family therapy ◆ Marital therapy ◆ Group therapy ◆ Therapy with children and adolescents, etc.

Therapy process

It is typical for the psychoanalyst to be positioned at the head of the patient and slightly behind so that the patient cannot see the therapist. This limits any kind of non-verbal communication between the two people. The patient is typically on the couch, relaxed, and ready to focus on the therapist's instruction, which facilitates free association. The roles of the patient and psychoanalyst are explicitly defined by Freud. The patient is an active participant, freely revealing all thoughts exactly as they occur and describing all dreams. The psychoanalyst is a shadow-person. He reveals nothing personal, nor does he give any directions to the patient. His verbal responses are for the most part brief and non-committal, so as not to interfere with the associative flow. He departs from this style of communication when an interpretation of behavior is made to the patient.

Some of the techniques used in psychoanalysis are free association, dream analysis, hypnosis, catharsis and abreaction therapy **(Figure 6.12)**.

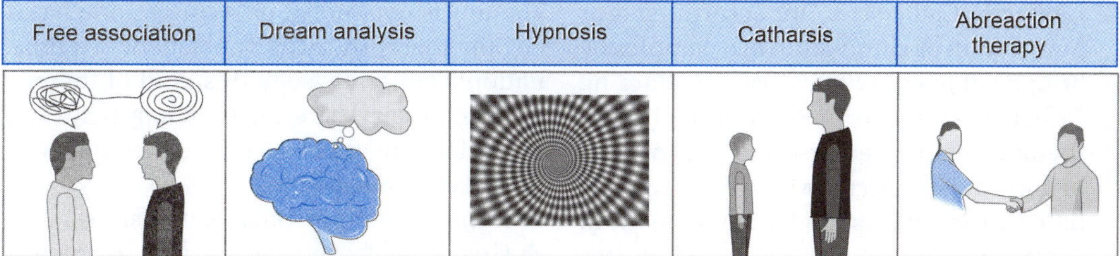

Figure 6.12: Techniques used in psychoanalysis

1. **Free association:** In free association, the patient is allowed to say whatever crosses his mind in response to a word that is given by the therapist. For example, the therapist might say 'mother' or 'blue' and the patient would give a response also typically one word to each of the words the therapist utters. The therapist then looks for a theme or pattern to the patient's responses. So, if the patient responds 'evil' to the word 'mother' or 'dead' to the word 'blue' the therapist might pick up one potential theme, but if the patient responds 'kind' and 'true' to the words 'mother' and 'blue' respectively, the therapist might hear a completely different theme. The theme may give the therapist an idea of the cause of patient's emotional disturbance.

2. **Dream analysis:** Freud believed that behavior is rooted in the unconscious and that dreams are a manifestation of the troubles people repress. A better way to get an idea of the problem is to monitor and interpret dreams. The patient is asked to keep a dream lag (incorporation into dreams the daytime experiences that have occurred approximately one week prior to the dream). Analysis of the patient's dreams helps to gain additional insight into his problem and the resistances. Thus, dreams symbolically communicate areas of intrapsychic conflict. The therapist then attempts to assist the patient to recognize his intrapsychic conflicts through the use of interpretation. The process is complicated by the occurrence of transference reactions. This refers to the patient's development of strong positive or negative feelings towards the analyst which represent the patient's past response to a significant other usually a parent. The therapist's reciprocal response to the patient is called countertransference. Such reactions must be handled appropriately before progress can be made. By termination of therapy, the patient is able to conduct his life according to an accurate assessment of external reality and is also able to relate to others uninhibited by neurotic conflicts. Psychoanalytical therapy is a long-term proposition. The patient is seen frequently, usually five times a week. It is therefore time-consuming and expensive.

3. **Hypnosis:** Hypnosis is an artificially induced state in which the person is relaxed and usually suggestible. It is a means for entering an altered state of consciousness in which desired changes in behavior and thinking can be brought about using visualization and suggestion. Relaxation procedure is guided by the therapist. Hypnosis can be induced in many ways such as by using a fixed point for attention, rhythmic monotonous instructions, etc.

   In hypnotherapy, relaxation is guided by the therapist who has been trained in techniques of trance formation and who then asks certain questions of the patient or uses guided imagery to help picture the situation in an effort to find the cause of the problem. At the end of the session, the therapist leaves some helpful hints for the patients. These are called posthypnotic suggestions and typically include positive, affirming statements for the patient to think about as well as instructions to help the person accomplish self-hypnosis.

4. **Catharsis:** Catharsis is, "the act of purging or purification or elimination of a complex by bringing it to consciousness and affording to expression". In psychoanalysis, the therapist helps the person to see the root of the problem and then by talking or some other means allows the patient to learn to evacuate this problem from the mind. This can take place in conjunction with other form of psychoanalysis.

These therapies are undertaken on a one-to-one basis between patient and the therapist. The nurse can be helpful in the treatment process by allowing the patient to talk about the experiences in therapy and by carefully documenting the responses of the patient.

5. **Abreaction therapy:** Abreaction is a process by which repressed material, particularly a painful experience or conflict is brought back to consciousness. The person not only recalls but also relives the material which is accompanied by an appropriate emotional response. It is most useful in acute neurotic conditions caused by extreme stress (post-traumatic stress disorder, hysteria, etc.). Although abreaction is an integral part of psychoanalysis and hypnosis it can also be used independently.

Abreaction can be brought about by a strong encouragement to relive the stressful events. The procedure is begun with neutral topics at first and gradually approaching areas of conflict. Although abreaction can be done with or without the use of medication, the procedure can be facilitated by giving a sedative drug intravenously. A safe method is the use of thiopentone sodium, 500 mg dissolved in 10 cc of normal saline. It is infused at a rate no faster than 1 cc/minute to prevent sleep as well as respiratory depression.

Individual Psychotherapy

Individual psychotherapy is a method of bringing change in a person by exploring his or her feelings, attitudes, thinking and behavior.

Therapy is conducted on a one-to-one basis, i.e., the therapist treats one patient at a time. Patients generally seek this kind of therapy based on their desire. Such therapy helps to:

❖ Understand themselves and their behavior
❖ Make personal changes
❖ Improve interpersonal relationships
❖ Get relief from emotional pain or unhappiness

Indications

Stress-related disorders, alcohol and drug dependence, sexual disorders and marital disharmony.

Therapy process

The patient is encouraged to discover for himself the reasons for his behavior. The therapist listens to the patient and offers explanation and advice when necessary. By this he helps the patient to come to a greater understanding of self and find a way of dealing with his problems. The relationship between the patient and the therapist proceeds through stages similar to those of the nurse–patient relationship: introduction, working and termination *(See Appendix 15 for Psychotherapy Format)*

Supportive Psychotherapy

In this, the therapist helps the patient to relieve emotional distress and symptoms without probing into the past and changing the personality. He uses various techniques such as:

❖ **Ventilation:** It is a free expression of feelings or emotions. Patient is encouraged to talk freely whatever crosses his mind.
❖ **Environmental modification/manipulation:** Improving the well-being of mental patients by changing their living condition.
❖ **Persuasion:** Here the therapist attempts to modify the patient's behavior by reasoning.
❖ **Re-education:** Educating the patient regarding his problems, ways of coping, etc.
❖ **Reassurance:** Reassurance is used to dispel apprehension and restore confidence and promote hope. However, care should be

taken against offering false reassurance and providing it prematurely even before the patient has fully opened up.

❖ **Explanation:** Explanation of the nature of symptoms and their causes is done by the therapist during the therapy. The choice of treatment and the likely outcome are explained to the patient.

❖ **Guidance:** Guidance involves offering direct advice on handling particularly difficult situation in patient's real life. He may be advised on how and when he should seek help in future.

Phases of Therapy

1. Initial phase focuses on assessment and relationship formation. Assessment encompasses full physical and psychiatric evaluation including level of motivation, patient's strengths and weaknesses. The therapist should be able to empathize with the patient in order to understand him better.

2. The working phase involves intense therapeutic activity with further exploration of the patient's problems and life situations. The various therapeutic techniques are applied and attempts are made to give the patient an insight into his problems.

3. The terminal phase intends to strengthen the patient's improvement and prepare him to end his treatment.

Behavior Therapy

It is a form of treatment for problems in which a trained person deliberately establishes a professional relationship with the patient, with an objective to remove or modify existing symptoms and promote positive personality, growth and development. Behavior therapy involves identifying maladaptive behaviors and seeking to correct these by applying the principles of learning derived from the following theories:

❖ Classical conditioning model by Ivan Pavlov (1936).

❖ Operant conditioning model by BF Skinner (1953).

Major assumptions of behavior therapy

Based on the above-mentioned theories following are the assumptions of behavior therapy:

❖ All behavior is learned (adaptive and maladaptive).

❖ Human beings are passive organisms that can be conditioned or shaped to do anything if correct responses are rewarded or reinforced.

❖ Maladaptive behavior can be unlearned and replaced by adaptive behavior if the person receives exposure to specific stimuli and reinforcement for the desired adaptive behavior.

❖ Behavioral assessment is focused more on the current behavior rather than on historical antecedents.

❖ Treatment strategies are individually tailored.

Behavior therapy is a short duration therapy which is cost-effective. The total duration of therapy is usually 6–8 weeks. Initial sessions are given daily, but the later sessions are spaced out. Unlike psycho-analysis where the therapist is a shadow person, in behavior therapy both the patient and therapist are equal participants. There is no attempt to unearth an underlying conflict and the patient is not encouraged to explore his past.

Behavior therapy techniques

Behavior therapy techniques are based on the classical and operant conditioning theories. These techniques help the client to change their behavior and promote psychological health. The commonly used techniques are presented in **Figure 6.13.**

1. **Systematic desensitization:** It was developed by Joseph Wolpe based on the behavioral principle of counter conditioning. In this, patients attain a state of complete relaxation who are then exposed to the stimulus that elicits the anxiety response. The negative reaction of anxiety is inhibited by the relaxed state, a process called reciprocal inhibition.

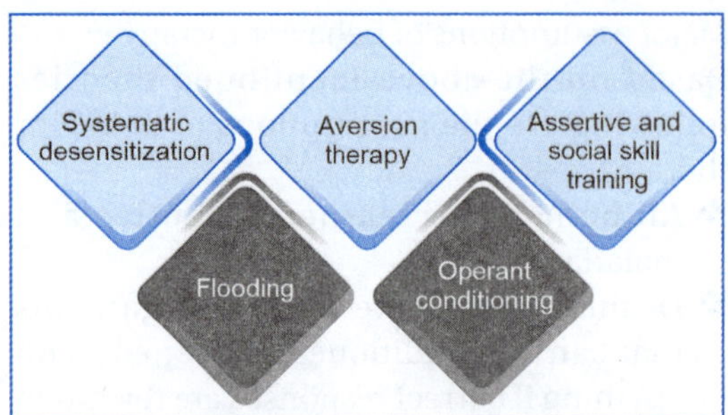

Figure 6.13: Behavior therapy techniques

It consists of three main steps:

a. *Relaxation training:* There are many methods which can be used to induce relaxation. Some of them are:
   - Jacobson's progressive muscle relaxation
   - Hypnosis
   - Meditation or yoga
   - Mental imagery
   - Biofeedback

b. *Hierarchy construction:* Here the patient is asked to list all the conditions which provoke anxiety. He is then asked to list them in descending order of anxiety provocation.

c. *Desensitization of the stimulus:* This can either be done in reality or through imagination. At first, the lowest item in hierarchy is confronted. The patient is advised to signal whenever anxiety is produced. With each signal he is asked to relax. After a few trials, patient is able to control his anxiety gradually.

   Indications:
   - Phobias
   - Obsessions
   - Compulsions
   - Certain sexual disorders

2. **Flooding:** The patient is directly exposed to phobic stimulus but escape is made impossible. Prolonged contact with the phobic stimulus, therapist's guidance and encouragement and his modeling behavior reduce anxiety.

Indication: Specific phobias

3. **Aversion therapy:** Pairing of the pleasant stimulus with an unpleasant response so that even in absence of the unpleasant response the pleasant stimulus becomes unpleasant by association. Punishment is presented immediately after a specific behavioral response and the response is eventually inhibited. Unpleasant response is produced by electric stimulus, drugs, social disapproval or even fantasy.

Indications:
   - Alcohol abuse
   - Paraphilias
   - Homosexuality
   - Transvestism

4. **Operant conditioning procedures for increasing adaptive behavior**

   a. *Positive reinforcement:* When a behavioral response is followed by a generally rewarding event such as food, praise or gifts, it tends to be strengthened and occurs more frequently than before the reward. This technique is used to increase desired behavior.

   b. *Token economy:* This program involves giving token rewards for appropriate or desired target behaviors performed by the patient. The token can later be exchanged for other rewards. For example, in inpatient hospital wards patients receive a reward for performing a desired behavior such as tokens which they may use to purchase luxury items or certain privileges.

5. **Operant conditioning procedures to teach new behavior**

   a. *Modeling:* Modeling is a method of teaching by demonstration wherein the therapist shows how a specific behavior is to be performed. In modeling, the patient observes other patients indulging in target behaviors and getting rewards for those behaviors. This will make the patient repeat the same behavior and earn rewards in the same manner.

   b. *Shaping:* In shaping the components of a particular skill the behavior is reinforced step-by-step. The therapist starts shaping by reinforcing the existing behavior. Once it is established, he reinforces the responses which are closest to the desired behavior and ignores the other responses. For example, to establish eye-to-eye contact the therapist sits opposite the patient and reinforces him even if he moves his upper body towards him. Once this is established he reinforces the person's head movement in his direction and this procedure continues till eye-to-eye contact is established.

c. *Chaining*: Chaining is used when a person fails to perform a complex task. The complex task is broken into a number of small steps and each step is taught to the patient. In forward chaining, one starts with the first step, goes on to the second step, then to the third and so on. In backward chaining, one starts with the last step and goes on to the next step in a backward fashion. Backward chaining is found to be more effective in training the mentally disabled.

6. **Operant conditioning procedures for decreasing maladaptive behavior**

   a. *Extinction/ignoring:* Extinction means removal of attention rewards permanently following a problem behavior. This includes actions like not looking at the patient, not talking to the patient, or having no physical contact with the patient, etc. following the problem behavior. This is commonly used when patient exhibits odd behavior.

   b. *Punishment*: Aversive stimulus (punishment) is presented contingent upon the undesirable response. The punishment procedure should be administered immediately and consistently following the undesirable behavior with clear explanation. Differential reinforcement of an adaptive or desirable behavior should always be added when punishment is being used for limiting an undesirable behavior. Otherwise, the problem behaviors tend to get maintained because of the lack of adaptive behaviors and skill defect.

   c. *Timeout*: Timeout method includes removing the patient from the reward or the reward from the patient for a particular period of time following a problem behavior. This is often used in the treatment of childhood disorders. For example, the child is not allowed to go out of the ward to play if he fails to complete the given work.

   d. *Restitution (over-correction)*: Restitution means restoring the disturbed situation to a state that is much better than what it was before the occurrence of the problem behavior. For example, if a patient passes urine in the ward, he would be required to not only clean the dirty area but also mop the entire/larger area of the floor in the ward.

   e. *Response cost:* This procedure is used with individuals who are on token programs for teaching adaptive behavior. When undesirable behavior occurs, a fixed number of tokens or points are deducted from what the individual has already earned.

7. **Assertiveness and social skill training:** Assertive training is a behavior therapy technique in which the patient is given training to bring about change in emotional and other behavioral pattern by being assertive. Patient is encouraged not to be afraid of showing an appropriate response, negative or positive, to an idea or suggestion. Assertive behavior training is given by the therapist, first by role play and then by practice in a real-life situation. Attention is focused on more effective interpersonal skills. Social skills training helps to improve social manners like encouraging eye contact, speaking appropriately, observing simple etiquette, and relating to people *(See Appendix 17 for Behavior Therapy Format)*

Cognitive Therapy

Cognitive therapy is a psychotherapeutic approach based on the idea that behavior

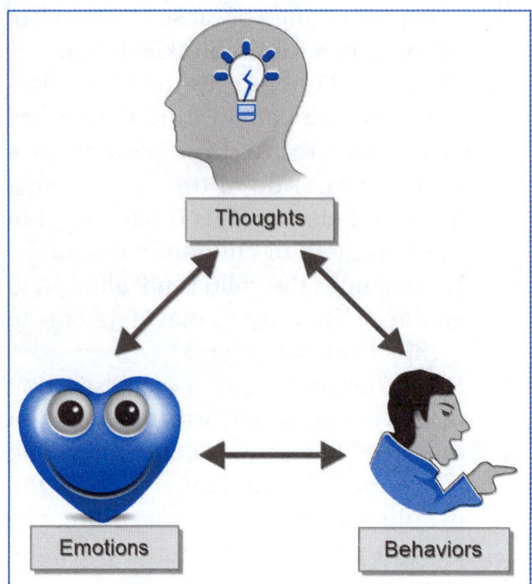

Figure 6.14: CBT approach

is secondary to thinking. It focuses on how patients think about themselves and their world, make changes in current ways of thinking, feeling and behaving **(Figure 6.14)**.

Indications

❖ Anxiety, eating disorders
❖ Personality disorders
❖ Suicidal thoughts or attempts
❖ Sexual disorders

It is used in individual, family and group settings and applicable to people of all ages and cultures.

Fundamental Assumptions

❖ Cognitive therapy is based on the premise that the way a person perceives an event rather than the event itself determines its relevance and the emotional response to it.
❖ The core sequential beliefs in CBT are triggered situation, thought process, provoked emotions, associated behavior and expressed physical reactions. For example, a stressful situation such as failure in the examination makes the person to think he is not capable to do the work, he feels sad and worthless, he withdraws from people and stops talking with others, feels tired, experiences loss of sleep and appetite.

❖ It is time limited, attempting to cause change rapidly and often within an established time frame.
❖ Therapeutic change can be affected through an alteration of idiosyncratic, dysfunctional modes of thinking leading to cognitive change.
❖ These therapies are based on the belief that patients are the architects of their own misfortune and have control over their thoughts and actions.
❖ They not only help the patient to overcome the problem for which he or she is seeking help but also help the patient to learn something about the process of therapy and develop therapeutic skills applicable to other problems.
❖ Cognitive therapy aims at altering the cognitions for effecting a change in behavior.
❖ It implies that all psychiatric disorders have some amount of cognition impairment and an improvement in it enhances patient's recovery.

Techniques of Cognitive Therapy

The four main groups of cognitive techniques are **(Figure 6.15)**:

1. **Techniques for stopping intrusive cognitions:** These methods aim at stopping intruding thoughts through distraction. Attention is directed to another mental act like doing mental arithmetic or copying a figure. The method of 'thought stopping' as done in obsessional ruminations is also tried.

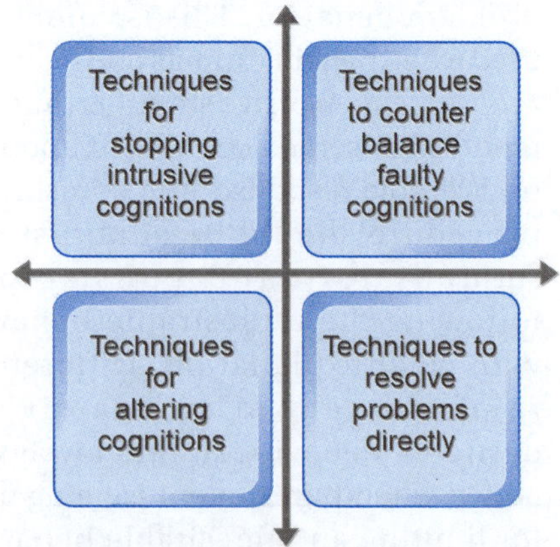

Figure 6.15: Cognitive therapy techniques

2. **Techniques to counterbalance faulty cognitions:** This involves counterbalancing intruding cognitions and the emotions provoked by them with another thought. As an example, when an anxious patient with chest pain becomes apprehensive thinking that he has a 'heart problem', he may be trained to think that it is only a muscular pain and does not relate to the heart.

3. **Techniques for altering cognitions:** These are aimed at changing the nature of cognitions. The patient is helped to identify 'maladaptive cognitions' and their 'logical errors'. Some errors which are not mutually exclusive and which occur in depression are as follows:

   o *Faulty inference*: It refers to making faulty interpretations of a situation or an event where there is no factual evidence to make such conclusions. For example, if a friend fails to respond to a letter sent by the person, he considers it as a sign of friend's hostility or dislike towards him.

   o *Overgeneralization*: This is making a general conclusion based on a single incident. An example is generalizing all students of a particular class as substandard based on poor marks scored by a single student.

   o *Magnification or minimization*: These are distorted evaluations. For example, a minor error is magnified or an important achievement is minimized in an unrealistically distorted manner.

   o *Unrealistic assumptions*: An example is the assumption that one can be happy only if one is a top scorer all the time.

4. **Techniques to resolve problems directly:** These involve several steps.

   a. Defining the problem more clearly.

   b. Dividing it into small subproblems which can be better managed.

   c. Finding out alternate methods of solving each subproblem.

   d. Considering the merits and demerits of each method.

   e. Selecting one method which is most advantageous at that instance.

Therapy Process

Therapy is result-oriented and defines goals so that progress towards them can be monitored. The therapist is a coach and teacher for the patients learning new skills. Therapist may help the patient identify situations in which undesired thoughts and actions occur and then assist with the development of alternatives.

Its overall goal is to increase self-efficacy or proficiency and sense of control over life. Patient must participate actively and be committed to the decision for change. The patient-therapist interaction is a goal-oriented collaborative partnership with a beginning, middle and an end.

Cognitive therapy helps people examine these beliefs, learn how they influence feelings and behaviors and identify and alter dysfunctional beliefs that predispose them to distort their experiences. By understanding the idiosyncratic ways the people perceive themselves, their experiences of the world and the future, the therapist can help the patient alter negative emotions, change their view of life experiences and behave more adaptively.

PSYCHOSOCIAL THERAPIES

Psychosocial therapy is a form of psychotherapy which emphasizes the interface between the patient and the patient environment. Therapy is structured and planned, and focused on achieving the specified goals for well-being of the patient.

❖ Psychosocial therapy is a specialized, formal interaction between the patient and the therapist. Therapist establishes and maintains therapeutic relationship to assist the patient in overcoming specific emotional, mental and social problems.

❖ Psychosocial therapy is a form of psycho-logical therapy designed to help an individual with emotional or behavioral disturbances adjust to situations that require social interaction with members of the family, work group, community and any other social unit.

—APA Dictionary of Psychology

❖ In this textbook commonly used psycho-social therapies such as group therapy, family therapy, therapeutic community, recreational therapy, art therapy and occupational therapies are described.

Group Therapy

Group psychotherapy is a treatment in which carefully selected people who are emotionally ill meet in a group guided by a trained therapist and help one another for personality change.

Meaning

* Group therapy is the treatment of multiple patients at the same time by one or more healthcare providers.
* Group therapy is an effective form of therapy in which a small number of people meet together under the guidance of a professionally trained therapist to help themselves and one another.

Indications

* People with emotional trauma.
* Person suffering with anxiety, depression, post-traumatic stress disorder.
* Individuals with alcohol disorder or substance abuse.
* Patients with personality disorders.

Contraindications

* Antisocial patients.
* Actively suicidal or severely depressed patients.
* Patients who are delusional and who may incorporate the group into their delusional system.
* Patients who are unable to participate due to their cognitive impairment.

Group Size

Optimal size for group therapy is 8–10 members with homogeneous group.

Frequency and Length of Sessions

Most group psychotherapists conduct group sessions once a week with each session lasting for about 45–60 minutes. Patients may receive therapy until they achieve relief from their symptoms and begin to develop a normal life; this can take anywhere from weeks to months or even years.

Stages of Group Therapy

Tuckman's model of group development suggests 5 stages of group therapy. These are presented in **Figure 6.16**.

Stage 1—Forming: During this stage patients exhibit feelings of anxiety and uncertainty concerning the group. The actual group interaction is low during this stage. Group members ask for information from each other and give information about themselves. Therapist's role at this stage is to educate the group and establish cohesiveness by discussing goals and expectations.

Stage 2—Storming: In this stage, competition and conflict in the relationship between group members and therapist start to develop.

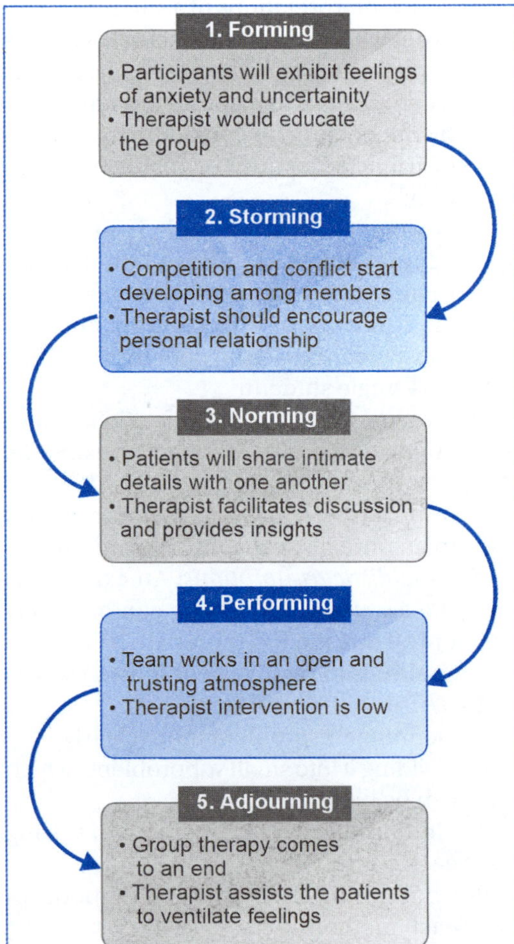

Figure 6.16: Stages of group therapy

Conflict starts to arise when individuals have to adjust their ideas, attitudes, feeling and beliefs to suit the group. The therapist should encourage patients to develop strong and personal relationships with one another. The reinforcement of goals and purpose of the group can help bring patients together.

Stage 3—Norming: During this phase the group members reach a consensus about group dynamics and the group perceives itself to be a part of the team. Patients' commitment to the group and its goals strengthen thereby improving group cohesiveness. During this phase the patients share intimate details with one another. The therapist should facilitate discussion and provide insights.

Stage 4—Performing: During this stage the team works in an open and trusting atmosphere. Patients are aware of each other's strengths and weaknesses and can help each other develop and grow. The therapist intervention is low as the group functions almost entirely on its own.

Stage 5—Adjourning: It is the final stage of group development which signifies that group therapy is coming to an end. The therapist should assist patients in voicing their feelings and facilitate discussion of closing topics.

Approaches to Group Therapy

The therapist's role is primarily that of a facilitator. He should:

- ❖ Provide a safe, comfortable atmosphere for self-disclosure.
- ❖ Use transference situations to develop insight into their problems.
- ❖ Protect members from verbal abuse or from scapegoating.
- ❖ Whenever appropriate provide positive reinforcement; it provides support to the ego and encourages future growth.
- ❖ Handle circumstantial patients, hallucinating and delusional patients in a manner that protects the self-esteem of the individual and also set limits on the behavior so as to protect other group members.
- ❖ Develop an ability to recognize when a group member is "fragile"; he should be approached in a gentle, supportive and non-threatening manner.
- ❖ Use silence effectively to encourage introspection and facilitate insight.
- ❖ Use laughter and a moderate amount of joking as it can act as a safety valve and at times also contribute to group cohesiveness.
- ❖ Employ role-play as it may help a member develop insight into ways in which he relates to others.

Therapeutic Factors Involved in Group Therapy

These involve sharing experiences, support to and from group members, socialization, imitation and interpersonal learning **(Figure 6.17)**.

- ❖ **Sharing experience:** This helps the patients to realize that they are not isolated and that others also have similar experiences and

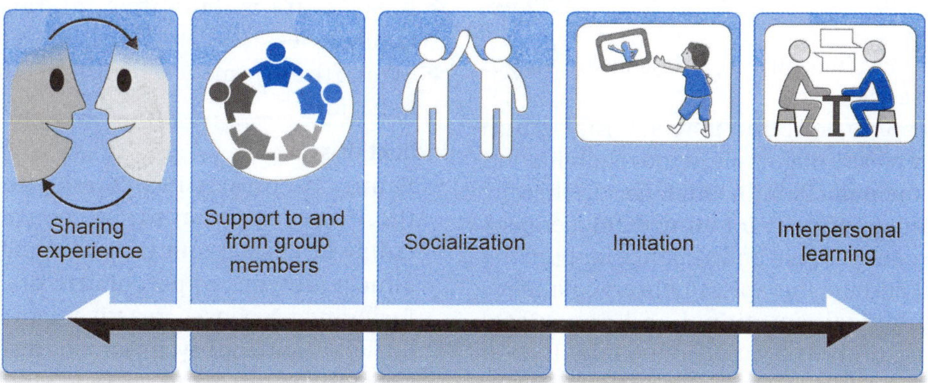

Figure 6.17: Therapeutic factors involved in group therapy

problems. Hearing from other patients that they have shared experiences is often more convincing and helpful than reassurance from the therapist.

❖ **Support to and from group members:** Receiving help from other group members can be supportive to the person helped. The sharing action of being mutually supportive is an aspect of the group cohesiveness that can provide a sense of belonging for patients who feel isolated in their everyday lives.

❖ **Socialization:** It is acquisition of social skills (for example, maintaining eye contact) within a group through comments that members provide about one another's deficiencies in social skills. This process can be helped by trying out new ways of interacting within the safety of the group.

❖ **Imitation:** It is learning from observing and adopting the behaviors of other group members. If the group is run well, patients imitate the adaptive behaviors of other group members.

❖ **Interpersonal learning:** It refers to learning through communicating with others whether it is verbal or non-verbal.

Some Useful Techniques in Group Therapy
❖ Reflecting or rewarding comments of group members.
❖ Asking for group reaction to one member's statement.
❖ Asking for individual reaction to one member's statement.
❖ Pointing out any shared feelings within the group.
❖ Summarizing various points at the end of the session.

In conclusion, one may say that group therapy plays a major role in the rehabilitation of the mentally ill individual. Group therapy gives an opportunity for immediate feedback from a patient's peer and a chance for both the patient and the therapist to observe patient's psychological, emotional and behavioral response towards a variety of people. Thus, it helps the patient to master communication and interpersonal skills, problem solving, decision making and assertive skills thus enabling him to re-enter the society's mainstream with a greater degree of confidence (*See Appendix 19 for Group Therapy Format*)

Family Therapy

Family therapy is an ideal counseling method for helping family members adjust to an immediate family member struggling with an addiction, psychological issues or mental health diagnosis. It can help individual family members build stronger relationships, improve communication and manage conflicts within the family system.

Meaning
❖ Family therapy is a type of treatment designed to help with issues that specifically affect families' mental health and functioning.
❖ Family therapy is a structured form of psychotherapy that seeks to reduce distress and conflict by improving the systems of interactions between family members.

Aims of Therapy
❖ Create a better home environment, solve family issues and understand the unique issues that a family might face.
❖ Improve communication among family members.
❖ Explore family dynamics and its relationship to psychopathology.
❖ Mobilize family's internal strength and functional resources.
❖ Restructure maladaptive interactional family styles.
❖ Strengthen family's problem-solving behavior.

Indications
❖ Family therapy is indicated whenever there are relational problems within a family or marital unit which can occur in almost all types of psychiatric problems including psychoses, reactive depression, anxiety disorders, psychosomatic disorders, substance abuse and various childhood psychiatric problems.

- ❖ Family therapy is the treatment of choice when there is a marital problem or sibling conflict.
- ❖ Family therapy may also be indicated when problems are caused by using one child as the scapegoat.
- ❖ Situational crises such as the sudden death of a family member, and maturational crises such as birth of the first child may cause sufficient stress to warrant family therapy.

Patient Referral

- ❖ Families may be referred for treatment by private physicians and agencies such as the school system, welfare board, parole officers, and judges.
- ❖ Some families are referred for therapy from emergency room psychiatric services after a visit caused by a crisis in the family such as a drug overdose.
- ❖ On discharge from a psychiatric hospital, a patient and his family may be referred for family therapy as part of follow up services.

Types of Family Therapy

Some of the commonly used family therapies are as follows **(Figure 6.18):**

1. **Family system therapy:** It focuses on helping members utilize the strengths of their relationships to overcome mental health problems.
2. **Functional family therapy:** It focuses on helping family members look for solutions while building trust and respect for each individual.
3. **Narrative family therapy:** It encourages each family member to tell his own story so as to understand and view problems more objectively than just seeing them through their own narrow lens.
4. **Psychoeducation:** It focuses on helping family members better understand mental health condition, treatment options, self-help approaches, etc.
5. **Supportive family therapy:** It focuses on creating a safe environment where family members can openly share what they are feeling and get support from their family.
6. **Multimodal approaches:** It focuses on the use of two or more methods.

Principles

Family therapy sees an individual's psychiatric symptoms as inseparably related to the family in which he lives. Thus, the focus of treatment is not the individual but the family. Main focus is on what goes on among the individuals rather than within one or more individuals.

- ❖ Therapist analyzes specific previous conflict situations and suggests alternative ways in which the family members could have responded to one another during the conflict.
- ❖ Therapist directly addresses the source conflict at a more abstract level as by pointing out pattern of interaction that the family might not have noticed.
- ❖ Family therapist is more interested in solving the problems rather than identifying the cause.

Guidelines for Conducting Family Therapy

Incorporating the following ground rules for therapy sessions will more likely result in productive appointments and greater gains when it comes to family relationships.

- ❖ Explain the reason for family therapy.
- ❖ Adhere to the timings of appointment.
- ❖ Intimate the location and duration of the session in advance.

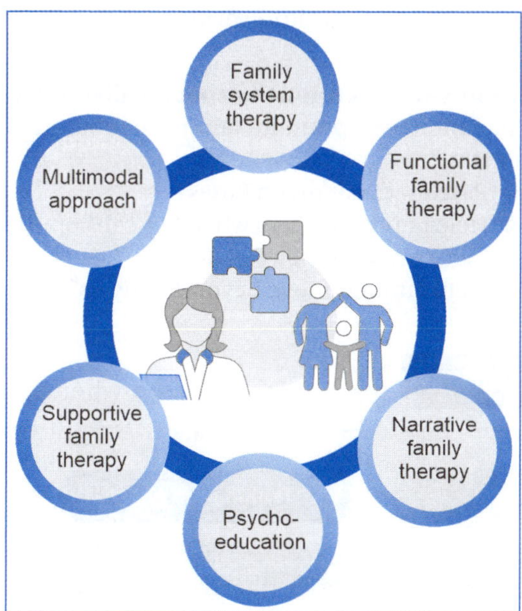

Figure 6.18: Types of family therapy

❖ Instruct the family members to await their turn to talk as everyone would be provided an opportunity.

❖ Inform the approximate number of family sessions in advance.

❖ Avoid verbal arguments or fights during the session.

❖ Inform members about the confidentiality of the contents of the sessions and record-keeping practices.

❖ Make a formal contract with the family about roles of therapist and family members.

Steps in Family Therapy

Most of family theorists identify the individual's problems as a symptom of trouble within the family. Main steps involved in family therapy are discussed under three phases: initial, middle and termination phase **(Figure 6.19)**.

1. *Initial Phase*

Initial phase includes family assessment, formulation of treatment plan and establishing formal contract.

❖ Family assessment includes three generation genogram, family functioning, information on different life cycle stages, parenting styles, life events, environmental stressors or illness in a family member and family functions.

❖ Assessment focuses on how the family has coped with problems and the process of transition from one stage to another.

❖ Once assessment is done the therapist draws the structural map which is a diagrammatic representation of the family system showing the different subsystems, its boundaries, power structures and relationships between people.

❖ Later the therapist presents the treatment plan to the family and negotiates with the members the plan and action they would like to take up at the present time.

❖ The time frame and modality of therapy is contracted with the family, and the therapy is put into force.

❖ A brief understanding of the family homeostasis is presented to the family in positive connotation appreciating the way in which the system is functioning.

2. *Middle Phase*

During this phase, based on nature of the disorder and the degree of pathology the choice of therapy technique is determined. Commonly used techniques are behavioral, psychodynamic and structural techniques.

❖ **Behavioral techniques:** Focus on skill training, example modeling, role playing, etc.

❖ **Psychodynamic technique:** Therapist works with the family to develop new emotional insights and explore novel ways of responding to the situation.

❖ **Structural techniques:** These methods focus on helping family members with boundaries and power dynamics within the family.

Family interventions to specific disorders: Techniques to promote family adaptation to illness:

❖ Psychoeducation on illness

❖ Help family to accept what they can control, focus on what they can do

❖ Help families move beyond "why us"

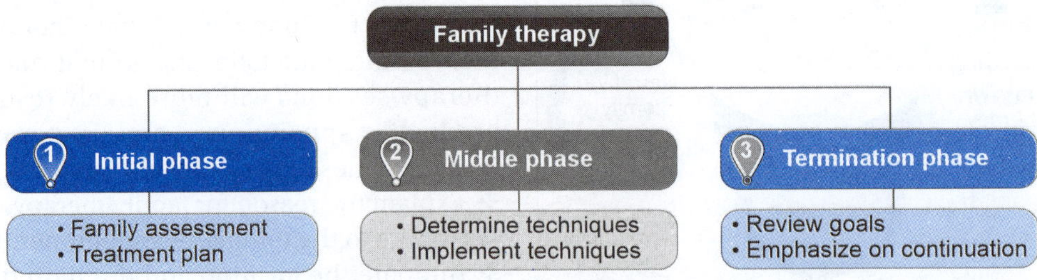

Figure 6.19: Steps in family therapy

❖ Facilitate them when grieving for inevitable losses.

❖ Set individual and family goals related to illness and to non-illness developmental events.

❖ Facilitate major family lifestyle changes.

Family interventions to schizophrenia:

❖ Psychoeducational interventions to increase family members' understanding of the disorder and their ability to manage the positive and negative symptoms of schizophrenia.

❖ Interventions related to expressed emotions, family resilience, reduction of stress, caregiver's burden, skill training and emotional support.

❖ Help family members to anticipate and solve problems, maintain reasonable expectations for patients.

Bipolar affective disorder:

❖ Educate family on early signs and symptoms of BPAD and medication management.

❖ Focus on management of mood swings of the patient, anger management and feelings of frustration.

Depression:

❖ Primary focus should be on low family support, ineffective communication, poor expression of affect, abuse and insecurity.

❖ Cognitive behavioral therapy and interpersonal interventions for depression.

Anxiety:

❖ Assist family members in using exposure, reward, relaxation and response prevention techniques to reduce patient's anxieties.

❖ Cognitive behavioral therapy.

Eating disorders: Interventions should help parents build effective and developmentally appropriate strategies for promoting and monitoring their child's eating behaviors.

Childhood disorders:

❖ Focus on development of effective parenting and contingency management strategies that will disrupt problematic family interactions associated with ADHD and ODD.

❖ Parents to be taught to use communication and social training tools that are adapted to the needs of their children and apply these techniques to their family interactions at home for autism spectrum disorder patients.

Substance misuse:

❖ Enhance coping abilities of family members.

❖ Eliminate the family factors that constitute barriers to treatment.

❖ Use family support to stay abstinence from substance use.

❖ Change characteristics of family environment that contribute to relapse.

❖ Encourage to join groups such as Alcohol anonymous, AI-Anon, AL-teen.

3. *Termination Phase*

❖ Review the initial goals of the therapy.

❖ Therapist describes new patterns or changes that have emerged.

❖ Emphasize on continuation of new patterns.

❖ Therapist negotiates new goals, new tasks or new interactions with the family that they will carry out for the future.

Therapeutic Community

The concept of therapeutic community was first developed by Maxwell Jones in 1953. He wrote a book entitled "Social Psychiatry" which was first published in England. Later on, when it was published in the United States, its title was changed to "Therapeutic Community."

Definition

Stuart and Sundeen defined therapeutic community as, "a therapy in which patient's social environment would be used to provide a therapeutic experience for the patient by involving him as an active participant in his own care and the daily problems of his community."

A therapeutic community is a drug free environment in which people with addictive problems live together in an organized and structured way in order to promote change and make possible a drug-free life in the outside society. The therapeutic community forms a miniature society in which residents and staff in the role of facilitators, fulfill distinctive roles and adhere to clear rules, all designed to promote the transitional process of the residents.

—Ottenberg, 1993

Objectives

- Use patient's social environment to provide a therapeutic experience for him.
- Enable the patient to be an active participant in his own care and become involved in daily activities of his community.
- Help patients solve problems, plan activities and develop the necessary rules and regulations for the community.
- Increase their independence and gain control over many of their own personal activities.
- Enable the patients become aware of how their behavior affects others.

Elements of Therapeutic Community

- Free communication
- Shared responsibilities
- Active participation
- Involvement in decision making
- Understanding of roles, responsibilities, limitations and authorities

Components of Therapeutic Community

The main components of a therapeutic community are daily community meetings, patient government, staff meetings and living and learning opportunities **(Figure 6.20).**

Daily community meetings

- These meetings are composed of 60–90 patients. All levels of unit staff are involved including administrative personnel. Acute patients are not involved in the meetings.
- Meetings should be held regularly for 60 minutes.
- Discussion should focus mainly on day-to-day life in the unit.
- During discussions patients' feelings and behaviors are examined by other members.
- Frank discussions are encouraged. These may take place with much outpouring of emotions and anger.

Patient government or ward council

- The purpose of patient government is to deal with practical unit details such as house-keeping functions, activity planning and privileges.
- A group of 5–6 patients will have specific responsibilities such as housekeeping, physical exercise, personal hygiene, meal distribution, a group to observe suicidal patients, etc. Staff members should always be available.
- All decisions should be fed back to the community through community meetings.

Staff meetings or review

A staff meeting should be held following each community meeting wherein the patients are excluded and only the staff are present. In this meeting the staff would examine their own responses, expectations, and prejudices.

Living and learning opportunities

Learning opportunities are to be provided within the social milieu which should provide realistic learning experiences for the patients.

Advantages of Therapeutic Community

- Patient develops harmonious relationships with other members of the community
- Gains self-confidence
- Develops leadership skills
- Learns to understand and solve problems of self and others
- Becomes sociocentric

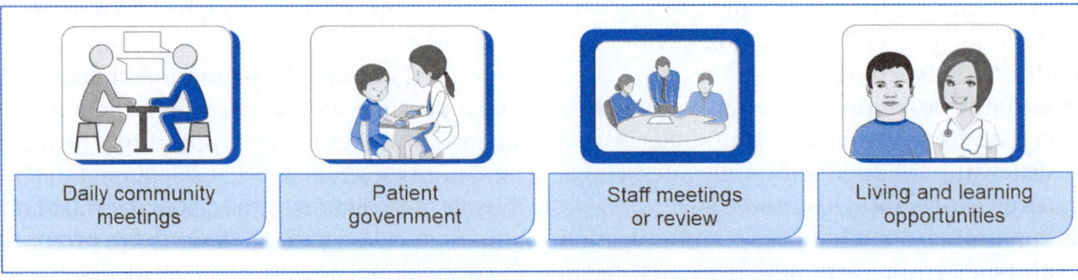

Figure 6.20: Components of therapeutic community

- Learns to live and think collectively with the members of the community.
- Lastly, therapeutic community provides opportunities to participate in the formulation of hospital rules and regulations that affect patient's personal liberties like bedtime, mealtime, weekend permission, control of radio or TV, social activities, late night privileges, etc.

Disadvantages of Therapeutic Community
- Role blurring between staff and patient
- Group responsibility can easily become nobody's responsibility
- Individual needs and concerns may not be met
- Patient may find the transition to community difficult

Role of the Nurse
- Providing and maintaining a safe and conflict free environment through role modeling and group leadership
- Sharing of responsibilities with patients
- Encouraging patient to participate in decision-making functions
- Assisting patients to assume leadership roles
- Giving feedback
- Carrying out supervisory functions

In conclusion, therapeutic community is an approach which is:
- Democratic as opposed to hierarchical
- Rehabilitative rather than custodial
- Permissive instead of limited and controlled

Recreational Therapy

Recreation is a form of activity therapy used in most psychiatric settings. It is a planned therapeutic activity that enables people with limitations to engage in recreational experiences.

Meaning
Recreational therapy or therapeutic recreation is the use of recreation by qualified professionals to promote independent functioning and to enhance the health and well-being of people with illness and disabling conditions.

Aims
- Encourage social interaction
- Decrease withdrawal tendencies
- Provide outlet for feelings
- Promote socially acceptable behavior
- Develop skills, talents and abilities
- Increase physical confidence and a feeling of self-worth

Points to be Kept in Mind
- Provide a non-threatening and non-demanding environment
- Provide activities that are relaxing and without rigid guidelines and time-frames
- Provide activities that are enjoyable and self-satisfying

Types of Recreational Activities
a. **Motor forms:** These can be further divided into fundamental and accessory. Among the fundamental forms are such games as hockey and football, while the accessory forms are exemplified by play activity and dancing.
b. **Sensory forms:** These can be either visual, e.g., looking at motion pictures, play, etc. or auditory such as listening to a concert.
c. **Intellectual forms:** These include reading, debating and so on.

Suggested Recreational Activities for Psychiatric Disorders
- **Anxiety disorders**: Aerobic activities like walking, jogging, etc.
- **Depressive disorder:** Non-competitive sports which provide outlet for anger like jogging, walking, running, etc.
- **Manic disorder:** One-to-one basis individual games like shuttle badminton, ball badminton, etc.
- **Schizophrenia:** Activities requiring concentration like chess, puzzles, social activities to give patient contact with reality like dancing, athletics.
- **Dementia:** Concrete, repetitious crafts and projects that breed familiarization and comfort.
- **Childhood and adolescent disorders:** It is better to work with the child on a one-to-one basis and give him a feeling

of importance. Employ activities such as playing, storytelling and painting. Adolescents fare better in groups; provide gross motor activities like sports and games to use up excess energy.

- ❖ **Mental retardation:** Activities should be according to the patient's level of functioning such as walking, dancing, swimming, ball playing, etc. *(See Appendix 18 for Recreational Therapy Format)*

Music Therapy

Music therapy is the functional application of music towards the attainment of specific therapeutic goals. Music therapy is facilitated by a trained therapist and is often used in rehabilitation centers, chronic psychiatric wards, etc.

Meaning

It is a type of expressive art therapy which uses music to improve and maintain the physical, psychological and social well-being of individuals. It involves a broad range of activities such as listening to music, singing and playing a musical instrument.

Indications in Psychiatry

- ❖ Depression
- ❖ Schizophrenia and other psychosis
- ❖ Substance use disorders
- ❖ Dementia
- ❖ Attention-deficit hyperactivity disorder
- ❖ Learning disorders
- ❖ Mental retardation

Advantages

- ❖ Improves fine motor skills by playing simple melodies on a piano or tapping out a rhythm on drum pads.
- ❖ Improves cognitive skills like learning, listening and attention span.
- ❖ Group drumming circles have been used to induce relaxation, provide an outlet for emotional expressions and foster social connectedness among members of a group.
- ❖ Music might be incorporated into guided imagery or progressive muscle relaxation techniques to enhance the effectiveness of these methods.

- ❖ Perceiving music helps a person understand the emotions that others are experiencing.

Types of Music Therapy

In general, there are two types of music interventions: active and receptive. These two types of interventions are usually combined during the treatment process. Music is conducted with individuals or in groups. It may be selected by the therapist or the participant in therapy.

- ❖ **Active interventions:** In this the participant is involved in making music with the therapist. For example, singing or playing a musical instrument.
- ❖ **Receptive interventions:** In this the participant listens and responds to music.

Dance Therapy

It is a psychotherapeutic use of movement which furthers the emotional and physical integration of the individual. Dance has been used to improve self-esteem and body image; lessen depression, fear and isolation; and express emotions.

Meaning

Dance/movement therapy (DMT) is a type of therapy that uses movement to help individuals achieve emotional, cognitive, physical and social integration.

Indications

- ❖ Anxiety
- ❖ Depression
- ❖ Eating disorders
- ❖ Poor self-esteem
- ❖ Post-traumatic stress disorder
- ❖ Dementia
- ❖ Autism
- ❖ Communication issues

Advantages

- ❖ It can be practiced in daycare centers, mental health, rehabilitation, medical settings and in nursing homes as well as old age homes.
- ❖ Helps in developing self-awareness, self-perception, relational abilities and mindfulness.

- As language is not a barrier it can be used to improve interaction and communication with people of all ages, couples, family and group therapy formats.
- Facilitates expression of feelings and aspects of personality.
- Fosters integration of physical, emotional and social experiences that result in a sense of increased self-confidence and contentment.
- Exercise through body movement maintains good circulation and muscle tone.
- Improves learning, clarifies personal values and helps to cope with a variety of psycho-physiologic dysfunctions.

Occupational Therapy

Occupational therapy is the application of goal-oriented, purposeful activity in the assessment and treatment of individuals with psychological, physical or developmental disabilities.

Goal

The main goal is to enable the patient achieve a healthy balance of occupations through the development of skills that will allow him to function at a level satisfactory to himself and others.

Settings

Occupational therapy is provided to children, adolescents, adults and elderly patients. These programs are offered in psychiatric hospitals, nursing homes, rehabilitation centers, special schools, community group homes, community mental health centers, day care centers, halfway homes and deaddiction centers.

Advantages

- Helps to develop social skills and provide an outlet for self-expression.
- Strengthens ego defenses.
- Develops a more realistic view of the self in relation to others.

Points to be Kept in Mind

- The patient should be involved as much as possible in selecting the activity.
- Select an activity that interests or has the potential to interest him.
- The activity should utilize patient's strengths and abilities.
- The activity should be of short duration to foster a feeling of accomplishment.
- If possible, the selected activity should provide some new experience for the patient.

Process of Intervention

It consists of six stages:

1. Initial evaluation of what patient can do and cannot do in a variety of situations over a period of time.
2. Development of immediate and long-term goals by the patient and therapist together. Goals should be concrete and measurable so that it is easy to see when they have been attained.
3. Development of therapy plan with planned intervention.
4. Implementation of the plan and monitoring the progress. The plan is followed until the first evaluation. If found satisfactory it is continued and altered if not.
5. Review meetings with patient and all the staff involved in treatment.
6. Setting further goals when immediate goals have been achieved; modifying the treatment program as relevant.

Types of Activities

1. **Diversional activities:** These activities are used to divert one's thoughts from life stresses or to fill time. For example, organized games.
2. **Therapeutic activities:** These activities are used to attain a specific care plan or goal. For example, basket making, carpentry, etc.

Suggested Occupational Activities for Psychiatric Disorders

- **Anxiety disorder:** Simple concrete tasks with no more than 3 or 4 steps that can be learnt quickly. For example, kitchen tasks, washing, sweeping, mopping, mowing lawn and weeding gardens.
- **Depressive disorder:** Simple concrete tasks which are achievable; it is important for the patient to experience success. Provide positive reinforcement after each achievement. For example, crafts, mowing lawn, weeding gardens.

- **Manic disorder:** Non-competitive activities that allow the use of energy and expression of feelings. Activities should be limited and changed frequently. Patient needs to work in an area away from distractions. For example, raking grass, sweeping, etc.
- **Schizophrenia (paranoid):** Non-competitive, solitary meaningful tasks that require some degree of concentration so that less time is available to focus on delusions. For example, puzzles, scrabble, etc.
- **Schizophrenia (catatonic):** Simple concrete tasks in which patient is actively involved. Patient needs continuous supervision, and at first works best on a one-to-one basis. For example, metal work, molding clay, etc.
- **Antisocial personality:** Activities that enhance self-esteem and are expressive and creative but not too complicated. Patient needs supervision to make sure each task is completed. For example, leather work, painting, etc.
- **Dementia:** Group activities to improve feeling of belongingness and self-worth. Provide those activities which promote familiar individual hobbies. Activities need to be structured, requiring little time for completion and not much concentration. Explain and demonstrate each task, then have patient repeat the demonstration. For example, cover making, packing goods, etc.
- **Substance abuse:** Group activities in which patient uses his talents. For example, involving patient in planning social activities, encouraging interaction with others, etc.
- **Children:** Playing, storytelling, painting, poetry, music, etc.
- **Adolescents:** Creative activities such as leather work, drawing, painting.
- **Mental retardation:** Repetitive work assignments are ideal; provide positive reinforcement after each achievement. For example, cover making, candle making, packaging goods, etc. *(See Appendix 16 for Occupational Therapy Format)*

ROLE OF A NURSE IN PSYCHOLOGICAL THERAPIES

The nurse has an important role in enhancing the therapeutic effects of activity therapies. Some points to be kept in mind are:

- Close co-ordination between the nursing staff and the activity therapy department is essential.
- By engaging in these activities, the nurse not only has an opportunity to support the therapeutic efforts of the recreational therapist but also has an invaluable opportunity to observe the patient in different settings.
- Through her observations of the patient's behavior during these activities, the nurse gains valuable information that she can subsequently utilize to therapeutic advantage in the working phase of the nurse–patient relationship.

- Physical therapies are treatment approaches that use physiologic or physical interventions to effect behavioral change.
- Psychopharmacology is the study of medications used to treat psychiatric disorders.
- Biological theories suggest that many of the psychiatric disorders are caused by dysregulation (imbalance) in the complex process of brain structures communicating with each other through neurotransmission.
- Nurses must understand general principles of psychopharmacology and have specific knowledge related to psychotropic drugs.

* Psychotropic drugs are classified as antipsychotics, antidepressants, mood stabilizers, anxiolytics and hyposedatives, antiepileptics, antiparkinsonian drugs and miscellaneous drugs.
* Antipsychotics are psychotropic drugs that are used for the treatment of psychotic symptoms. Antipsychotics are typical and atypical.
* Typical antipsychotics work by inhibiting dopaminergic neurotransmission. Atypical antipsychotics work by blocking D2 dopamine receptors as well as serotonin receptor antagonist action.
* The main indicators for antipsychotic drugs are management of schizophrenia, mania and depression with psychotic symptoms, behavioral problems in childhood disorders, eating and organic psychiatric disorders.
* The most common side-effects of conventional antipsychotic medication include anticholinergic effects, photosensitivity and extrapyramidal side-effects.
* Antidepressants are drugs used for treatment of depressive illness. These are also called mood elevators or thymoleptics.
* Mood stabilizers are used for the management and treatment of bipolar affective disorders (having disturbance in mood including mania and depression).
* Lithium was the first mood stabilizer and the first-line treatment option in the treatment of mania.
* Carbamazepine and sodium valproate are anticonvulsant drugs used as mood stabilizers.
* Anxiolytics are also called minor tranquilizers with most of them belonging to the benzodiazepine group of drugs.
* In clinical practice anticholinergic drugs have their primary use as treatments for medication-induced movement disorders.
* Miscellaneous drugs include drugs used in deaddiction, child psychiatry, eating disorders, stimulants, vitamins, calcium channel blockers, etc.
* Commonly used deaddiction drugs are antabuse and anticraving drugs.
* Commonly used medications in child psychiatry are clonidine and methylphenidate.
* ECT is a form of treatment wherein a seizure is artificially induced in an anesthetized patient by passing an electric current through electrode applied to the patient's head.
* Electroconvulsive therapy is treated like a minor surgical procedure that requires pre-treatment, intratreatment and post-treatment nursing care.
* Psychological therapies refer to a variety of treatments that aim to help an individual to identify and manage disturbed thoughts, emotions and behavior.
* Psychotherapy is referred to as a systemic treatment primarily employing verbal communication as the means of treatment aimed at relieving the patient's symptoms and helping him to understand and modify his conduct so as to lead a well-adjusted life.
* Some of the techniques used in psychoanalysis are free association, dream analysis, hypnosis, catharsis and abreaction therapy.
* Individual psychotherapy is a method of bringing about change in a person by exploring his or her feelings, attitudes, thinking and behavior.
* In supportive psychotherapy, the therapist helps the patient to relieve emotional distress and symptoms without probing into the past and changing the personality.

- ❖ Behavior therapy involves identifying maladaptive behaviors and seeking to correct these by applying the principles of learning theories.
- ❖ Cognitive therapy is a psychotherapeutic approach based on the idea that behavior is secondary to thinking.
- ❖ Psychosocial therapy is a form of psychotherapy which emphasizes the interface between the patient and the patient environment.
- ❖ Group psychotherapy is a treatment in which carefully selected people who are emotionally ill meet in a group guided by a trained therapist and help one another for personality change.
- ❖ Family therapy is an ideal counseling method for helping family members adjust to an immediate family member struggling with an addiction, psychological issues or mental health diagnosis.
- ❖ Therapeutic community is a therapy in which patient's social environment would be used to provide a therapeutic experience for the patient by involving him as an active participant in his own care and the daily problems of his community.
- ❖ Recreational therapy is a planned therapeutic activity that enables people with limitations to engage in recreational experiences.
- ❖ Music therapy is the functional application of music towards the attainment of specific therapeutic goals.
- ❖ Dance therapy is the psychotherapeutic use of movement which furthers the emotional and physical integration of the individual.
- ❖ Occupational therapy is the application of goal-oriented, purposeful activity in the assessment and treatment of individuals with psychological, physical or developmental disabilities.

REVIEW QUESTIONS

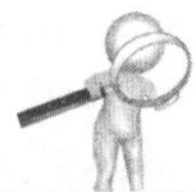

Long Essays

1. List the physical therapies used in psychiatry. Explain indications, contra-indications, mechanism of action, side effects and nurses' responsibility for antipsychotics.
2. Role of a nurse in administration of psychotropic drugs.
3. Define ECT. Explain indications, contra-indications, side effects and role of a nurse in ECT management.
4. Describe therapeutic community.
5. What is occupational therapy? Explain suggested occupational therapies for psychiatric patients.
6. Explain alternative therapies in psychiatry and role of a nurse.
7. What is the meaning of group therapy? Explain stages of group therapy and therapeutic factors involved in group therapy.
8. Describe indications, contraindications and side-effects of lithium. Explain nurses' responsibility for a patient receiving lithium.

Short Essays

1. Classification of psychotropic drugs
2. Classification of antipsychotic drugs
3. EPS
4. Neuroleptic malignant syndrome

5. Mood stabilizing drugs
6. Lithium
7. Drugs used in treatment of anxiety
8. Psychological therapies
9. Psychoanalytical therapy
10. Abreaction therapy
11. Individual psychotherapy
12. Family therapy
13. Group therapy
14. Steps in family therapy

Short Answers

1. Drug-induced Parkinsonism
2. Akathisia
3. Dystonia
4. Complications of ECT
5. Dream analysis
6. Behavior therapy
7. Aversion therapy
8. Token economy
9. Psychodrama
10. Major assumptions of behavior therapy
11. Systematic desensitization
12. Meditation

Fill in the Blanks

1. Antianxiety drugs are also called as ________.
2. ________ is a drug of choice for mania
3. A major adverse effect of clozapine is ________.
4. The binding sites of neurotransmitters are called ________.
5. Main side effect of typical antipsychotics is ________.

State the Following Statements are True or False

1. Psychoanalysis is a form of psychotherapy developed by Sigmund Freud.
2. Aversion therapy means the desirable behavior is paired with an unpleasant stimulus.
3. A blood lithium level of less than 2.0 mEq/L may be associated with toxicity.
4. Drug-induced parkinsonism is an extra-pyramidal symptom.
5. Diazepam is an anxiolytic drug.
6. Fluoxetine is an antipsychotic drug.

Multiple Choice Questions

1. **What is a receptor?**
   a. Binding site for neurotransmission
   b. Separates two neurons
   c. Situated in vesicles
   d. Releases chemicals

2. **What is a synapse?**
   a. Binding site for neurotransmission
   b. Separates two neurons
   c. Situated in vesicles
   d. Releases chemicals

3. **Haloperidol is a/an:**
   a. Antipsychotic   b. Mood stabilizer
   c. Antidepressant   d. Anticoagulant

4. **After three days of taking haloperidol the patient shows restlessness, becomes fidgety and is unable to sit still. Which of the following extrapyramidal symptoms is the patient experiencing?**
   a. Drug-induced Parkinsonism
   b. Acute dystonia
   c. Akathisia
   d. Tardive dyskinesia

5. **A patient is on clozapine drug for the past 2 weeks. He reports fever, sore throat and general weakness. Which of the following nursing intervention is most appropriate?**
   a. Inform the patient to take broad spectrum antibiotics
   b. Discontinue the therapy
   c. Inform the patient to check WBC count
   d. Both b and c

6. **Which of the following is a major side effect of typical antipsychotics?**
   a. Tardive dyskinesia
   b. Thyroid abnormality
   c. Weight gain
   d. Headache

7. **Which of the following drug needs a WBC level checked periodically?**
   a. Lithium
   b. Clozapine
   c. Olanzapine
   d. Diazepam

8. **A schizophrenia patient who is on Haloperidol since one week exhibits muscular spasms and involuntary movements of neck and jaw. The nurse interprets these findings as:**
   a. Acute dystonia
   b. Tardive dyskinesia
   c. Akathisia
   d. Drug-induced parkinsonism

9. **Atypical antipsychotics include:**
   a. Haloperidol and clozapine
   b. Chlorpromazine and trifluoperazine
   c. Risperidone and olanzapine
   d. Fluphenazine and haloperidol

10. **The treatment of choice for extrapyramidal symptom such as tardive dyskinesia is to:**
    a. Administer antianxiety drugs as per order
    b. Administer sedatives as per order
    c. Discontinue the drugs
    d. Administer anticholinergic drugs as per order

11. **Which of the following receptors are blocked by tricyclic antidepressants?**
    a. Dopamine
    b. Norepinephrine
    c. GABA
    d. Anticholinergic

12. **Which of the following instructions should the nurse include while imparting health education to a patient who has been prescribed lithium?**
    a. Restrict fluid intake to one liter daily
    b. Maintain a fluid intake of 2.5–3 liters daily
    c. Restrict sodium intake
    d. Maintain potassium levels

13. **A patient is on chlorpromazine drug. On assessment the patient demonstrates a** shuffling gait, stooped posture, drooling and ataxia. The nurse concludes that the patient has developed:
    a. Tardive dyskinesia
    b. Drug-induced Parkinsonism
    c. Dystonia
    d. Akathisia

14. **Therapeutic levels of Lithium are:**
    a. 0.5–1.5 mEq/L
    b. 0.6–1.0 mEq/L
    c. 0.8–1.2 mEq/L
    d. 1.0–2.0 mEq/L

15. **One of the side effects of an antipsychotic drug is abnormal, irregular choreoathetoid movements of the mouth muscles. It is termed as:**
    a. Akathisia
    b. Tardive dyskinesia
    c. Agranulocytosis
    d. Acute dystonia

16. **Which of the following is the nurse's correct interpretation when the patient has serum lithium level 2.0 mEq/L?**
    a. The levels are below therapeutic range; inform the physician
    b. The levels are within therapeutic range; do nothing
    c. The levels are elevated; patient should be assessed for lithium toxicity manifestations
    d. The levels are slightly elevated; do nothing

17. **Medications that affect psychic function are:**
    a. Mood stabilizers
    b. Psychotropic drugs
    c. Antidepressants
    d. Anxiolytics

18. **Autonomic side-effects are:**
    a. Dry mouth, constipation, cycloplegia
    b. Weight gain, jaundice, dermatitis
    c. Photosensitivity, renal failure, jaundice
    d. Agranulocytosis, tachycardia, hypotension

19. **Exclude the antidepressant drug from the following:**
    a. Chlorpromazine
    b. Clomipramine
    c. Clozapine
    d. Chlordiazepoxide

20. **Patients on MAOI's should be advised not to ingest __________ rich foods to prevent hypertensive crisis.**
    a. Thiamine
    b. Tyramine
    c. Tyrosine
    d. Thyroxine

21. **Signs and symptoms of lithium toxicity include:**
    a. Constipation, dry mouth, drowsiness
    b. Dizziness, thirst, dysuria, arrhythmias
    c. Ataxia, tinnitus, blurred vision, diarrhea
    d. Ataxia, muscle weakness, nausea and vomiting

22. **In which of the following relaxation techniques does the patient relax major muscle groups in a fixed order beginning with small muscle groups of the feet and working towards the head or vice-versa:**
    a. Biofeedback therapy
    b. Guided imagery
    c. Progressive muscle relaxation
    d. Meditation

23. **Contraindications of lithium are:**
    a. Renal diseases
    b. Thyroid diseases
    c. Pregnancy
    d. All of the above

24. **__________ Indicates lithium toxicity.**
    a. 0.8–1.2 mEq/L
    b. 0.8–1.5 mEq/L
    c. 0.6–1.0 mEq/L
    d. >2.0 mEq/L

25. **Benzodiazepines reduce anxiety by acting on which of the following neurotransmitter?**
    a. GABA
    b. Sertraline
    c. Noradrenaline
    d. Dopamine

26. **Which of the following condition is a primary indication for ECT?**
    a. Major depression
    b. Simple schizophrenia
    c. Anxiety disorder
    d. Phobic disorder

27. **Which of the following is a contra-indication for ECT?**
    a. Brain tumor
    b. Major mental illness
    c. General weakness
    d. Extreme sadness

28. **Which of the following problem would a nurse need to address immediately in post-ECT recovery period?**
    a. Excessive sleepiness
    b. Disorientation
    c. Urinary incontinence
    d. Changes in vital signs

29. **A patient with which of the following disorders would a nurse need to prepare for ECT?**
    a. A 35-year female patient with somatoform disorder
    b. A 65-year male patient with dementia
    c. A 40-year female patient with hypomania
    d. A 32-year female patient with major depressive disorder

30. **Which of the actions would be most appropriate for a patient scheduled for ECT at 10 AM?**
    a. Providing clear liquid diet
    b. Insert indwelling urinary catheter
    c. Administering atropine medication
    d. Administering diazepam medication

31. **Which of the following conditions is a contraindication of ECT treatment?**
    a. Osteoporosis
    b. Diabetes mellitus
    c. Recent myocardial infarction
    d. Use of multiple medications

32. **The patient has just awakened from an electroconvulsive therapy treatment. The most appropriate nursing action at this time would be to:**
    a. Arrange for the patient's diet to be served
    b. Orient the patient
    c. Observe the patient for signs of suicidal behavior
    d. Observe the patient for hallucinatory behavior

33. **Elements of therapeutic community include all, *except:***
    a. Free communication
    b. Shared responsibilities
    c. Active participation
    d. Free association

34. **Who developed the psychoanalytic theory?**
    a. Sigmund Freud
    b. Maxwell Jone
    c. Aaron Beck
    d. Albert Ellis

35. **Techniques used in psychoanalysis include all, *except:***
    a. Free association
    b. Dream analysis
    c. Abreaction therapy
    d. Psychotherapy

36. **Cognitive techniques include all, *except:***
    a. Abreaction therapy
    b. Thought stopping techniques
    c. Problem resolving techniques
    d. Counterbalance faulty cognitions

37. **The optimal size for group therapy is:**
    a. 15–20 members
    b. 8–10 members
    c. 20–25 members
    d. 15–25 members

38. **Which of the following is a specialized type of group therapy?**
    a. Psychodrama
    b. Psychotherapy
    c. Supportive psychotherapy
    d. Behavior therapy

39. **Relaxation therapies include all, *except:***
    a. Meditation
    b. Deep breathing exercise
    c. Yoga
    d. Catharsis

40. **Behavior therapy techniques include all, *except:***
    a. Modeling
    b. Exposure and response prevention
    c. Reinforcement schedules
    d. Free association

41. **Systematic desensitization consists of the following steps, *except:***
    a. Relaxation training
    b. Hierarchy construction
    c. Desensitization of stimulus
    d. Resolving unconscious conflicts

42. **Which of the following is a technique used in hypnosis?**
    a. Flooding
    b. Questioning
    c. Suggestion
    d. Desensitization

43. **The theory of operant conditioning was proposed by:**
    a. Ian Pavlov
    b. Watson
    c. BF Skinner
    d. Harry Stock Sullivan

44. **Which of the following is the correct meaning of cognitive therapy?**
    a. Helps the people examine beliefs, learn how they influence thinking and behavior
    b. Helps the people to learn adaptive behavior
    c. Helps the people to unlearn maladaptive behaviors
    d. Helps the people to learn new skills

45. **Mr D is suffering with obsessive thoughts of contamination and involved in rituals of hand washing. To treat these obsessive rituals, Mr D refrains from carrying them out despite their strong urges to do so. Which of the following technique is the therapist using?**

a. Response prevention
b. Flooding
c. Exposure
d. Relaxation training

46. A nurse wants to teach eye to eye contact maintenance behavior to a child. The nurse sits opposite the patient and reinforces the responses which are closest to the desired behavior and ignores the other responses. Which of the following technique is the nurse using?
a. Modeling   b. Chaining
c. Shaping   d. Response cost

47. Which of the following therapy takes the form of a group, where individuals share similar problems and psychopathologies?
a. Supportive psychotherapy
b. Group psychotherapy
c. Structured therapy
d. Family therapy

48. In which of the following behavioral techniques do participants receive tokens for engaging in adaptive behavior which at a later time can be exchanged for a variety of desired items?
a. Token economy
b. Response cost
c. Positive reinforcement
d. Negative reinforcement

49. All psychiatric disorders have cognitive and behavioral components. Which of the following is an important goal of cognitive behavior therapy?
a. Teaching adaptive skills
b. Reducing client's maladaptive behavior
c. Challenge client's irrational thought process
d. Help client reduce their fear responses to phobic stimuli

50. In a therapeutic community, patient participates in the decision making and problem solving processes that affects the management of the treatment setting. This refers to:
a. An autocratic form of staff government
b. A structured form of staff involvement
c. A democratic form of self-government
d. A structured form of patient involvement

ANSWER KEY

Fill in the Blanks

1. Anxiolytics	2. Lithium	3. Agranulocytosis	4. Receptors	5. Extrapyramidal symptoms

State the Following Statements are True or False

1. True	2. True	3. False	4. True	5. True	6 False

Multiple Choice Questions

1. a	2. b	3. a	4. c	5. d	6. a	7. b	8. a	9. c	10. d
11. b	12. b	13. b	14. c	15. b	16. c	17. b	18. a	19. b	20. b
21. d	22. c	23. d	24. d	25. a	26. a	27. a	28. d	29. d	30. c
31. c	32. b	33. d	34. a	35. d	36. a	37. b	38. a	39. d	40. d
41. d	42. c	43. c	44. a	45. a	46. c	47. b	48. a	49. c	50. c

Community Mental Health Nursing

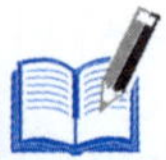

CHAPTER OUTLINE

- Concept, Importance and Scope of Community Mental Health
- Attitudes, Stigma and Discrimination Related to Mental Illness
- Prevention of Mental Illness
- Community Mental Health Services
- Mental Health Agencies—Government At National Level
- Community Mental Health Nursing

Community mental health as a treatment philosophy was mandated by the Community Mental Health Centers Act of 1963, thus bringing about the shift of mental healthcare from the institution to the community, and heralding the era of deinstitutionalization. This shift dramatically changed the methods of treating mental illness in past few years.

CONCEPT, IMPORTANCE AND SCOPE OF COMMUNITY MENTAL HEALTH

Community mental health means providing services to the persons and families with mental illness within the community using community resources. The community settings may be any home setting, religious place, schools, or any other place in community. Community Mental Health Services (CMHS) is a common development in mental health services worldwide. It positively affects reducing to utilize other services, reducing stigma, improving help-seeking attitudes, and promoting mental health.

Concept of Community Health Services

- ❖ Community mental health focuses on detection, prevention, early treatment, and rehabilitation of mentally ill individuals.
- ❖ It provides mental health services using community resources and the primary health care system.
- ❖ It goes "beyond the hospital-based care and treatment" by including programs for mental health promotion, prevention, and treatment of mental disorders.
- ❖ Inclusion of psychosocial support available in the community (religious groups, self-help groups, faith healers, local bodies, etc.)
- ❖ It also includes rehabilitation plans for persons with significant disability due to intellectual disability and recovering substance abusers and chronic mentally ill patients.
- ❖ It focuses on prevention of harm from alcohol and substance use.
- ❖ Develops linkages with primary health care system and tertiary care hospitals.
- ❖ Plans for stigma removal.
- ❖ Protection of the human rights of mentally ill persons.

Scope of Community Health Services

- ❖ Creating knowledge and awareness about the mental health delivery services in the community
- ❖ Promoting acceptability of services
- ❖ Reducing the treatment gap

❖ Reducing stigma
❖ Improving patient satisfaction with treatment and continuity of treatment
❖ Reducing violence in the community and schools due to mental health issues
❖ Enhancing the status of mental health within public health
❖ Facilitating psychosocial support for mentally ill individuals
❖ Providing treatment for mentally ill using primary health care system
❖ Providing rehabilitative services
❖ Participating in mental health promotion activities

Community Mental Health Initiatives

❖ Mental health services for disaster-affected populations
❖ School mental health programs
❖ Media and helpline programs
❖ Self-help groups
❖ Crisis intervention services
❖ Halfway home and day care centers
❖ Home based community program
❖ Community based rehabilitation
❖ Extension programs by satellite clinics
❖ Faith healers
❖ Telepsychiatry
❖ Tele Mental Health Assistance and Networking Across States (Tele-MANAS)

Importance of Community Mental Health Services

❖ To promote and maintain mental health of family through preventive and promotive interventions.
❖ To enhance the potentials of community people and use their strength to provide essential competence for positive mental health.
❖ To educate the family members regarding identification of various stressors and coping mechanisms to deal with problems.
❖ To help the family members to recognize that the social, cultural and situational aspects have an influence on behavior and how it can affect the individual persons' behavior in the family.

❖ To teach community people to monitor their mental health and that of community.

ATTITUDES, STIGMA AND DISCRIMINATION RELATED TO MENTAL ILLNESS

An individual's values and personal beliefs affect his attitude about mental illness, the mentally ill and treatment of mental illness. There still exists a stigma surrounding individuals who need or use psychiatric mental health services. The need continues for public education to modify or alter misconceptions about mental illness and people with mental disorders.

General Attitude Towards the Mentally Ill

❖ In general, the community responds to the mentally ill through denial, isolation and rejection. There is also a lack of understanding of mental illness as any other illness, and a lack of tendency to reject both the patients and those who treat them.
❖ Mentally ill are viewed as people with no capacity for understanding.
❖ People believe mental illness cannot be cured and even if the patient does get better complete physical rest is considered essential.
❖ The mentally ill are by and large perceived as aggressive, violent and dangerous.

Stigma and Discrimination Related to the Mentally Ill

Stigma refers to the discrediting, devaluing, and shaming of a person because of the characteristics or attributes that they possess. Generally, stigma leads to negative social experiences such as isolation, rejection, marginalization, and discrimination.

Stigma is a set of negative and unfair beliefs that a society or group of people have about something.

A stigma is a negative and often unfair social attitude attached to a person or group, often placing shame on them for a perceived deficiency or difference to their existence.

Prejudice means to prejudge and generally implies prejudgment based on erroneous beliefs or incomplete information.

Discrimination is manifested as prejudice in behaviors that endorse differential treatment of people with mental and substance use disorders.

Causes of Stigma

- Stigma often comes from lack of understanding or fear. Some people believe people with mental health problems are dangerous when in fact they are not.
- Inaccurate or misleading media representations of mental illness are one of the main causes. Media reports often link mentally ill people with violence or portray people with mental health problems as dangerous, criminal, evil or disabled and unable to live a normal life.

Types of Stigma

Stigma can come from self, society, employers, media and even from friends and family members.

- **Public stigma**: It involves the negative or discriminatory attitudes that others have about mental illness. It occurs when the general public supports a prejudice about a stigmatized group.
- **Self-stigma**: It refers to the negative attitudes, internalized shame that people with mental illness have about their own condition. It occurs when a member of a stigmatized group internalizes the negative views held by the general public.
- **Institutional stigma**: It involves policies of government and private organizations that intentionally or unintentionally limit opportunities for people with mental illness. Examples include lower funding for mental illness research or fewer mental health services relative to other health care.

Harmful Effects of Stigma and Discrimination

Stigma and discrimination can contribute to worsening of symptoms and reduced likelihood of getting treatment. Following are the effects of stigma on individual and others:

- Reduced hope

- Lower self-esteem
- Increased psychiatric symptoms
- Difficulties with social relationships
- Reduced likelihood of staying with treatment
- More difficulties at work
- Reluctance to seek help or treatment and less likely to stay with it
- Social isolation
- Lack of understanding by family, friends, co-workers or others
- Fewer opportunities for work or other social activities or trouble finding housing
- Bullying, physical violence or harassment
- Health insurance that does not adequately cover mental illness treatment

Addressing Stigma

The National Alliance on Mental Illness (NAMI) suggested following strategies to reduce stigma.

- Talk openly about mental health such as sharing on social media
- Educate yourself and others by responding to misperceptions or negative comments by sharing facts and experiences
- **Be conscious of language:** Remind people that words matter
- **Encourage equality:** Equality between physical and mental illness. Draw comparisons to how they would treat someone with cancer or diabetes
- Show compassion for those with mental illness
- **Be honest about treatment:** Normalize mental health treatment just like other health care treatment
- Let the media know when they are using stigmatizing language presenting stories of mental illness in a stigmatizing way
- **Choose empowerment over shame:** Fight stigma by choosing to live an empowered life
- **Get treatment:** Do not let the fear of being labeled with a mental illness. Treatment can provide relief by identifying what is wrong and reducing symptoms
- **Don't let stigma create self-doubt and shame:** Stigma does not just come from

others. Seeking counseling, educating about condition, connecting with others who have mental illness can help to gain self-esteem and overcome destructive self-judgment

❖ **Do not isolate yourself:** Reach out to people to whom you trust for the compassion, support and understanding

❖ **Do not equate yourself with illness:** You are not an illness. So instead of saying "I'm bipolar" say "I have bipolar disorder". Instead of calling yourself a schizophrenic say "I have schizophrenia"

❖ **Join a support group:** Join local and national groups such as National Alliance on Mental Illness (NAMI) which offers local programs and internet resources that help reduce stigma by educating people who have mental illness

❖ **Speak out against stigma:** Consider expressing opinions at events, in letters to the editor or on the internet. It will help to instill courage in others who are facing similar challenges and educate the public about mental illness

MODELS OF PREVENTIVE PSYCHIATRY AND ROLE OF A NURSE

In the 1960s, psychiatrist Gerald Caplan described levels of prevention specific to psychiatry. He described *primary prevention* as an effort directed towards reducing the incidence of mental disorders in a community. *Secondary prevention* refers to decreasing the duration of disorder while *tertiary prevention* refers to reducing the level of impairment **(Figure 7.1)**.

Primary Prevention

Primary prevention seeks to prevent the occurrence of mental disorders by strengthening individual, family and group coping abilities.

Role of a Nurse in Primary Prevention

Community mental health nurses are in a key position to identify individual, family and group needs, conflicts and stressors. Thus, they play a major role in identifying high-risk groups and preventing the occurrence of mental illness in them. Some interventions include:

1. Individual-centered intervention

❖ Antenatal care to the mother and educating her regarding the adverse effects of irradiation, certain drugs and prematurity

❖ Ensuring timely and efficient obstetrical assistance to guard against the ill effects of anoxia and injury to the newborn at birth

❖ Dietary corrections to those infants suffering from metabolic disorders

❖ Correction of endocrine disorders

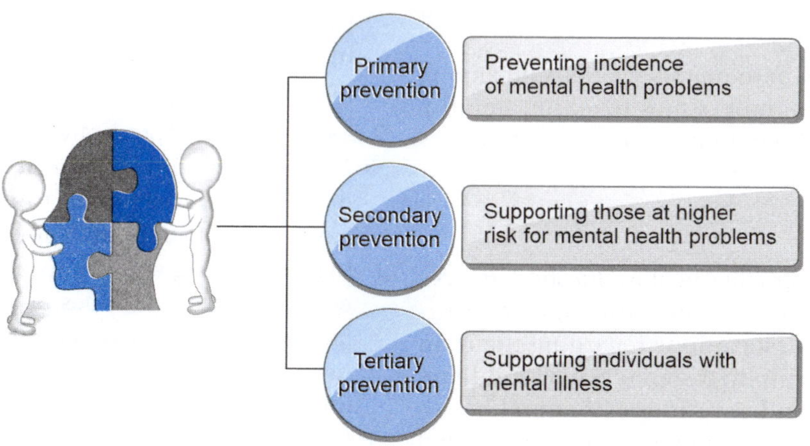

Figure 7.1: Levels of prevention (This paradigm was developed by Bloom, 1979)

- Liberalization of laws regarding termination of unwanted pregnancy
- Training programs for physically and mentally handicapped children like blind, deaf, mute and mentally subnormal, etc.
- Counseling the parents of physically and mentally handicapped children with particular reference to the nature of defects. The parents need to accept and emotionally support the child and be satisfied with limited goals in the field of achievement
- Fostering bonding behaviors. Explaining the importance of warm, accepting, intimate relationship and avoiding prolonged separation of mother and child are essential

2. Interventions oriented to the school child
- Teaching growth and development to parents and teachers
- Identifying problems related to poor scholastic performance and emotional disturbances among school children and giving timely intervention. School teachers can be taught to recognize the beginning symptoms of problems and referring to appropriate agencies

3. Family-centered interventions to ensure harmonious relationship
- Educating parents about appropriate disciplinary measures
- Promoting open health communication in families
- Rendering crisis counseling to parents of physically and mentally handicapped children
- Ensuring harmonious relationship among family members and teaching healthy adaptive techniques to cope with stress producing events

4. Interventions oriented to keep families intact
- Extending mental health education services at Child Guidance Clinics; at parent-teacher associations regarding the triad relationship between teacher, child and parent; and at various extramural health agencies regarding integration of mental health into general health practice

- Strengthening social support for the frustrated aged and helping them to retain their usefulness
- Promoting educational services in the field of mental health and mental hygiene
- Developing parent-teacher associations
- Rendering home-maker services—In the event of mother's prolonged absence from home due to illness or other reasons, a public health nurse can be arranged for providing basic services
- Providing marital counseling for those experiencing marital problems

5. Interventions for families in crisis
In developmental crisis situations such as the child passing through adolescence, birth of a new baby, retirement or menopause, death of a wage earner in the family, desertion by the spouse, etc. crisis intervention can be provided at:
- Mental hygiene clinics
- Psychiatric first-aid centers
- Walk-in clinics

6. Mental health education
- Conduct mass health education programs through film shows, flash cards and appropriate audio-visual aids regarding prevention of mental illnesses and promotion of mental health in the community
- Educate health workers regarding prevention of mental illness so that they can function effectively in all the areas of prevention

7. Society-centered preventive measures
- **Community development:** Culturally deprived families need biological and psychosocial supplies. They need better hygienic living conditions, proper food, education, health facilities, and recreational facilities. Otherwise psychopathy, alcoholism, drug addiction, crime and mental illness will result in such situations
- Collection and evaluation of epidemiological, biostatistical data

Secondary Prevention

Secondary prevention targets people who show early symptoms of mental health disruption but regain premorbid level of functioning through aggressive treatment.

Role of a Nurse in Secondary Prevention

- **Early diagnosis and case finding**: This can be achieved by educating the public, community leaders, industrialists, Mahila Mandals, Balwadis, etc. on how to recognize early symptoms of mental illness, and case findings through screening and periodic examination of population at risk, monitoring of patients, etc. Thus, in clinics, schools, home healthcare and the work place, community mental health nurses detect early signs of increased levels of anxiety, decreased ability to cope with stress and failure to perceive self, the environment and/or reality accurately and provide direct services as appropriate.
- **Early reference**: The public should be educated to refer these cases to proper hospitals as soon as they recognize early symptoms of mental illness.
- **Screening programs**: Simple questionnaires should be developed to identify the symptoms of mental illness, and administration of the same in the community for early identification of cases. These questionnaires can be simplified in local languages, and used widely in the colleges, schools, industries, etc.
- **Early and effective treatment for patient and family members as relevant**: Counseling services should be provided to caregivers of mentally ill patients.
- **Training of health personnel**: Orientation courses should be provided to health workers to detect cases in the course of their routine work.
- **Consultation services**: Nurses working in general hospitals may come across various conditions such as puerperal psychosis, anxiety states, peptic ulcer, ulcerative colitis, bronchial asthma, etc. These basic care providers need guidance and consultation to deal with these conditions in an effective manner.
- **Crisis intervention**: If crisis is not tackled in time it may lead to mental disorders or even suicide. Sometimes anticipating the crisis situation and guiding the individual in time can help them to cope with the crisis situation in a better way.

Tertiary Prevention

Tertiary prevention targets those with mental illness and helps to reduce the severity, discomfort and disability associated with their illness. In these terms, community mental health nurses play a vital role in monitoring the progress of discharged patients in halfway homes, houses, etc., especially with regard to their medication regimen, coordination of care, etc.

Role of a Nurse in Tertiary Prevention

- Family members should be involved in the treatment program actively so as to ensure effective follow-up.
- Occupational and recreational activities should be organized in the hospital so as to prevent idling.
- Community based programs can be launched through meeting with family members when the need for discharge from the hospital should be emphasized. These programs can be implemented through day hospitals, night hospitals, after care clinics, halfway homes, ex-patient hostels, foster care homes, etc. Follow-up care can be handed over to community health nurses.
- There should be constant communication between the community health nurses and the mental health institution regarding follow-up of the discharged patient. The ultimate aim of the hospital and community-based programs is to re-socialize and remotivate the patient for a functional role in the community, consistent with his resources.
- There are a wide range of services that need to be provided to patients as part of the tertiary prevention program. Nurses need to be familiar with the agencies in the

community that provide these services. Collaborative relationships between mental healthcare providers and community agencies are absolutely essential if rehabilitation is to succeed.

❖ An important intervention in the maintenance of patients in their own homes in the community is the Training in Community Living (TCL) program, designed by 'Stein and Test'. In this model, when a person is referred for hospital admission the staff goes to the community with him rather than his going to the hospital to be with the staff. This real-world experience with the patient enables the nurse to assess accurately the skills that the person needs to learn and to mutually agree on realistic goals.

❖ Another aspect of community life that is more difficult to assess accurately and deal with effectively, is the stigma attached to mental illness. Many patients and their families try to avoid stigma by keeping the nature of the person's illness a secret. The need for secrecy places additional stress on the family system because there is always the fear that the truth will be revealed. Nurses in the community are in a key position to monitor community attitudes and help in fostering a realistic attitude towards the mentally ill.

❖ For some patients, the emotional climate of the family to which they return can have a significant effect on their adjustment, and eventually recovery from the debilitating effects of chronic mental illness. Families sometimes view mental illness as a weakness of character that can be overcome by exertion of moral effort. This type of familial attitude may result in guilt on the part of the patient who believes that he has disappointed his significant others. Guilt leads to increased anxiety and decreased self-esteem. These are the conditions that interfere with a high level of functioning. Therefore, nurses working with families need to foster healthy attitudes towards the mentally ill member.

MENTAL HEALTH SERVICES AVAILABLE AT PRIMARY, SECONDARY AND TERTIARY LEVEL INCLUDING REHABILITATION AND NURSES' RESPONSIBILITIES

Mental health services include public awareness, early identification, treatment for illness, family education, long-term care, rehabilitation and ensuring human rights of mentally ill persons. Mental health services are delivered through mental hospitals located at central and state level. These can also be delivered through district and taluk hospitals, and primary health centers. Private and non-governmental organizations are also involved in delivering mental health care.

Primary Level

The primary level mental health services are available at sub-centers, primary health centers, community mental health centers and psychiatric hospitals/nursing homes.

Role of Medical Officer in Primary Health Center Related to Mental Health Care

❖ Impart skills to team members
❖ Ensure supplies
❖ Support and supervision of other health care personnel
❖ Initiate community involvement
❖ Provide treatment for mentally ill persons
❖ Monitoring work of health personnel

Effective measures to care for mentally ill persons at this level are:

❖ Correct diagnosis with explanation
❖ Avoiding unnecessary investigations
❖ Listening to the patient
❖ Teaching relaxation techniques
❖ Guidance about daily routines and activities
❖ Mobilizing family resources
❖ Use of medicines for short periods and formulation of groups of patients for self-help

Staff Nurse's Role

❖ First aid
❖ Nursing care of outpatients and inpatients
❖ Mental health education

Multipurpose Health Workers Role
- ❖ Identification of cases
- ❖ First aid
- ❖ Referral
- ❖ Follow-up
- ❖ Mental health education

Community Health Guides or Any Volunteer Role
- ❖ Identification of cases
- ❖ Referral
- ❖ Follow-up
- ❖ Mental health education

Secondary Level

Secondary level mental health services are available at general hospital psychiatric units, government and private psychiatric hospitals and voluntary organizations.

Activities of Psychiatric Hospitals

Psychiatric hospitals have become part of a continuum of mental health services available to patients and their families which offer a variety of treatments for psychiatric disorders. Their activities include:
- ❖ Outpatient treatment
- ❖ Inpatient treatment
- ❖ Education and training
- ❖ Research
- ❖ Rehabilitation
- ❖ Referral
- ❖ Follow-up
- ❖ Mental health education
- ❖ Community outreach programs

Tertiary Level

Tertiary level mental health services are available at rehabilitation centers of Government and private psychiatric hospitals, voluntary organizations, non-governmental mental health organizations.

Activities
- ❖ Rehabilitation
- ❖ Family and patient mental health education
- ❖ Community outreach programs
- ❖ Follow-up
- ❖ Training and education
- ❖ Research

Other Mental Health Services Available for Psychiatric Patients

Partial hospitalization (Day care centers, Day hospitals): Partial hospitalization is an innovative alternative to hospitalization. Individuals in partial hospitalization program attend structured programming throughout the day and return home in the evenings. The main goal is development of skills that help patients better manage their symptoms. Patients are generally referred to partial hospitalization when they are experiencing acute psychiatric symptoms that are difficult to manage but do not require 24–hour care. It is ideally suited to most of the psychiatric syndromes particularly chronic psychotic disorders, neurotic conditions, personality disorders, drug and alcohol dependence and mental retardation.

Partial hospitalization has the advantages of lesser separation from families, more involvement in the treatment program and a lessening of patient's preoccupation with the illness which may be intensified by full hospitalization **(Box 7.1)**.

Quarterway homes: This is a place usually located within the hospital campus itself but not having the regular services of a hospital. There may not be routine nursing staff or routine rounds and most of the activities of the place are taken care of by the patients themselves.

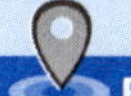

BOX 7.1: Main day care centers in India
- ❑ Sanjivini, New Delhi
- ❑ SCARF (Schizophrenia Research Foundation), Chennai, has started a day care center called "BAVISHYA" in 1985
- ❑ Anugraha Day Care Center, Chennai
- ❑ Association of the Friends of Mentally Ill, Mumbai
- ❑ Institute of Mental Health, Ahmedabad
- ❑ Psychiatric Center, Kolkata
- ❑ NIMHANS, Bengaluru
- ❑ Dharwad Institute of Mental Health and Neurosciences, Dharwad, Karnataka
- ❑ The Richmond Fellowship Society, Bengaluru
- ❑ Kripamayee Institute of Mental Health, Miraj

Halfway homes: A halfway home is a transitory residential center for mentally ill patients who no longer need the full services of a hospital but are not yet ready for a completely independent living. It attempts to maintain a climate of health rather than of illness, and to develop and strengthen individual capacities. At the same time it enables the recognition of problems that require medical attention and permits the discovery of conditions in the community which are acting adversely on the individual. Thus, halfway homes have a major role in the rehabilitation of the mentally ill individual.

Objectives

❖ To ensure a smooth transition from hospital to the family
❖ To integrate the individual into mainstream society

Activities

Community mental health nurses play a vital role in monitoring the progress of discharged patients in halfway homes especially with regard to their medication regimen and co-ordination of care. Some of the interventions carried out in halfway homes include:

❖ **Assessment:** It includes following types of assessment:
  ○ *Clinical assessment*: Assessing for residual psychiatric symptoms which may affect his ability to function
  ○ *Social assessment:* Assessing for family support, attitude of family members and economic status of the family
  ○ *Psychological assessment:* Assessing self-esteem, confidence, patient's level of motivation
  ○ *Vocational assessment:* Assessing physical strength, hand coordination, attention, concentration, etc.
❖ Remediating disabilities through supportive interventions.

Outcomes

Expected outcomes include successful return of the patients to their homes, prevention of relapses, economic self-sufficiency made possible through vocational counseling and self-employment programs.

Nurses need to be familiar with the various halfway homes available in the community as collaboration with such facilities is absolutely essential for successful rehabilitation **(Box 7.2)**.

Self-help Groups

A self-help group is a voluntary group of persons who share common needs or problems which are not addressed by other segments of the society. They meet at regular intervals and interact face-to-face with each other. They share their experiences, strategies, successes and failures and find solutions to their problems. Members can be a great source of support to each other.

Characteristics

❖ A distinguishing characteristic of self-help groups is their homogeneity.
❖ SHG members have similar disorders and share their experiences good or bad, successful or unsuccessful with one another.
❖ Self-help groups are based on the premise that 'people who have experienced a

---

BOX 7.2: List of halfway homes available in India

❑ Medico-Pastoral Association, Bengaluru
❑ Atmashakti Vidyalaya, Bengaluru
❑ Richmond Fellowship, Bengaluru
❑ Puraskara After Care Home, Bengaluru
❑ Cadabam's Home for the Mentally Disabled, Bengaluru
❑ Family Fellowship Society for Psychosocial Rehabilitation, Bengaluru
❑ Raju Rehabilitation Foundation, Bengaluru
❑ YWCA Halfway Home for Mentally Ill, Chennai
❑ Dr Boaz's Rehabilitation Center, Chennai
❑ Dr Dhairyan's Psychotherapy and Rehabilitation Center, Chennai
❑ Sowkya Halfway Home at Madurai
❑ Delhi Psychosocial Rehabilitation Society
❑ Paripurnata Halfway Home, West Bengal
❑ Society for Mental Health, Kerala

particular problem are able to help others who have the same problem".

❖ Self-help groups emphasize cohesion which is exceptionally strong in these groups. Because the group members have similar problems and symptoms, they develop a strong emotional bond. But each group may have its unique characteristics to which the members can attribute magical qualities of healing.

Functions

❖ One of their most important functions is to demonstrate to individuals that they are not alone in having a particular problem.
❖ The members work together using their strengths to gain control over their lives. By doing so they educate each other, provide mutual support and alleviate the sense of alienation usually felt by people drawn to this kind of group.
❖ Sharing each other's experiences not only helps the members by providing mutual support but also by generating alternate ways to view and resolve problems. Thus, they help in overcoming maladaptive patterns of behavior or states of feeling that traditional mental health professionals have not generally dealt with successfully.
❖ These groups prevent physical, emotional and social problems and breakdowns; improve an individual's or a family's quality of life; and provide the education necessary to develop the member's potential further.

Strategies

❖ Group leaders include promotion of dialogue, self-disclosure and encouragement among members. Concepts used in support groups include psychoeducation, self-disclosure and mutual support.
❖ The processes involved in self-help groups are social affiliation; learning self-control; and modeling methods to cope with stress and acting to change the social environment.

Examples

Alcoholics Anonymous (AA), Association for Mentally Disabled (AMEND), Narcotic Anonymous, An alliance for the mentally ill (AASHA), Bipolar India, etc.

Suicide prevention centers: There are many suicide prevention centers in India in the voluntary sector doing good work and helping those in need. Some of them are:

❖ Helping Hands and MPA in Bengaluru
❖ Sneha in Chennai
❖ Sahara in Mumbai
❖ Sanjivini and Sumaitri in New Delhi

Others

❖ Community group homes
❖ Large homes for long-term care
❖ Hostels
❖ Home care programs
❖ District rehabilitation centers (**Figure 7.2**)

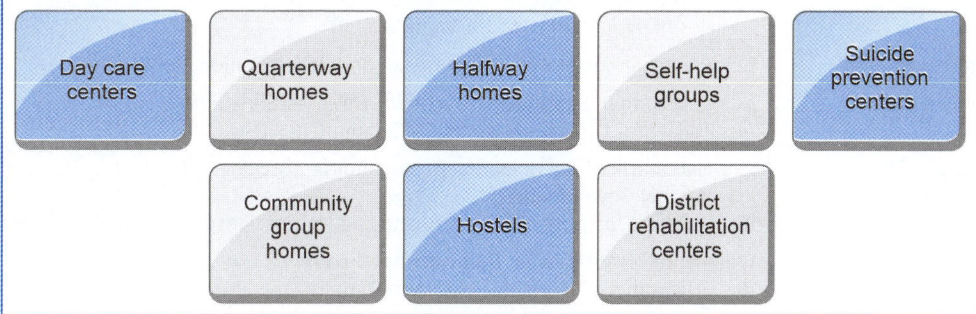

Figure 7.2: Other mental health services

MENTAL HEALTH AGENCIES: GOVERNMENT AND VOLUNTARY, NATIONAL AND INTERNATIONAL

Mental health agency is any private or public facility that is licensed by state government or central government as a mental health treatment facility. It includes a psychiatric hospital, a psychiatric unit of a general hospital, residential treatment center for mentally ill individuals, etc.

Mental health services are delivered through mental hospitals at Central, State and District levels **(Table 7.1)**.

Mental Health Agencies—Government at National Level

According to the Press information Bureau, Government of India, Ministry of health and Family welfare 2014, there are 3,800 psychiatrists, 898 clinical psychologists, 850 psychiatric social workers and 1,500 psychiatric nurses in the country. There are three centrally run mental health institutions, 40 state run mental hospitals **(Table 7.2)** and 398 departments of psychiatry in various medical colleges across the country equipped to treat patients suffering from mental illness.

TABLE 7.1: Mental health services at various levels in India	
Central level	◆ National level hospitals, e.g., NIMHANS, Bengaluru
State level	◆ State level hospitals, e.g., Dharwad Institute of Mental Health and Neurosciences, Dharwad, Karnataka ◆ National Mental Health Programme
District level	◆ General hospital psychiatric units ◆ District Mental Health Programme
Local level	◆ Primary health centers ◆ Community mental health centers ◆ Sub-centers

TABLE 7.2: State-wise list of mental hospitals	
Name of the state/UT	**Name of the hospital and place**
Andhra Pradesh	1. Government Hospital for Mental Care, Visakhapatnam
Assam	2. Lokopriya Gopinath Bordoloi Institute of Mental Health, Tezpur (Central Government)
Bihar	3. Institute of Mental Health, Bhojpur
Jharkhand	4. Central Institute of Psychiatry, Kanke, Ranchi (Central Government) 5. Ranchi Institute of Neuropsychiatry and Allied Science (RINPAS), Ranchi
Delhi	6. Institute of Human Behavior and Allied Sciences (IHBAS), Delhi
Goa	7. Institute of Psychiatry and Human Behavior, Panaji
Gujarat	8. Hospital for Mental Health, Bhuj 9. Hospital for Mental Health, Jamnagar 10. Hospital for Mental health, Ahmedabad 11. Hospital for Mental Health, Vadodara
Himachal Pradesh	12. Himachal Hospital of Mental Health and Rehabilitation, Boileauganj
Jammu & Kashmir	13. Government Hospital for Psychiatric Diseases, Srinagar 14. Psychiatric Diseases Hospital GMC, Jammu
Karnataka	15. National Institute of Mental Health and Neurosciences (NIMHANS), Bengaluru (Central Government) 16. Dharwad Institute of Mental Health and Neurosciences (DIMHANS), Dharwad
Kerala	17. Mental Health Center, Thiruvananthapuram 18. Government Mental Health Centre, Thrissur 19. Government Mental Health Centre, Kozhikode

Contd...

Contd...

Name of the state/UT	Name of the hospital and place
Madhya Pradesh	20. Gwalior Manasik Arogyashala, Gwalior 21. Mental Hospital, Indore
Maharashtra	22. Regional Mental Hospital, Nagpur 23. Regional Mental Hospital, Pune 24. Regional Mental Hospital, Thane 25. Regional Mental Hospital, Ratnagiri
Meghalaya	26. Meghalaya Institute of Mental Health and Neurosciences, Shillong 27. Modern Psychiatric Hospital, Agartala
Nagaland	28. Mental Hospital, Kohima
Odisha	29. Mental Health Institute, Cuttack
Punjab	30. Dr Vidyasagar Punjab Mental Hospital, Amritsar
Rajasthan	31. Psychiatric Center, Jaipur 32. Mental Hospital, Jodhpur
Tamil Nadu	33. Institute of Mental Health, Chennai
Telangana	34. Institute of Mental Health, Hyderabad
Uttar Pradesh	35. Institute of Mental Health and Hospital, Agra 36. Mental Hospital Bareilly, Bareilly 37. Mental Hospital, Varanasi
West Bengal	38. Lumbini Park Mental Hospital, Kolkata 39. Institute of Mental Care, Purulia 40. Mental Hospital Berhampore, Berhampore 41. The Mental Hospital, Kolkata 42. Institute of Psychiatry, Kolkata 43. Calcutta Pavlov Hospital, Kolkata

The details of mental health institutes in the country are given below:

Mental Health Agencies—International

Some of the mental health agencies at the international level are World Health Organization, The United Nations Educational Scientific and Cultural Organization (UNESCO), The World Federation for Mental Health (WFMH), The Internal Society for Mental Health Online (ISMO), National Alliances for the Mentally Ill (NAMI).

COMMUNITY MENTAL HEALTH NURSING

Community mental health—psychiatric nursing is the application of specialized knowledge to populations and communities to promote and maintain mental health and to rehabilitate populations at risk that continue to have residual effects of mental illness.

Psychiatric nursing in the community setting differs markedly from its hospital counterpart. The community setting requires that the psychiatric nurse possesses knowledge about a broad array of community resources and be flexible in approaching problems related to individual psychiatric symptoms, family and support systems and basic living needs such as housing and financial support **(Box 7.3)**.

Goals of Community Mental Health Nursing

❖ To provide prevention activities to populations for the purpose of promoting mental health
❖ To provide interventions as early as possible
❖ To provide corrective learning experiences for patient-groups who have deficits and disabilities in the basic competencies

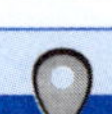

BOX 7.3: Community mental health-psychiatric nurse attributes

- Awareness of self, personal and cultural values
- Non-judgmental attitude
- Flexibility
- Problem solving skills
- Ability to cross service systems such as work with schools, other healthcare providers, employers, etc)
- Knowledge of community resources
- Willingness to work with the family or significant others identified by the patient as support people
- Understanding of the social, cultural and political issues that affect mental health and illness
- Knowledge of political activism

needed to cope in society, and to help individuals develop a sense of self-worth and independence

- ❖ To anticipate when populations become at risk for particular emotional problems and to identify and change social and psychological factors that diversely affect people's interaction with their environments
- ❖ To develop innovative approaches to primary prevention activities
- ❖ To assist in providing mental health education to populations about mental health and illness and to teach people how to assess their mental health

Community Mental Health Nursing Process

Assessment

The key aspects of assessment include:

- ❖ Impairments directly due to the psychiatric disorder such as persistent hallucinations, negative symptoms, social withdrawal, under-activity and slowness
- ❖ Secondary social disadvantages such as unemployment, poverty and homelessness as well as the stigma attached to psychiatric illness
- ❖ Personal reactions to illness such as low self-esteem and hopelessness, poor motivation and capacity for self-management and performance of social roles

- ❖ Unpredictable behavior, risk of harm to self and others and liability to relapse
- ❖ Financial position of the patient
- ❖ Availability of community resources
- ❖ Social circumstances to which the patient is likely to return to

The expected outcome of the assessment is a detailed outline of the person's present functioning, highest level of functioning and the needed services.

Intervention

Community psychiatric nurses must approach interventions with flexibility and resourcefulness to meet the broad range of needs of the patients with continued mental deficits. Interventions cannot be directed only towards discrete psychiatric symptoms but must also facilitate patient's access to various community resources providing for basic needs such as housing, nutrition, etc.

Since people suffering from mental illness often remain in or return to the community following treatment, nurses must be able to assess the presence of continued mental health problems and plan and implement interventions within the confines of the resources available in the community.

Carr, et al. (1984) have identified the following roles for nurses working in community mental health services **(Figure 7.3)**:

Consultative role: This means giving advice to other professionals in the community about the type and level of nursing care required for a given patient group.

Clinician role: Providing direct nursing care to the patients in the community.

Therapeutic role: Employing psychotherapeutic and behavioral methods for management of patients.

Assessor/researcher role: The nurse may assess the care given to the patient/patient group, and may also assess the outcome of ongoing care programs.

Educator: Creating awareness in the community about mental health and mental illness with special focus on vulnerable groups.

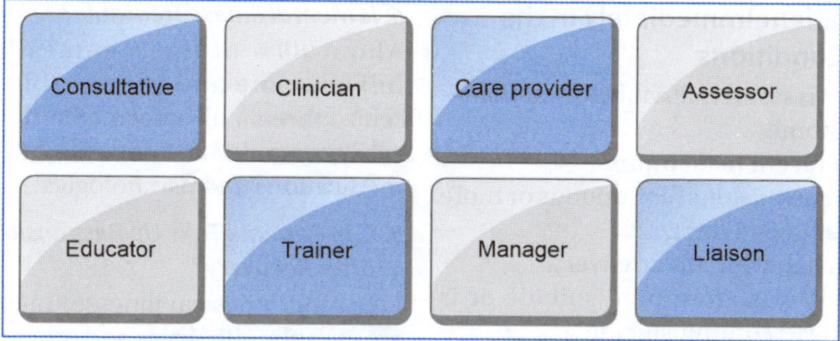

Figure 7.3: Roles of community mental health nurse

Trainer/manpower facilitators: Training of para professionals, community leaders, school teachers and other care-giving professionals in the community.

Manager/administrator: Management of resources, planning and co-ordination.

Domiciliary care: Services are provided to the patient by visiting their homes. Services like administration of medications, assessment of the level of functioning and improvement of patients, monitoring of side-effects of drugs, counseling of patients and family members are offered at the patient's home setting.

Liaison role: Nurses working in the community help the patients and the family members by bridging the gap between the patient and the hospital, patient and the employers and also by networking in the community for resource development.

Preventive roles: These preventive roles are under primary, secondary and tertiary levels.

Other areas of community health psychiatric nursing are:
* Social skills training
* Anxiety management and relaxation
* Assertive training
* Bereavement counseling
* Group meetings
* Community out-reach work services
* Childcare services
* Adult care and elderly care services

Tips for Working in the Community

Identification of patients in the community: Talk to important people like, village panchayat members, local leaders, teachers, educated youth, members of service agencies like Angawadi, Mahila Mandals, etc. and request them to tell you about individuals:
* Who talk nonsense and act in a manner considered strange or abnormal
* Who have become very quiet and do not talk or mix with other people
* Who claim to hear voices or see things that others cannot hear or see
* Who are suspicious and claim that others are trying to harm them
* Who have become unusually cheerful, crack jokes and say that they are very wealthy and superior to others when it is not really so
* Who have become very sad lately and cry without reason
* Who talk about suicide or have made an attempt at suicide
* Who get possessed by God or spirit or who are said to be the victims of black magic or evil power
* Who are dull, mentally not grown up like others of their age and slow since birth

When you visit homes, enquire about members suffering from mental illness. Ask the above-mentioned questions tactfully without offending them and obtain information about the existence of a patient among them in that family, neighborhood or their relatives.

When you go to a school, enquire from teachers and students about children who suffer from fits, behavioral and learning problems.

Refer the Patient Immediately in the Following Conditions

* The patient is severely ill, violent or unmanageable at home
* History of recent head injury
* Repeated convulsions (continuous or more than three times a day)
* Disturbed behavior after delivery
* The patient has attempted suicide or is threatening to commit suicide
* Disturbed behavior in people with known diabetes or hypertension
* People who show abnormal behavior after taking alcohol or any other intoxicating substances

Follow-up care with special emphasis on medication regimen, improvement made, and side-effects, patient's occupational function.

Be Prepared to Answer Certain Common Questions Asked Regarding Mental Illness

1. Is Mental Illness Hereditary?

The role of genetic factors is well established only in some psychiatric illnesses (for example, schizophrenia, mania and depression). It is also not true that if a family member is suffering from schizophrenia the other members will always develop the same illness. The chances though are more likely, factors such as personality and environment play an equally important role.

2. Is Mental Illness Contagious?

Mental illnesses do not spread through contact of any form. Individual genetic vulnerability or predisposition and precipitating factors play an important role in disease occurrence.

3. Do Ghosts, Black Magic, Curse Cause Mental Illness?

Many people do not consider mental illness as an illness but possession by a ghost or supernatural power. Causation of most of the mental illnesses is well known for which specific methods of treatment are available.

4. Is Mental Illness Treatable?

About 80% of the mental illnesses are fully curable and preventable. Excluding schizophrenia, all other mental illnesses can be easily controlled and prevented through proper medications and psychological therapies.

5. Can Patients Take Up Responsibilities after Recovery?

Like other physical illnesses mental illnesses are curable with drugs and other physical and psychological methods.

Depression and mania are self-limiting illnesses, lasting from 6 to 9 months. Anxiety neurosis, hysteria etc., are fully curable and preventable disorders. If schizophrenia is managed early and correctly, the patient may become socially and occupationally normal within few weeks.

6. Can Marriage Cure Mental Illness?

A mentally ill person can get worse if he gets married when ill as marriage can become an additional stress. A patient who has recovered can get married and live a normal life like any other person.

A nurse can play an important role in community by making the public aware of some important principles related to mental illness:

* Mental illnesses like physical illness can be easily treated with medications and psychological methods.
* The treatment of mental illness is not just confined to drugs; it also includes many other psychological therapies like behavior modification therapy, counseling, activity therapy, family therapy, group therapy, etc.
* Continuity of treatment is more important for curing mental illnesses. Treatment should never be tampered without the advice of a psychiatrist.
* In majority of mental illnesses, for example, mania, depression and other neurotic disorders like dissociative disorder, patients recover completely without any residual effect if the treatment is taken on a regular basis.

❖ Early detection and prompt treatment for mental illnesses results in better improvement in psychiatric patients enabling them to lead socially productive lives.

REMEMBER

❖ Do not give false assurances or make false promises; just tell them you will do your best to help them

❖ Do not make any decisions for the family

❖ Do not criticize or blame

❖ See that they develop confidence in their abilities

❖ Do not let them become dependent on you

❖ Avoid half-hearted attempts; hard work yields good results

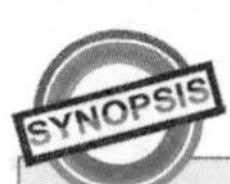

❖ Community mental health means providing services to the persons and families with mental illness within the community using community resources.

❖ In general, the community responds to the mentally ill through denial, isolation and rejection. There is also a lack of understanding of mental illness as any other illness, and a lack of tendency to reject both the patients and those who treat them.

❖ In the 1960s, psychiatrist Gerald Caplan described levels of prevention specific to psychiatry.

❖ He described primary prevention as an effort directed towards reducing the incidence of mental disorders in a community. Secondary prevention refers to decreasing the duration of disorder while tertiary prevention refers to reducing the level of impairment.

❖ Mental health services are delivered through mental hospitals located at central and state level. These also can be delivered through district and taluk hospitals, and primary health centers. Private and non-governmental organizations are also involved in delivering mental health care.

❖ Individuals in partial hospitalization program attend structured programming throughout the day and return home in the evenings.

❖ A halfway home is a transitory residential center for mentally ill patients who no longer need the full services of a hospital but are not yet ready for a completely independent living.

❖ Mental health agency is any private or public facility that is licensed by state government or central government as a mental health treatment facility.

❖ Voluntary organizations are a valuable community resource for mental health. They are often more sensitive to the local realities than centrally driven programs.

❖ Community mental health—psychiatric nursing is the application of specialized knowledge to populations and communities to promote and maintain mental health and to rehabilitate populations at risk that continue to have residual effects of mental illness.

REVIEW QUESTIONS

Long Essays

1. List levels of prevention. Describe role of a nurse in prevention of psychiatric disorders.
2. Enumerate the therapeutic activities of a nurse in community mental healthcare.
3. Explain in detail about mental health services available for mentally ill patients.

Short Essays

1. Mental health services available at various levels.
2. Scope of community mental health services.
3. Explain general attitude of people towards mentally ill individuals.

Short Answers

1. Goals of community mental health nursing
2. List the roles of a nurse in primary prevention
3. List the roles of a nurse in tertiary prevention

Give the Meaning of the Following

Stigma, discrimination, day care centers, self-help groups, halfway homes

Fill in the Blanks

1. Primary prevention is aimed at __________.
2. Secondary prevention is aimed at __________.
3. Tertiary prevention is aimed at __________.

State the Following Statements are True or False

1. Tertiary prevention targets on normal individuals who are living in the community.
2. Secondary prevention targets on individuals who are at risk for developing mental illness.
3. Stigma and discrimination can contribute to worsening of symptoms.
4. Primary prevention efforts are directed towards reducing disability among mentally ill people.
5. Self-help groups are voluntary organizations.

Multiple Choice Questions

1. **The follow-up and disability management is a part of:**
   a. Primary prevention
   b. Secondary prevention
   c. Tertiary prevention
   d. Dextra prevention

2. **The main aim of primary prevention is:**
   a. Strengthening individual, family and group coping abilities
   b. Helping mentally ill patients to regain premorbid level of functioning through treatment
   c. Helping to reduce the discomfort and disability associated with illness
   d. Enable the patient to achieve maximum range of interest and activity

3. **The main aim of secondary prevention is:**
   a. Strengthening individual, family and group coping abilities
   b. Helping mentally ill patients to regain premorbid level of functioning through treatment
   c. Helping to reduce the discomfort and disability associated with illness
   d. Enable the patient to achieve maximum range of interest and activity

4. **The main aim of tertiary prevention is:**
   a. Strengthening individual, family and group coping abilities

b. Helping mentally ill patients to regain premorbid level of functioning through treatment

c. Helping to reduce the discomfort and disability associated with illness

d. Enabling the patient to achieve maximum range of interest and activity

5. **The main aim of psychiatric rehabilitation is:**

a. Strengthening individual, family and group coping abilities

b. Helping mentally ill patients to regain premorbid level of functioning through treatment

c. Helping to reduce the discomfort and disability associated with illness

d. Enabling the patient to achieve maximum range of interest and activity

6. **Halfway homes are:**

a. Located within the hospital campus wherein patients take care of themselves

b. Transitory residential centers to integrate the individual into main stream of life

c. Innovative alternative to hospitalization with only day treatment program

d. Located within the hospital campus to reduce the disability of the patient

7. **Which of the following belongs to liaison role?**

a. Helping the patients and family members by bridging the gap between the patient and the hospital

b. Services are provided to the patient by visiting the home

c. Training the paraprofessionals in the community regarding management of psychiatric patients

d. Creating awareness in the community about mental illness

8. **In which of the following groups do members suffering from similar disorders share their experiences, strategies, successes and failures and find solutions to their problems**

a. Voluntary groups

b. Community groups

c. Self-help groups

d. Professional groups

🔒 ANSWER KEY

Fill in the Blanks

| 1. Prevention of incidence of mental health problems | 2. Supporting high risk individuals | 3. Supporting individuals with mental illness | | |

State the Following Statements are True or False

| 1. False | 2. True | 3. True | 4. False | 5. True |

Multiple Choice Questions

| 1. c | 2. a | 3. b | 4. c | 5. d |
| 6. b | 7. a | 8. c | | |

Psychiatric Emergencies and Crisis Intervention

CHAPTER OUTLINE

- ❑ Types of Psychiatric Emergencies—Attempted Suicide, Violence/Aggression, Stupor, Substance Intoxication and Withdrawal, Panic Attacks, Hysterical Attacks, Victims of Disaster, Rape Victim, Neuroleptic Malignant Syndrome, Serotonin Syndrome, Drug Toxicity
- ❑ Crisis—Characteristics, Types, Signs and Symptoms, Phases, Process, Intervention, Techniques, Modalities of Crisis Intervention

Psychiatric emergency is a condition wherein the patient has disturbances of thought, affect and psychomotor activity leading to a threat to his existence (suicide), or threat to the people in the environment (homicide). This condition needs immediate intervention to safeguard the life of the patient, bring down the anxiety of the family members and enhance emotional security to others in the environment.

Meaning

A psychiatric emergency is an acute disturbance of thought, mood, behavior of a patient which causes sudden distress to the individual/others and sudden disability or death thus requiring immediate management.

TYPES OF PSYCHIATRIC EMERGENCIES AND THEIR MANAGEMENT

Psychiatric emergencies do not mean that patients are suffering from only psychiatric disorders. They may be present due to medical conditions or conditions unrelated to medical field like disaster, rape, etc. Psychiatric emergencies may be classified as major where there is a danger to life either of the patient or to others in his environment or minor where there is no threat to life but causes severe incapacitation **(Table 8.1)**.

TABLE 8.1: Types of psychiatric emergencies		
Major emergencies	**Minor emergencies**	**Medical emergencies**
• Attempted suicide • Violence/aggression	• Stupor • Substance intoxication and withdrawal • Panic attacks • Hysterical attacks • Transient situational disturbances • Epileptic furor • Rape victim • Victims of disaster	• Neuroleptic malignant syndrome • Serotonin syndrome • Over dose of common psychiatric medications

Initial Approach during Emergency

* Initial approach to the patient should be warm, direct and concerned.
* A quick evaluation to identify the nature of condition and institution of care on the basis of seriousness is essential.
* Emergency staff should have basic knowledge of handling psychiatric emergencies.
* Medicolegal cases need to be registered separately and informed to the concerned officer.
* Hospital security must be adequate to control violent and dangerous patients.
* History and clinical findings should be recorded clearly in the emergency file.
* Patient's condition and plans of management should be explained in simple language to both the patient and family members.

Attempted Suicide

Suicide is a type of deliberate self-harm defined as an intentional human act of killing oneself. An attempted suicide is a suicidal act with non-fatal outcome. Suicide intent is an intention to end one's life through the act of suicidal behavior. Died by suicide is the recommended language which is preferred over the phrase 'committed suicide'. In psychiatry, a suicidal attempt is considered to be one of the commonest emergencies **(Box 8.1)**.

Risk Factors for Suicide

According to National Crime Records Bureau 2022, a total of 1,64,033 suicides were reported in the country in 2021. India reported a rate of 12 per 1 lakh population. Suicide is common in all level of people. Some important risk factors for suicide are presented in **Figure 8.1**.

Patient Characteristics

* **Age**
  o Males above 40 years of age
  o Females above 55 years of age
* **Sex**
  o Men have greater risk of completed suicide.
  o Suicide is three times more common in men than in women.
  o Women have higher rate of attempted suicide.
* Being unmarried, divorced, widowed or separated
* Recent losses
* History of trauma or abuse
* Individuals from higher or lower class show a greater tendency as compared to those from middle-class.

Conditions Associated with Suicidal Ideation

* Having a definite suicidal plan
* History of previous suicidal attempts
* Depression
* Schizophrenia
* Bipolar affective disorder
* Post traumatic stress disorder
* Substance abuse
* Borderline personality disorder

Physical Disorders

Patients with incurable or painful physical disorders like cancer and AIDS.

Psychosocial Factors

* Failure in examination
* Dowry harassment
* Marital problems
* Loss of loved object
* Isolation and alienation from social groups
* Financial and occupational difficulties

Suicidal Tendency in Psychiatric Wards

Certain psychiatric disorders where the patient may develop suicidal tendencies include:

BOX 8.1: Case vignette—Attempted suicide

Ms A, 45-year-old female, divorced, living alone is admitted to hospital the previous day due to over dose of lorazepam (30 tablets of 2 mg). She has not been attending to her duties for the past 2 weeks. She acknowledges feelings of depression since last fortnight, insomnia, anorexia and loss of weight. She says she wanted to die, had been thinking of suicide for the past week and planned the overdose. She is unhappy that the attempt failed. She states that 'nobody can help me' and sees no way to help herself. She denies having any close friends or relations, hobbies or activities. She views death as a "relief".

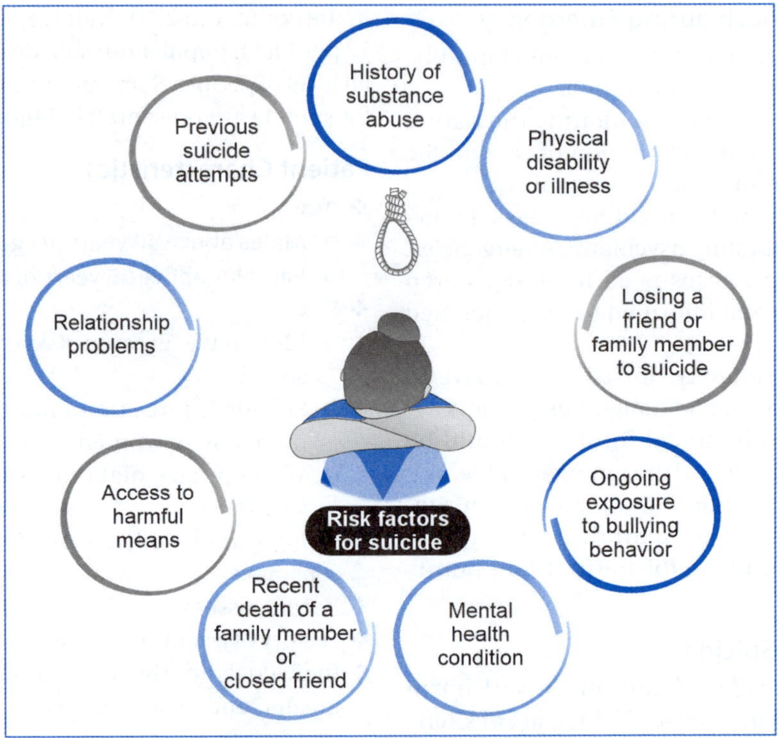

Figure 8.1: Risk factors for suicide

❖ **Major depression**: This is one of the commonest conditions associated with a high risk of suicide. Suicide in a major depressive episode is due to pervasive and persistent sadness; pessimistic cognitions concerning the past, present and future; delusions of guilt, helplessness, hopelessness and worthlessness; and derogatory voices urging him to take his life. The risk of suicide is more when the acute phase has passed and the characteristic psychomotor retardation has improved. This is so because the patient has more energy to carry out his suicidal plans now, though he might have been harboring them for quite some time. Feelings of loneliness, worthlessness, helplessness and hopelessness often result in intense feelings of depression, anger or hostility directed towards oneself. If no one is available to talk or listen to negative feelings a suicide attempt may occur in an effort to seek help or end as emotional conflict.

❖ **Schizophrenia**: Major risk factors among schizophrenics include the presence of associated depression, young age and high levels of premorbid functioning (especially during college education). People in this risk group are more likely to realize the devastating significance of their illness more than other groups of schizophrenic patients do, and see suicide as a reasonable alternative.

❖ **Mania**: Manic patients occasionally commit suicide. This is usually the result of grandiose ideation. The patient believes that he is a great person, or wishes to prove his supernatural powers. With this intent in mind, he may carry out some dangerous activity that can cost him his life.

❖ **Drug or alcohol abuse**: Suicide among alcoholics can be due to depression in the withdrawal phase. Also, the loss of friends and family, self-respect, status, and a general realization of the havoc alcohol has created in his life can cause the individual to wish to die.

- ❖ **Personality disorder**: Individuals with histrionic and borderline traits may occasionally attempt suicide.
- ❖ **Organic conditions**: Conditions such as delirium and dementia due to changes of mood like anxiety and depression may also induce suicidal tendency.

Management

- ❖ Be aware of certain signs which may indicate that the individual may commit suicide
  - ○ Suicidal threat
  - ○ Writing farewell letters
  - ○ Giving away treasured articles
  - ○ Making a will
  - ○ Closing bank accounts
  - ○ Appearing peaceful and happy after a period of depression
  - ○ Refusing to eat or drink
- ❖ Monitoring patient's safety needs
  - ○ Take all suicidal threats or attempts seriously and notify psychiatrist
  - ○ Search for toxic agents such as drugs/alcohol
  - ○ Do not leave the drug tray within the reach of patient, ensure daily medication is swallowed
  - ○ Remove sharp instruments such as razor blades, knives, glass bottles from his environment
  - ○ Remove straps and clothing such as belts, neckties
  - ○ Do not allow the patient to bolt his door on the inside, make sure somebody accompanies him to the bathroom
  - ○ Patient should be kept under constant observation and never left alone
  - ○ Have good vigilance especially during morning hours
  - ○ Spend time with him, talk to him, and allow him to ventilate his feelings.
  - ○ Encourage him to talk about his suicidal plans/methods
- ❖ If suicidal tendencies are very severe, sedation should be given as prescribed.

- ❖ Encourage verbal communication of suicidal ideas as well as his/her fear and depressive thoughts. A 'no suicidal' pact may be signed between the patient and the nurse. It is a written agreement that the patient will not act on suicidal impulses but will approach the nurse to talk about it.
- ❖ Enhance self-esteem of the patient by focusing on his strengths rather than weaknesses. His positive qualities should be emphasized with realistic praise and appreciation. This fosters a sense of self worth and enables him to take control of his life situation.

Management of Attempted Suicide in the Inpatient Unit

- ❖ Assess for vital signs, check airway and clear it, if necessary
- ❖ If pulse is weak, start IV fluids
- ❖ Turn patient's head and neck to one side to prevent regurgitation and swallowing of vomitus
- ❖ Emergency measures to be instituted in case of self-inflicted injuries

Management of Shock

- ❖ Transfer the patient to medical center immediately.
- ❖ If there is no evidence of life, leave the body in the same position/room in which it was found (in case of suicide move the patient from common living area, for example, dining room or TV room).
- ❖ In case, the patient has attempted suicide by jumping, do not leave the body in a place which is visible to other patients of the ward.
- ❖ Inform authorities, record the incident accurately.
- ❖ Contact local guardian and inform them.
- ❖ Place an attendant outside the room where the body is kept.
- ❖ Once the patient is transferred to mortuary or police custody, clean the place with disinfectant solution.
- ❖ Hand over the patient's properties to the concerned authorities/relatives.

❖ Carry out the institutional formalities for death certificate.

❖ The senior staff should discuss the incident in detail with all the staff and reassure them. The discussion should include possible lapses and preventive measures that need to be undertaken.

❖ Care for other patients should include the following:
  ○ Transfer all the patients away from the incident location
  ○ Keep the patients in the center engaged by games and other recreational activities
  ○ Serve food and medication to patients earlier than schedule
  ○ Observe for any change in the behavior, inform the psychiatrist

World Suicide Prevention Day is celebrated on 10th September. Section 115 of the Mental Health Care Act 2017 decriminalized the attempt to die by suicide, thereby reducing further stress on the victim.

Violence/Aggression

Anger is a normal human emotion. However, when anger leads to aggression and violence, the situation requires immediate intervention and de-escalation **(Box 8.2)**.

Meaning of Violence

Violence is a severe form of aggressiveness. During this stage, patient is irrational, unco-operative, delusional and assaultive.

Warning Signs of Violence

❖ Tense or angry facial expression
❖ Restlessness
❖ Increased speech
❖ Prolonged eye contact
❖ Verbal threats or violent gestures
❖ Verbalization of anger or violent feelings

Psychiatric Disorders Associated with Violent Behavior

❖ Schizophrenia especially paranoid
❖ Mania
❖ Antisocial personality
❖ Alcohol intoxication or withdrawal
❖ Substance withdrawal
❖ Post traumatic stress disorder
❖ Organic psychiatric disorders like, delirium, dementia, Wernicke Korsakoff's psychosis

Management

❖ An excited patient is usually brought tied up with a rope or in chains. The first step should be to remove the chains. A large proportion of aggression and violence is due to the patient feeling humiliated at being tied up in this manner.

❖ Talk to the patient and see if he responds. Firm and kind approach by the nurse is essential.

❖ Assure the patient about his physical safety

❖ Usually, sedation is given. Common drugs used are: diazepam 10–20 mg IV; haloperidol 10–20 mg; chlorpromazine 50–100 mg IM.

❖ Once the patient is sedated, collect history carefully from relatives; rule out the possibility of organic pathology. In particular check for history of convulsions, fever, recent intake of alcohol, fluctuations of consciousness.

❖ Carry out complete physical examination.

❖ Send blood specimens for hemoglobin, total cell count, etc.

❖ Look for evidence of dehydration and malnutrition. If there is severe dehydration, IV drip may be started.

❖ Remove potentially dangerous objects. Have less furniture in the room and remove sharp instruments, ropes, glass items, ties, strings, match boxes, etc., from patient's vicinity. Caution the patient when there is possibility of an accident.

BOX 8.2: Case vignette—Aggressive behavior

A 50-year-old man is brought to psychiatric emergency with hands tied. He is tremulous, agitated and aggressive, demanding immediate attention, speaking loudly, excited, having stared looks, flushed face, flared nostrils, hands are clenched. He is pushing the furniture with legs, slamming objects and uncooperative.

❖ Keep environmental stimuli such as lighting and noise levels to a minimum; assign a single room; limit interaction with others

❖ Stay with the patient as hyperactivity increases to reduce anxiety level and foster a feeling of security

❖ If the patient is not calmed by talking down and refuses medication, restraints may become necessary.

❖ Following application of restraints, observe patient every 15 minutes to ensure that nutritional and elimination needs are met. Also observe for any numbness, tingling or cyanosis in the extremities. It is important to choose the least restrictive alternative as far as possible for these patients.

❖ Approach towards the agitated and aggressive patient should be through verbal de-escalation. Encourage the patient to 'talk out' his aggressive feelings rather than acting them out.

❖ Redirect violent behavior with physical outlets such as exercise, outdoor activities.

❖ Guidelines for self-protection when handling an aggressive patient:
  ○ Never see a potentially violent person alone
  ○ Keep a comfortable distance away from the patient (arm length)
  ○ Be prepared to move, a violent patient can strike out suddenly
  ○ Maintain a clear exit route for both the staff and patient
  ○ Be sure the patient has no weapons in his possession before approaching him
  ○ If patient is having a weapon ask him to keep it on the table or floor rather than fighting with him to take it away
  ○ Keep a pillow, mattress or blanket wrapped around the arm between you and the weapon
  ○ Distract the patient momentarily to remove the weapon (throwing water in the patient's face, yelling, etc.)
  ○ Give prescribed antipsychotic medications

Stupor

Stupor is a clinical syndrome of akinesis and mutism but with relative preservation of conscious awareness. Stupor may be caused by schizophrenia (catatonic), affective disorder (depressive or very rarely manic stupor) or hysteria (dissociative stupor) or by neurological conditions.

Characteristics

❖ Patient is mute, motionless and unresponsive to stimuli but otherwise completely conscious, aware and alert

❖ Catatonic stupor is suggested by negativism, waxy flexibility and other movements

❖ Depressive stupor by tearfulness and a sad expression

❖ Dissociative stupor by closed eyes and resistance to passive eye-opening

❖ There is risk of starvation and severe dehydration as these patients refuse to eat or drink

Management

❖ Ensure patent airway
❖ Administer IV fluids
❖ Collect history and perform physical examination
❖ Draw blood for investigations before starting any treatment
❖ Pass NG tube and feed through it
❖ Other care is same as that for an unconscious patient

Substance Intoxication and Withdrawal

Alcohol, cocaine and phencyclidine are the substances that most commonly lead to violent behavior. Delirium tremens is an acute condition resulting from withdrawal of alcohol. Alcohol withdrawal can be life threatening and seizure can occur. Delirium tremens starts within 7 days of withdrawal usually within 24 to 72 hours.

Management

❖ Keep the patient in a quiet and safe environment away from stimulation

- ❖ Sedation is usually given with diazepam 10 mg or lorazepam 4 mg IV followed by oral administration
- ❖ Maintain fluid and electrolyte balance
- ❖ Reassure patient and family

Panic Attacks

Episodes of acute anxiety and panic can occur as a part of psychotic or neurotic illness. The patient will experience palpitations, sweating, tremors, feelings of choking, chest pain, nausea, abdominal distress, fear of dying, paresthesia, chills or hot flushes. This mimics ischemic heart attack or serious medical condition.

Characteristics
- ❖ White knuckled
- ❖ Heart pounding terror
- ❖ People feel like they are going mad
- ❖ Fear and feeling of dying
- ❖ Most of these attacks last only a few minutes

Management
- ❖ Give reassurance first, calm the patient and relatives
- ❖ Search for causes and rule out ischemic heart disorder
- ❖ Teach breathing and relaxation exercises and positive self-talk
- ❖ Diazepam 10 mg or lorazepam 2 mg may be administered

Hysterical Attacks

A hysteric may mimic abnormality of any function which is under voluntary control. The common modes of presentation may be:
- ❖ Hysterical fits
- ❖ Hysterical ataxia
- ❖ Hysterical paraplegia

   All presentations are marked by a dramatic quality and sadness of mood.

Management
- ❖ Hysterical fit must be distinguished from genuine fits. (*See* Page No. 139 for differences between hysterical and epileptic seizures)
- ❖ As hysterical symptoms can cause panic among relatives, explain to the relatives the psychological nature of symptoms. Reassure that no harm would come to the patient.
- ❖ Help the patient realize the meaning of symptoms and help him find alternative ways of coping with stress.
- ❖ Suggestion therapy with IV pentothal may be helpful in some cases.

Victims of Disaster

Victims of disaster are people who have survived from an unexpected, overwhelming stress which is beyond normally what is expected in life, for example earthquake, flood, riots and terrorism. Anger, frustration, guilt, numbness and confusion are common features in these people.

Management
- ❖ Treatment for life-threatening physical problems
- ❖ In selected cases, benzodiazepines are prescribed to reduce anxiety and induce sleep
- ❖ Referral to mental health service, if required
- ❖ Educate the victims that these emotional reactions are normal reactions to an extraordinary and abnormal situation, and are to be expected under the circumstances. Educate about the available services
- ❖ Teach coping strategies to avoid the development of crises. For example, strategies to be taught can include how to request information, access resources and obtain support
- ❖ Group therapy
- ❖ Critical Incident Debriefing (CID) is a special technique which is used to lessen the discomfort of the disaster victims.
- ❖ CID includes five phases: Fact, thought, reaction, reaching and reentry:
    - ○ In the *fact phase,* each participant is involved and encouraged to share his or her perception of the incident. Group members describe the incident, new information and pieces of information are integrated into a more understandable whole
    - ○ The *thought phase* builds on this information by asking participants to

reflect on the incident and share what they were feeling personally during the difficult times of crisis.

- In *reaction phase,* participants are asked to evaluate the impact of emotional aspects of the incident (for example, what was the worst part of the incident for you). Previously not discussed and less acceptable feelings are allowed to emerge in a safe environment. Knowing that other people are experiencing the same feelings makes them realize that these feelings are normal behavioral responses to abnormal circumstances. This brings a lot of relief to people who are under intense stress. Participants discuss stress related symptoms they had during the incident or are experiencing currently.
- The *teaching phase,* focuses on specific cognitive, emotional and spiritual strategies to reduce stress and ways to enhance group support.
- In the final *re-entry phase,* the facilitator encourages questions and summarizes the process. Finally, individuals are referred to further counseling, if needed.

Rape Victim

Rape is an unlawful sexual intercourse or other forms of sexual penetration carried out against a person without their consent.

Signs and Symptoms

Acute disorganization characterized by self-blame, fear of being killed, feeling of degradation and loss of self-esteem, feelings of depersonalization and derealization, recurrent intrusive thoughts, anxiety and depression are commonly seen. Long-term psychological effects like post-traumatic stress disorders (PTSD) can occur in some cases.

Management

- Be supportive, reassuring and non- judg-mental
- Physical examination for any injuries
- Give morning after pill to prevent possible pregnancy
- Send samples for STD and HIV infection
- Explain to the patient the possibility of PTSD, sexual problems like vaginismus and anorgasmia which may appear later

Neuroleptic Malignant Syndrome

Neuroleptic malignant syndrome is rare but most serious of these symptoms. It occurs in a small minority of patients taking neuroleptics, especially high potency compounds. It is a hypermetabolic reaction to dopamine antagonists, primary antipsychotic drugs such as phenothiazines and butyrophenones. Usually occurs early in treatment.

Signs and Symptoms

- Muscle rigidity
- Hyperpyrexia
- Tachycardia
- Hypertension
- Tachypnea
- Change in mental status and autonomic dysfunction

Management

The drug should be stopped immediately. Treatment is symptomatic and includes cooling the patient, maintaining fluid and electrolyte balance and treating infections. Diazepam can be used for muscle stiffness. The drug dantrolene is used to treat malignant hyperthermia. Bromocriptine, amantadine and L-dopa have been used to treat neuroleptic malignant syndrome. Treatment is usually in ICU.

Serotonin Syndrome

It occurs when serotonergic agents are used in combination with MAOI inhibitors. A sudden buildup of serotonin in the body may lead to life-threatening condition.

Symptoms

- Hyperthermia
- Diaphoresis
- Excitement or confusion
- Hyperreflexia
- Hypotension
- Tremor

Management

- ❖ Stop the drug immediately
- ❖ Monitor vital signs
- ❖ Administer IV fluids
- ❖ Severe hyperthermia may require sedation

Drug Toxicity

Drug overdosage may be accidental or suicidal. In either case, all attempts must be made to find out the drug consumed. A detailed history should be collected and symptomatic treatment instituted.

A common case of drug poisoning is lithium toxicity. The symptoms include drowsiness, vomiting, abdominal pain, confusion, blurred vision, acute circulatory failure, stupor and coma, generalized convulsions, oliguria and death.

Management

- ❖ Administer O_2
- ❖ Start IV line
- ❖ Assess for cardiac arrhythmias
- ❖ Refer for hemodialysis
- ❖ Administer anticonvulsants

Psychiatric nurses should meet patients' needs during emergency. They need to show confidence, empathy and knowledge in dealing with emergency conditions. The goal is to evaluate the problem quickly and develop a plan of care that is clinically sound, attends to the patient's perceived needs and effectively utilizes available resources.

CRISIS

Crisis can be viewed as an integral component of everyday life situations. A crisis may influence people's lives in different ways. As a consequence of a crisis experience, the individual may go down to a lower or less healthy level of functioning than what was before the crisis, or he may resume the same level of functioning by repressing the crisis and the related emotions. On the other hand, he may function at a healthier level than prior to the crisis, because the challenge of a crisis can bring out new strengths, skills and coping mechanisms.

Intervention at a crisis is extremely important to prevent mental illness because long-standing problems make the person totally incapable of handling the situation. If proper guidance is provided at the correct time, the victim will come out of it and be better equipped to handle future problems in life.

Definition

Crisis is an acute emotional upset; it is manifested in the inability to cope emotionally, cognitively or behaviorally and to solve problems as usual.   **—Hoff, 2009**

Crisis is a state of disequilibrium resulting from the interaction of an event with the individual's or family's coping mechanisms, which are inadequate to meet the demands of the situation, combined with the individual's or family's perception of the meaning of the event.   **—Taylor, 1982**

A crisis is a perception or experiencing of an event or situation as an intolerable difficulty that exceeds the person's current resources and coping mechanisms.

—James and Gilliland, 2005

A crisis is a period of psychological disequilibrium, experienced as a result of a hazardous event or situation that constitutes a significant problem that cannot be remedied by using familiar coping strategies.

—Robert 2000

Characteristics of Crisis

A crisis occurs when individuals are confronted with problems that cannot be solved. The following are characteristics of crisis events:

- ❖ The event is unexpected.
- ❖ It creates uncertainty.
- ❖ It is perceived as threatening.
- ❖ There is an apparent inability to modify or reduce the impact of stressful events.
- ❖ There is a high level of subjective discomfort such as fear tension or confusion.
- ❖ The crisis is personal in nature and can vary from person to person.

Crisis Proneness

Hendricks (1985) suggests that certain individuals are more prone to crisis than others. The list of characteristics often found in individuals who are regarded as being more susceptible to crisis are presented in **Box 8.3**.

It is important to note that individual personality traits must also be considered in conjunction with these characteristics. Crisis is defined by the individual; what is a crisis for one is merely an occurrence for another. This factor is a critical component that must be evaluated in relation to crisis prone characteristics as well as personality traits.

Types of Crises

A crisis is an unforeseen event that causes restlessness within the individual. Different types of crises can occur among individuals all of which require to be adept to the situation to keep working toward the goals. There are three types of crises commonly occurring in individuals **(Figure 8.2)**.

Maturational Crisis

Maturation is a transition point where an individual moves into a successive stage often generating disequilibrium. Maturational crisis is a stage in a person's life where adjustment and adaptation to new responsibilities and life patterns are necessary. Individuals are required to make cognitive and behavioral changes and integrate those physical changes that accompany development.

The extent to which individuals experience success in the mastery of these tasks depends on previous successes, availability of support systems, influence of role models and acceptability of new role by others.

The transitional periods or events that are most commonly identified as having increased crisis potential are adolescence, marriage, parenthood, midlife and retirement.

Situational Crisis

A situational crisis is one that is precipitated by an unanticipated stressful event that creates disequilibrium by threatening one's sense of biological, social or psychological integrity. Examples of events that can precipitate situational crises are premature birth, status and role changes, death of a loved one, physical or mental illness, divorce, change in

> **BOX 8.3:** Crisis proneness characteristics
>
> - Dissatisfaction with employment or lack of employment
> - History of unresolved crisis
> - History of substance abuse
> - Poor self-esteem, unworthiness
> - Superficial relationship with others
> - Difficulty in coping with everyday situations
> - Underutilization of resources and support systems
> - Aloofness and lack of caring

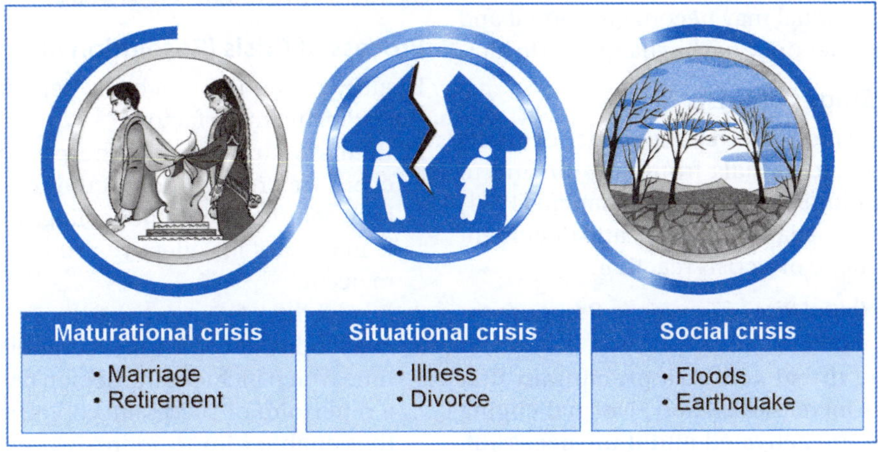

Figure 8.2: Types of crises

geographic location, an accident, financial loss, unexpected pregnancy, etc.

Social Crisis

Social crisis is accidental, uncommon, and unanticipated and results in multiple losses and radical environmental changes. Social crises include natural disasters like floods, earthquakes, violence, nuclear accidents, mass killings, contamination of large areas by toxic wastes, wars, etc. This type of crisis is unlike maturational and situational crisis because it does not occur in the lives of all people.

Because of the severity of the effects of social crisis, coping strategies may not be effective. Individuals confronted with social crisis usually do not have previous experience from which to draw expertise. Support systems may be unavailable because they may also be involved in similar situations. Mental health professionals are called upon to act quickly and provide services to large number of people and in some cases, the whole community.

Signs and Symptoms of Crisis

- ❖ The individual experiences a heavy burden of free-floating anxiety.
- ❖ The anxiety may be manifested through depression, anger and guilt. The victim will attempt to get rid of the anxiety using various coping mechanisms, healthy or unhealthy.
- ❖ The individual may become incapable of even taking care of his daily needs and may neglect his responsibilities.
- ❖ The individual may become irrational and blame others for what has happened to him.

Phases/Stages of Crisis

A crisis situation involves a sequence of events that leads individuals from equilibrium to disequilibrium and back again. Caplan (1964) is the first clinician to describe and document the four stages of a crisis reaction.

Phase I—Initial Rise of Tension in Response to an Event

Perceived threat acts as a precipitant that generates increased anxiety. Normal coping strategies are activated and if unsuccessful, the individual moves into Phase II.

Phase II—Increased Tension

Ineffectiveness of the Phase I coping mechanism leads to further disorganization. The individual experiences a sense of vulnerability and increased tension disrupting daily living. The individual may attempt to cope with the situation in a random fashion. If the anxiety continues and there is no reduction, the individual enters Phase III.

Phase III—Redefining the Crisis

With continued failure of the individual's efforts, a further rise in tension acts as a stimulus for mobilization of emergency and novel problem-solving measures. At this stage, the problem may be redefined, the individual may resign himself to the problem or he may find a solution to it. The individual is most amenable to assistance in this phase. New problem-solving measures may also affect a solution. Return to precrisis level of functioning may occur. If problem solving is unsuccessful, further disorganization occurs and the individual is said to have entered Phase IV.

Phase IV—Psychological Breakdown

If the problem continues, the tension mounts beyond a further threshold resulting in a major breakdown in the individual's mental and social functioning. Severe to panic levels of anxiety with profound cognitive, emotional and physiological changes may occur. Referral for further treatment is necessary.

Process of Crisis (Resolution of Crisis)

Healthy resolution of a crisis depends upon the following three factors:

1. Realistic appraisal of the precipitating event, i.e., recognition of the relationship between the event and feelings of anxiety is necessary for effective problem solving to occur.
2. Availability of support systems.
3. Availability of coping measures over a lifetime which includes the person developing a repertoire of successful coping strategies that enable him to identify and resolve stressful situations (**Box 8.4**).

Ms Kamala had moved from a small village to the nearest town to seek employment. She was unable to evacuate the town before the floods hit. She stayed temporarily at the shelter where other disaster responders were placed. Although Kamala was deeply affected by the pain and suffering that surrounded her, she had a clear plan of action. She resolved to quit the job and return closer to her family. She took a rented vehicle and reached the home town where she searched for a new job. Soon her crisis was over.

Mr John was also placed in the same shelter home after the sudden flooding and evacuation. He lost everything in floods including his home, parents and property. He was overwhelmed and unclear about the direction his life would take in the following few months. In the face of this crisis, he displayed complete hopelessness and helplessness and a crisis therefore became a trauma for him.

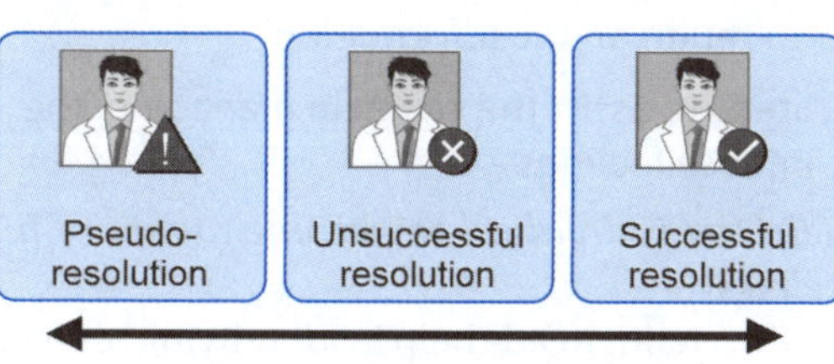

Figure 8.3: Resolution of crisis

There are three ways in which the individual may resolve the crisis **(Figure 8.3)**:

Pseudo-resolution

In this, the individual uses repression and pushes out of consciousness the incident and the intense emotions associated with it, resulting in the individual functioning at the same earlier level. But in future, if and when a crisis occurs, the repressed feelings may surface and influence the feelings aroused by the new crisis. In such a situation, the particular crisis may be more difficult to resolve because the feelings associated with the earlier crisis are neither expressed nor handled at that time.

Unsuccessful Resolution

In this, the victim uses pathological adaptation at any phase of crisis resulting in a lower level of functioning. The victim, rather than accepting the loss and reorganizing his life, keeps ruminating over the loss. An example is prolonged grief reaction which results in depression.

Successful Resolution

In this, the victim may go through the various phases of crisis but reaches Phase III where various coping measures are utilized to resolve the crisis situation. The individual develops better skills and problem-solving ability which can be and will be used in various crisis situations in future.

Crisis Intervention

Crisis intervention is a technique used to help an individual or family to understand and cope with the intense feelings that are typical of a crisis. This intervention provides opportunities for clients to learn new coping skills while identifying, mobilizing and enhancing those they already possess. Nurses function as part of the interdisciplinary team in the use of crisis intervention as a therapeutic modality. Nurses may employ crisis techniques in their work with high-risk groups such as patients with chronic diseases, new parents and bereaved persons. Nurses may also use crisis intervention in dealing with intra group staff issues and patient management issues.

Aims of Crisis Intervention Technique

❖ To provide a correct cognitive perception of the situation
❖ To assist the individual in managing the intense and overwhelming feelings associated with the crisis

Principles of Crisis Intervention

❖ Be specific, use concise statements and avoid overwhelming the patient with irrelevant questions or excessive detail
❖ Encourage the expression of feelings
❖ A calm, controlled presence reassures the person that the nurse can help
❖ **Listen for facts and feelings:** Seeking clarification, paraphrasing and reflection are effective strategies

❖ Allow sufficient time for the individuals involved to process information and ask questions

❖ Help patients legitimize feelings by letting them know that others in similar situations have experienced comparable emotions

❖ Clarify distortions by getting the persons to look at the situation realistically, focus on what can be changed versus what cannot

❖ Empower the person by allowing him to make informed choices

❖ Assist the person in confronting reality

❖ Encourage the person to focus on one implication at a time

Intervention

Crisis intervention is a short-term management technique designed to reduce potential permanent damage to an individual affected by a crisis. The steps involved in crisis intervention are presented in **Figure 8.4**.

1. Steps to provide a correct cognitive perception

Assessment of the situation

❖ This may be achieved by direct questioning with a purpose to identify the problem and the people involved.

❖ It is necessary to identify the support systems available and to know the depth in which the individual's feelings are affected.

❖ Assessment should also be done to identify the strengths and limitations of the victim.

Defining the event

❖ The victim at times may not be able to identify the precipitating event because of the possible denial or the reluctance to talk about it.

❖ It may be necessary for the therapist to review the details of the incidents in the past 2 to 4 weeks in order to identify the event that precipitated the crisis. Such a review will help the victim becoming aware of the precipitating event.

Develop a plan of action

❖ The victim and the people closely associated with him should have an active involvement in developing the plan of action.

❖ The therapist must be aware that the victim may not be in a condition to mentally comprehend complicated information due to the overwhelming anxiety experienced by him. The instructions given by the therapist must be simple and clear, and too much information should not be given at a time. The instructions may have to be written down as the victim may not be able to retain all the information.

2. Steps to assist the victim in managing the intense feelings

Help the individual to become aware of his feelings

❖ The victim needs help in identifying his own feelings, which is the first step in handling them.

❖ The therapist should use appropriate communication technique for the victim to be comfortable in expressing his feelings without the fear of being judged or criticized.

❖ The therapist should also be efficient in observing verbal and nonverbal behavior of the victim enabling him to make a careful assessment of his feelings.

Figure 8.4: Crisis intervention

Help the individual to attain mastery over his feelings

❖ The individual should be given adequate support and guidance through the therapeutic process for handling feelings associated with the crisis. However, special care should be taken not to give any false reassurance.

❖ He should not in any way be encouraged to blame others as it will only let him escape from taking any responsibility.

❖ Care must be taken to ensure that the individual does not develop too much dependence on the therapist, which is unhealthy.

❖ After the victim and the support groups, prepare the plan of action under the guidance of the therapist, it should be discussed with the victim and the concerned others so as to have a clear understanding of the methods of implementation of the plan.

❖ To improve coping with the situation necessary environmental manipulation must be done in physical or interpersonal areas.

❖ It is advisable for the patient to fix up another appointment with the therapist within a week so as to assess the effectiveness of the plan, and if need be, revise and modify it.

Techniques of Crisis Intervention

❖ **Catharsis**: Release of feelings that takes place as the patient talks about emotionally charged areas.

❖ **Clarification**: Encouraging the patient to express more clearly the relationship between certain events.

❖ **Manipulation**: Using the patient's emotions, wishes or values to benefit the patient in the therapeutic process.

❖ **Reinforcement of behavior**: Giving the patient positive reinforcement to adaptive behavior.

❖ **Support of defenses**: Encouraging the use of healthy, adaptive defenses and discouraging those that are unhealthy or maladaptive.

❖ **Increasing self-esteem**: Helping the patient to regain feelings of self-worth.

❖ **Exploration of solutions**: Examining alternative ways of solving the immediate problem.

Geriatric Considerations

Older persons who were most successful at adapting to losses earlier in life will cope more adaptively with the losses and grief inherent in aging. The elderly persons who experienced more losses are unable to complete the grief process resulting in bereavement overload. Such people are less able to adapt and re-integrate physical and mental health and are prone to depressive disorders.

Role of a Nurse in Crisis Intervention

Nurses respond to crisis situations on a daily basis. Crisis can occur in any unit, e.g., in general hospitals, home settings, community health centers, schools, offices, and in private practice. Indeed, nurses may be called upon to function as crisis helpers in any situation. Knowledge of crisis intervention techniques is thus an important clinical skill for all nurses regardless of the setting or practice specialty.

Nursing assessment

The first step in crisis intervention is assessment. During this phase, the nurse collects data regarding the following factors:

❖ Precipitating event or stressor

❖ Patient's perception of the event or stressor

❖ Nature and strength of the patient's support systems, coping resources

❖ Level of psychological stress the patient is suffering from and the degree of impairment he is experiencing

❖ Patient's previous strengths and coping mechanisms

During this phase, the nurse begins to establish a positive working relationship with the patient.

Nursing diagnoses

The primary nursing diagnoses in crisis intervention are:

❖ Ineffective individual coping refers to the inability to ask for help, solve the problems or meet role expectations.

❖ Ineffective family coping occurs when the family's support system is not successful and its social or economic wellbeing is threatened.

❖ Altered family processes result when family members are unable to adapt to the traumatic experience constructively.

Post-traumatic response is a sustained painful response to an overwhelming traumatic event.

Planning

In planning, the previously collected data is analyzed and specific interventions proposed. During this phase, the nurse undertakes the following activities:

❖ Dynamics underlying the present crisis are formulated.

❖ Alternative solutions to the problem are explored.

❖ Steps for achieving the solutions are identified.

❖ Environmental support needed to help the patient is decided upon.

❖ Coping mechanisms to be developed and those to be strengthened are identified.

Implementation

The following interventions are carried out to resolve crisis:

❖ **Environmental manipulation**: Environmental manipulation includes interventions that directly change the patient's physical or interpersonal situation. These interventions may remove stress and provide situational support. For example, a patient having difficulty in his job may take a week of sick leave so that he can be temporarily removed from that stress situation.

❖ **General support**: Nurses uses warmth, acceptance, empathy and reassurance to provide general support to the patient.

❖ **Generic approach**: The generic approach is designed to reach high-risk individuals and large groups as quickly as possible. It applies a specific method to all individuals faced with a similar type of crisis (for example, in social disasters). Debriefing is a method of generic approach. In debriefing method, disaster victims are helped to recall events and clarify traumatic experiences. It attempts to place the traumatic event in perspective, allows the individual to relive the event in a factual way, encourages group support, and provides information on normal reaction to critical events. The goal of debriefing is to prevent resulting maladaptive responses that might emerge if the trauma is suppressed.

❖ **Individual approach**: The individual approach is a type of crisis intervention similar to the diagnosis and treatment of a specific problem in a specific patient. It is particularly useful in combined situational and maturational crises and also beneficial when symptoms include homicidal and suicidal risk. The nurse must use the intervention that is most likely to help the patient develop an adaptive response to the crisis.

❖ **Evaluation**: The nurse and the patient review the changes that have occurred. The nurse should give credit for successful changes to the patient so that he realizes their effectiveness and that the learning from the crisis may help in coping with such future incidents. If the goals are not met, the nurse and the patient can return to the first step assessment and continue through the phases again.

Modalities of Crisis Intervention

Community-based crisis intervention modalities are based on the philosophy that the healthcare team must be active and go out to the patients rather than wait for the patients to come to them. Nurses working in these modalities intervene in a variety of community settings ranging from patient's home to street corners **(Figure 8.5)**.

Mobile Crisis Programs

Mobile crisis teams provide front-line interdisciplinary crisis intervention to individuals, families and communities. The nurse who is a member of the mobile crisis team should be able to provide onsite assessment, crisis management, treatment, referral and educational services to patients,

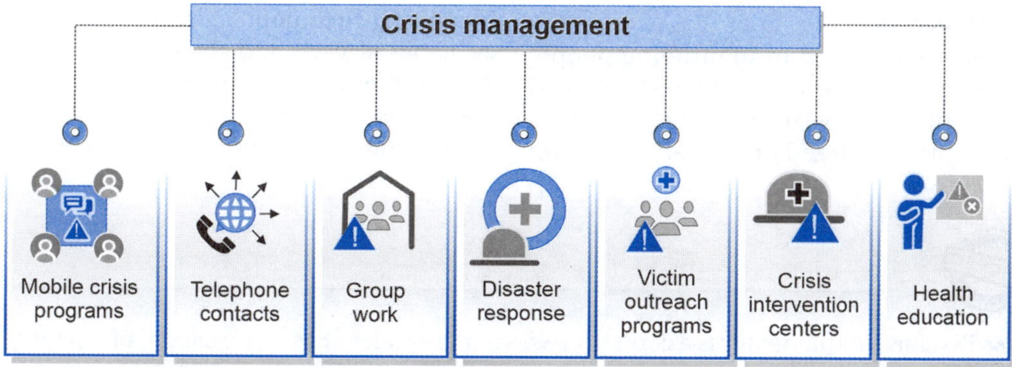

Figure 8.5: Modalities of crisis intervention

families and the community at large. Nurses are thus able to ensure mental healthcare for even the most underserved populations efficiently and cost effectively.

Telephone Contacts

Crisis intervention is sometimes practiced by telephone rather than through face-to-face contacts. The nurse should have effective listening skills to provide crisis intervention to victims.

Group Work

People who have common traits on stressors form a group. It provides an opportunity for the members to express common concerns and experiences, foster hope and build mutual support. Nurse's role in the group is active, focal and focused on the present. The nurse and the group help the patient solve the problem and reinforce new problem-solving behavior.

Disaster Response

As a part of the community nurses are called upon when an adventitious or social crisis strikes the community. Floods, earthquakes, airplane crashes, fires, nuclear accidents, etc., precipitate large number of crises. The nurse has an important role in dealing with psychosocial problems of disaster victims. The nurse participates in crisis operations and acts as a case finder for persons suffering from psychosocial stress. It is important that nurses in the immediate post disaster period go to places where victims are likely to gather such as hospitals, shelters, morgues. During this period, nurses use the generic approach of crisis intervention so that as many people as possible can receive help in a short duration of time.

Victim Outreach Programs

Victim outreach programs use crisis intervention techniques to identify the needs of victims and then to connect them with appropriate referrals and other resources.

Nurses work in victim outreach programs where victims are often seen immediately after the crisis. These victims need thorough evaluation, empathic support, information and help from the larger social networking system.

Crisis Intervention Centers

Crisis intervention centers provide emergency psychiatric care and counseling to victims experiencing extreme stress or conflict and to those involved in suicide attempts or drug or alcohol abuse. These centers which are usually self-contained units within a hospital or community healthcare center provide services 24 hours a day. These are delivered either directly on the premises or over the telephone. The primary objective of crisis intervention centers is to help the person cope with immediate problem and offer guidance and support for long-term therapy.

Health Education

Nurses are involved in identifying people who are at high risk for developing crisis and teaching them the necessary coping strategies. The public too needs to be educated on identifying such population, be aware of the available services and change their attitude. This will encourage the people to obtain information and seek services on how to deal with potential crisis producing problems.

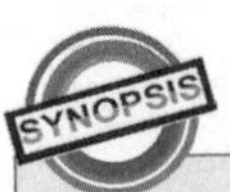

- Psychiatric emergency is a condition wherein the patient has disturbances of thought, affect and psychomotor activity leading to a threat to his existence (suicide), or threat to the people in the environment (homicide).
- Major emergencies in psychiatry are attempted suicide, violent and aggression behavior. Minor emergencies are stupor, substance intoxication, panic attacks, hysterical attack, transient situational disturbances, epileptic furor, rape victim and victims of disaster. Medical emergencies are neuroleptic malignant syndrome, serotonin syndrome, over dose of common psychiatric medications.
- An attempted suicide is a suicidal act with non-fatal outcome. Suicide intent is an intention to end one's life through the act of suicidal behavior.
- Risk factors for suicide attempt are major depression, schizophrenia, mania, drug or alcohol abuse, personality disorder and organic conditions.
- Violence is a severe form of aggressiveness. During this stage, patient is irrational, unco-operative, delusional and assaultive.
- Psychiatric disorders associated with violence behavior are schizophrenia, mania, antisocial personality, alcohol intoxication, substance withdrawal, PTSD and organic psychiatric disorders.
- Stupor is a clinical syndrome of akinesis and mutism but with relative preservation of conscious awareness.
- Stupor may be caused by schizophrenia (catatonic), affective disorder (depressive or very rarely manic stupor) or hysteria (Dissociative stupor) or by neurological conditions.
- Episodes of acute anxiety and panic can occur as a part of psychotic or neurotic illness.
- A hysteric may mimic abnormality of any function which is under voluntary control.
- Victims of disaster are people who have survived from an unexpected, overwhelming stress which is beyond normally what is expected in life, for example, earthquake, flood, riots and terrorism. Anger, frustration, guilt, numbness and confusion are common features in these people.
- Rape is an unlawful sexual intercourse or other forms of sexual penetration carried out against a person without their consent.
- Neuroleptic malignant syndrome is a hypermetabolic reaction to dopamine antagonists, primary antipsychotic drugs such as phenothiazines and butyrophenones.
- Crisis is an acute emotional upset; it is manifested in the inability to cope emotionally, cognitively or behaviorally and to solve problems as usual.
- There are three types of crises: maturational, situational and social crisis
- Caplan identified four phases of crisis, phase 1—initial rise of tension in response to an event, phase 2—increased tension, phase 3—redefining the crisis, phase 4—psychological breakdown.

❖ Crisis intervention includes assessment of the situation, defining the event, developing a plan of action, helping the individual to become aware of his feelings, helping the individual to attain mastery over his feelings.

❖ Technique of crisis intervention includes catharsis, clarification, manipulation, reinforcement, support of defenses, increasing self esteem, exploration of solutions.

❖ Various modalities of crisis intervention are mobile crisis programs, telephone contacts, group work, disaster response, victim outreach programs, crisis intervention centres and health education.

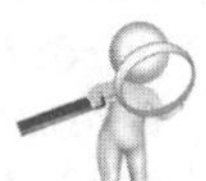

REVIEW QUESTIONS

Long Essays

1. List the common psychiatric emergencies. Describe nursing management for an attempted suicide patient.
2. Explain management of aggressive patient.
3. Role of a nurse in crisis intervention.

Short Essays

1. Risk factors for suicide
2. Suicide attempt prevention in psychiatric wards
3. Modalities of crisis intervention

Short Answers

1. Types of crises
2. Maturational crisis
3. Techniques of crisis intervention

Give the Meaning of the Following

Stupor, drug toxicity, crisis, catharsis, manipulation.

Fill in the Blanks

1. __________ is a transition point where an individual moves into a successive stage often generating disequilibrium.
2. __________ crisis is one that is precipitated by an unanticipated stressful event.
3. ________ crisis is accidental, uncommon and unanticipated and results in multiple losses.
4. ________ is the technique used to help an individual to understand and cope with the intense feelings of crisis.
5. ________ is a severe form of aggression.

State the Following Statements are True or False

1. Psychiatric emergency causes sudden distress to individual and others.
2. Anger is a normal human emotion.
3. Neuroleptic malignant syndrome is a common side effect of antipsychotics.
4. Crisis creates certainty.
5. Marriage is an example of situational crisis.

Multiple Choice Questions

1. **Following are the initial approaches during a psychiatric emergency, *except*:**
   a. Quick evaluation to identify the condition
   b. Initial approach should be warm and direct
   c. Hospital security should be adequate to control violent patients
   d. Initial focus should be on control of emotions

2. **All are psychiatric emergencies, *except*:**
   a. Major depression with suicidal attempt
   b. Manic excitement

   c. Chronic schizophrenia with blunt affect

   d. Alcohol intoxication

3. **While planning nursing process for a patient who is at risk for suicide, which of the following is a priority area for providing care?**
   a. Sleep
   b. Nutrition
   c. Self-esteem
   d. Safety

4. **Which one of the following is a commonest condition associated with high risk of suicide?**
   a. Hypomania
   b. Major depression
   c. Chronic schizophrenia
   d. Drug abuse

5. **In major depressive patients, which of the following is a risk factor for suicide tendency?**
   a. Psychomotor retardation
   b. Pessimistic cognition
   c. Stress situation
   d. Drug-induced sedation

6. **In schizophrenia, patients which of the following is a risk factor for suicide tendency?**
   a. Unable to control drug side effects
   b. Poor social support
   c. Lack of understanding about disease
   d. Associated depression

7. **In mania patients, which of the following is a risk factor for suicide tendency?**
   a. Hyperactive behavior
   b. Grandiose ideas
   c. Poor social support
   d. Stress from the situation

8. **Following are all signs of suicide tendencies, *except*:**
   a. Expressing suicidal ideas
   b. Writing farewell letters
   c. Appearing peaceful and happy
   d. Eating adequate food and having proper sleep

9. **Which of the following is an appropriate nursing intervention for suicidal patient?**
   a. Report to the unit doctor
   b. Ignore patient's suicidal comments
   c. Reassure the patient that suicidal thoughts will be reduced
   d. Teach healthier problem solving skills

10. **Patient tells you that "I am just a burden, everyone will be happy if I die". From this statement of the patient, the nurse is aware that:**
    a. Suicide talk is an attention getting tool
    b. Suicide is an impulsive act; it is not thought out
    c. Suicidal talk or ideation can lead to suicide behavior
    d. Suicidal people seldom really attempt suicide

11. **Which methods would a nurse use to determine a patient's potential risk for suicide?**
    a. Do not focus much on suicidal ideations
    b. Question the patient directly on suicidal thoughts
    c. Divert the patient's mind by asking future plans
    d. Observe the patient continuously

12. **Nursing supervisor tells you that Ms Uma must be placed on suicide precaution. The first intervention you begin is:**
    a. Place Ms Uma in a locked room
    b. Begin one-to-one observation at least every 15 minutes
    c. Allow Ms Uma what she wanted to do
    d. Isolate Ms Uma from others

13. **The following disorders contribute to aggressive behavior in a patient, *except*:**
    a. Delirium
    b. Acute mania episode
    c. Agitated depression
    d. Generalized anxiety disorder.

14. **Following are all appropriate nursing interventions for aggressive patients, *except*:**
a. Encourage the patient to talk out his aggressive feelings
b. Keep environmental stimuli to a minimum
c. Use punishment strategies
d. Remove hazardous objects and substances from patient vicinity

15. **A 20-year-old female is sexually assaulted on her way back home. Rape is an example of:**
a. Situational crisis
b. Maturational crisis
c. Social crisis
d. Adventitious crisis

16. **The primary goal of crisis intervention is to:**
a. Help the patient express his/her feelings
b. Identify stressors
c. Help the patient return to precrisis level
d. Support the family members

17. **Unanticipated stressful event leads to a _______ crisis.**
a. Maturational
b. Situational
c. Social
d. Multiple

18. **Retirement is a _______ crisis.**
a. Maturational
b. Situational
c. Social
d. Multiple

19. **Floods are an example of _______ crisis.**
a. Maturational
b. Situational
c. Social
d. Multiple

20. **Healthy resolution of crisis depends upon all of the following factors, e*xcept:***
a. Realistic appraisal of the precipitating event
b. Availability of support system
c. Availability of adaptive coping measures
d. Availability of medical facilities

21. **As per Caplan, which of the following phase is associated with successful crisis resolution?**
a. Phase 1   b. Phase 2
c. Phase 3   d. Phase 4

22. **Following are all adaptive coping techniques, *except*:**
a. Positive self-talk
b. Assertiveness
c. Time management
d. Expecting sympathy from others

23. **Which of the following nursing intervention is more appropriate to provide a correct cognitive perception of the situation to a crisis patient?**
a. Assessment of the situation
b. Defining the problem
c. Develop a plan of action
d. All of the above

24. **Which of the following nursing intervention assists the crisis victim in managing the intense feelings?**
a. Help the victim to identify his own feelings
b. Develop a plan of action
c. Provide health education
d. Encourage the victim to focus on one problem at a time

25. **The most important assessment data for the nurse to gather from a patient in crisis would be:**
a. Eating habits
b. Strength and limitations
c. Work habits
d. Economical background

26. **Which factors are most essential for the nurse to assess when providing crisis intervention for a patient?**
a. Anxiety level
b. Communication and coping skills
c. Patient's perception of triggering event and availability of resources
d. Level of depression

ANSWER KEY

Fill in the Blanks

1. Maturation	2. Situational	3. Social	4. Crisis intervention	5. Violence

State the Following Statements are True or False

1. True	2. True	3. False	4. False	5. False

Multiple Choice Questions

1. d	2. c	3. d	4. b	5. b
6. d	7. b	8. d	9. d	10. c
11. b	12. b	13. d	14. c	15. a
16. c	17. b	18. a	19. c	20. d
21. c	22. d	23. d	24. a	25. b
26. c				

Forensic Psychiatry/Legal Aspects

A psychiatric nurse is in the ward 24 hours of the day, and the final responsibility of the ward management is on the nurse. She should therefore be well-versed in legal aspects of care and treatment of the mentally ill. This knowledge helps her to guide the patients and relatives in matters related to rights of the patient and other aspects of mental health care. The legal and ethical context of care is important for all psychiatric nurses because it focuses concern on the rights of patients and the quality care they receive. The knowledge of legal aspects sensitizes the nurse on ethical decision making resulting in better care.

OVERVIEW OF INDIAN LUNACY ACT 1912 AND THE MENTAL HEALTH ACT 1987

The Indian Lunacy Act 1912 is derived from English lunacy Act, 1890 and contains 8 chapters and 100 sections **(Table 9.1).** It was enacted to govern reception, detention and care of lunatics and their property and to consolidate and amend the laws relating to lunacy. The enactment of ILA of 1912 was followed by opening of many new asylums, an improvement in the general conditions of asylums and an increase in awareness regarding the prevailing situation of lunatics in such asylum.

TABLE 9.1: Indian Lunacy Act chapters

Chapters	Description
Chapter I	Preliminary information and definitions
Chapter II	Reception of lunatics
Chapter III	Admission, treatment and discharge
Chapter IV	Proceedings of lunacy in presidency town
Chapter V	Proceedings of lunacy outside presidency town
Chapter VI	Establishment of asylums
Chapter VII	Expenses of lunatics
Chapter VIII	Power of state government to make rules

The Indian Mental Health Act (IMHA) 1987 came into effect in April 1993. This Act replaces the Indian Lunacy act 1912. This Act consolidates and amends the laws relating to the treatment and care of mentally ill persons, to make better provision with respect to their property and affairs and for matters connected therewith or incidental thereto. The Act is divided into 10 chapters consisting of 98 sections **(Table 9.2)**.

During the past century there has been a paradigm shift in delivering care to persons with mental illness in India **(Figure 9.1)**.

MENTAL HEALTH CARE ACT (MHCA) 2017

In India, the MHCA 2017 was passed on April 7, 2017 and enforced on May 29, 2018. This is an Act to provide for mental healthcare and services for persons with mental illness and to protect, promote and fulfill the rights of mentally ill persons during delivery of mental healthcare services and for matters connected therewith or incidental thereto.

Reasons for Enactment

The Government of India ratified the United Nations Convention on the Rights of Persons with Disabilities (UNCRPD) in 2007. The convention requires the laws of the country to align with the convention. The Mental Health Act, 1987 does not adequately protect the rights of persons with mental illness. To fulfill this obligation of the UNCRPD, the new Mental Health Care Bill was set in process.

TABLE 9.2: Indian Mental Health Act chapters	
Chapters	**Description**
Chapter I	Preliminary information and definitions
Chapter II	Establishment of central and state mental health authorities
Chapter III	Establishment and maintenance of psychiatric hospitals/nursing homes
Chapter IV	Procedure for admission and detention in psychiatric hospitals/nursing homes
Chapter V	Inspection, discharge, leave of absence and removal of mentally ill persons
Chapter VI	Judicial inquisition regarding alleged mentally ill person possessing property, custody of his person and management of his property
Chapter VII	Liability to meet cost of maintenance of mentally ill persons detained in psychiatric hospital or psychiatric nursing home
Chapter VIII	Protection of human rights of mentally ill persons
Chapter IX	Penalties and procedures
Chapter X	Miscellaneous

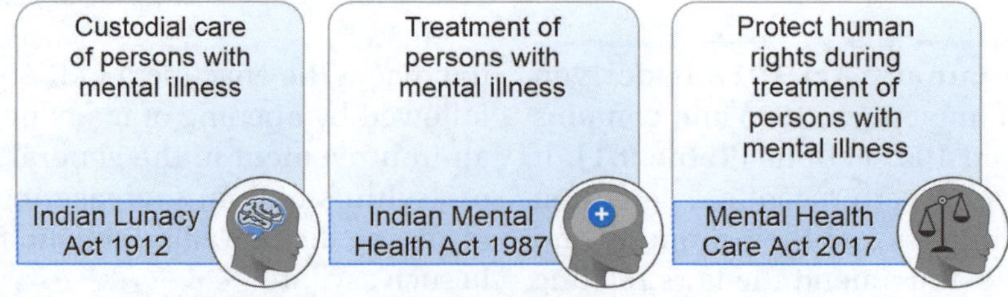

Figure 9.1: Paradigm shift in mental health acts

Key Features of MHCA

This act clearly articulates the mental capacity, advance directive, nominated representative and rights of person with mental illness (PWMI). Key features of act are presented in **Figure 9.2**.

- This act states the right to live life with dignity and no discrimination on basis of sex, religion, culture and caste.
- Every person shall have a right to confidentiality in respect of his/her illness and treatment.
- Every person shall have the right to access mental healthcare and treatment. This right is meant to ensure that services be accessible, affordable and of good quality.
- The act also assures free quality treatment for homeless persons or for those belonging to below poverty line (BPL).
- A mentally ill person shall have the right to make an advance directive that states how he wants to be treated for the illness during a mental health situation and who his nominated representative shall be.
- Every mental health establishment has to be registered with the relevant central or state mental health authority.
- A person with mental illness shall not be subjected to electroconvulsive therapy (ECT) without the use of muscle relaxants and anesthesia. ECT therapy will not be performed for minors. Sterilization shall not be performed in such patients; they will neither be put into solitary confinement nor isolation.
- Suicide is decriminalized. An attempted suicide will not be considered as punishable, which earlier included imprisonment up to a year and/or fine. Now the suicide attempt will be presumed as a result of severe stress and the person will not be subjected to investigation or prosecution.
- Insurers are now bound to provide medical insurance to persons with mental illnesses for treatment on the same basis as available for treatment of physical illnesses.

Description of the Act

MHCA takes a paradigm shift from its predecessor as it moves from discriminating and criminalizing the mentally ill to acknowledging and providing them their rights during the delivery of treatment and care. It includes 16 chapters and 126 sections **(Table 9.3)**.

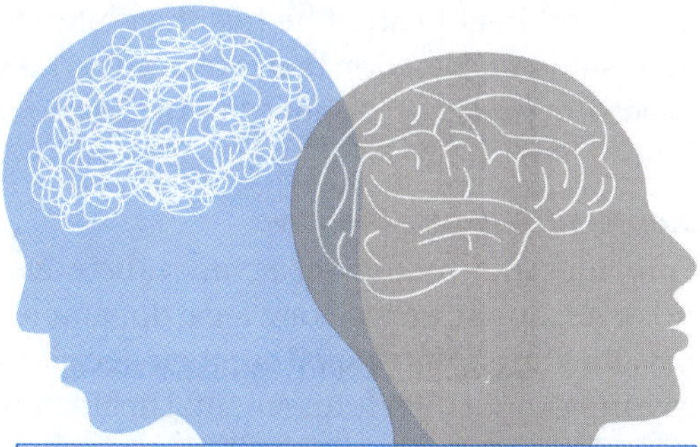

Figure 9.2: Key features of MHCA

TABLE 9.3: Chapters of Mental Health Care Act	
Chapters	**Description**
Chapter I	Preliminary information on definitions, short titles, extent and commencement
Chapter II	Mental illness and capacity to make mental healthcare and treatment decision
Chapter III	Advance directives
Chapter IV	Nominated representative
Chapter V	Rights of person with mental illness
Chapter VI	Duties of appropriate government
Chapter VII	Central mental health authority
Chapter VIII	State mental health authority
Chapter IX	Finance, accounts and audit
Chapter X	Mental health establishments

Contd...

Contd...

Chapters	Description
Chapter XI	Mental health review boards
Chapter XII	Admission, treatment and discharge
Chapter XIII	Responsibilities of other agencies
Chapter XIV	Restriction to discharge functions by professionals not covered by profession
Chapter XV	Offences and penalties
Chapter XVI	Miscellaneous

Chapter I: Preliminary Information

It contains preliminary information on definitions, short titles, extent and commencement. Some of the definitions included in this Act are:

- **Mental illness**: Means a substantial disorder of thinking, mood, perception, orientation or memory that grossly impairs judgment, behavior, capacity to recognize reality or ability to meet the ordinary demands of life, mental conditions associated with the abuse of alcohol and drugs but does not include mental retardation.
- **Minor**: Means a person who has not completed the age of 18 years.
- **Care giver**: Means a person who resides with a person with mental illness and is responsible for providing care to that person and includes a relative or any other person who performs this function either for free or for remuneration.
- **Informed consent**: Means consent given for a specific intervention, without any force, undue influence, fraud, threat, mistake or misrepresentation and obtained after disclosing to a person adequate information including risks and benefits of and alternatives to the specific intervention in a language and manner understood by the person.
- **Prisoner with mental illness**: Means a person with mental illness who is an undertrial or convicted of an offence and detained in a jail or prison.

- **Mental health nurse**: Means a person with a diploma or degree in general nursing or diploma or degree in psychiatric nursing recognized by the Indian Nursing Council.
- **Clinical psychologist**: Having a recognized qualification in clinical psychology from an institution approved and recognized by the Rehabilitation Council of India.
- **Psychiatric social worker**: Means a person having a postgraduate degree in social work and a master of philosophy in psychiatric social work obtained from any university recognized by the University Grants Commission.
- **Psychiatrist**: Means a medical practitioner possessing a postgraduate degree or diploma in psychiatry awarded by a university recognized by the UGC/National Board of Examinations/Indian Medical Council.

Chapter II: Mental Illness and Capacity to Make Mental Healthcare and Treatment Decisions

It deals with mental illness and the capacity to make mental healthcare and treatment decisions. Every person, including a person with mental illness shall be deemed to have the capacity to make decisions regarding his mental healthcare if he has the ability to understand information that is relevant to take a decision on the treatment or admission or personal assistance.

Chapter III: Advance Directive

It provides information on advance directives (Ads). Advance directives are legal documents that allow any adult to spell out their decisions in writing about their future mental healthcare when they become mentally ill. These include the way he/she wishes to be treated or not to be treated, individual whom he wants to appoint as nominated representative. A person with mental illness may revoke, amend or cancel AD many times. The legal guardian shall have right to make an advance directive in writing in respect of a minor, till such time he attains majority. An example for advance directive is given in **Box 9.1**.

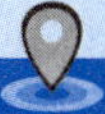

I have been suffering with schizophrenia for the past 10 years and living alone. I wish to be cared for as under:

- I want to wear my own cloths in the hospital
- I do not want to be administered electro convulsive therapy
- I do not want to be physically restrained

Chapter IV: Nominated Representative

It details on appointment, revocation or alteration of nominated representative (NR) and duties of nominated representative. Nominated representative is a person who is appointed by a person with mental illness to discharge treatment related decisions **(Box 9.2).**

Chapter V: Rights of Persons with Mental Illness

It describes rights of persons with mental illness. These include

- ❖ Right to access mental health care (Section 18)
- ❖ Right of confidentiality and to live with dignity
- ❖ Right to community living (Section 19)
- ❖ Right to protection from cruel, inhuman and degrading treatment (Section 20)
- ❖ Right to equality and non-discrimination (Section 21)
- ❖ Right to information (Section 22)
- ❖ Restriction on release of information in respect to mental illness (right to confiden-tiality) (Section 23)
- ❖ Right to access medical records (Section 24)
- ❖ Right to personal contacts and communi-cation (Section 25)
- ❖ Right to legal aid (Section 26)

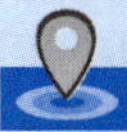

- Appointed by the PMI
- Consented to be nominated representative
- Competent to discharge functions
- Not a minor
- Provide support in making treatment decisions
- Apply to the MHE for support admission
- Apply to concerned board for discharge

- ❖ Right to make complaints about deficiencies in provision of services.
- ❖ Women with child should be separated for the safety of the child and it should be reviewed every 15 days.

Chapter VI: Duties of Appropriate Government

It explains the duties of appropriate government. The government has to plan, design and implement programs for the promotion of mental health and preventive programs, creating awareness about mental health and illness and reducing stigma associated with mental illness. Appropriate government should also take measures as regards human resource development and training, etc.

Chapters VII and VIII: Central and State Mental Health Authority

It deals with establishment of Central Mental Health Authority (CMHA) and State Mental Health Authority (SMHA). These authorities are meant for regulations and co-ordination of mental health services under the central and state governments. The composition of central and state authorities includes secretary, joint secretaries, director general of health services, directors of the central institutions for mental health, psychiatric social worker, clinical psychologist, mental health nurse, mentally ill individuals, caregivers of persons with mental illness, NGOs, etc.

Chapter IX: Finance, Accounts and Audits

It describes finance, accounts and audit information. The CMHA fund shall be constituted by any grants and loans made to the authority by the central government. CMHA shall prepare every year an annual report of all the activities and all the transactions which it shall submit to central government.

Chapter X: Mental Health Establishments

It deals with mental health establishments. No person or organization shall establish or run a mental health establishment unless it has been registered with the authority under the provision of this act. The Act provides guidelines for the establishment of new institutions.

Chapter XI: Mental Health Review Board

It includes mental health review boards to be established by state mental health authority. If any of the mental health establishments violate the provisions of this act, an application can be submitted to the board by patient with mental illness, his nominated representative or any person. Then the board proceeding will be conducted which is equivalent to judicial proceedings. The board shall have power to register, alter, modify or cancel advance directives, appointment of nominated representative, decide on application regarding admission, adjudicate complaints regarding deficiencies at mental health establishment, visit and inspect prison.

Chapter XII: Admission, Treatment and Discharge

It deals with admission, treatment and discharge. Admission is classified into two types: independent and supported admission **(Figure 9.3)**.

1. Independent admission

It is performed for those who have the capacity to make a decision on treatment, who is not a minor, he/she requests for their own admission (Section 86) **(Box 9.3)**. Admission is considered only if the attending mental health professional opines that mental illness is severe enough requiring admission, if the patient is likely to get benefitted from the admission and the patient capacity is intact. Person with

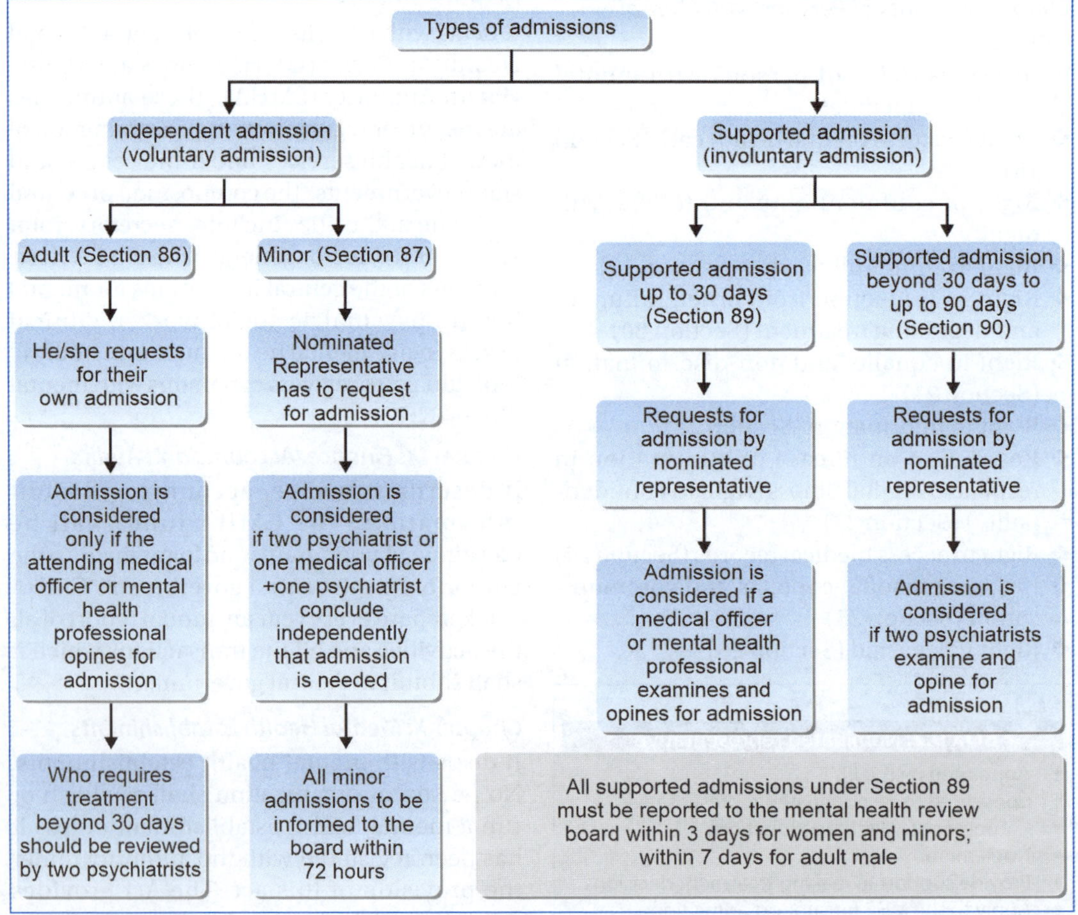

Fig. 9.3: Types of admission

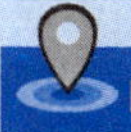

Mrs Reena, 24 years has mania, her symptoms worsened over the past two weeks. She approaches the nearest mental healthcare setting and requests for admission.

mental illness (PMI) must abide by the rules or bylaws of the mental health establishment, no treatment must be given without informed consent of PMI. Patient should be discharged at his or her own will **(Figure 9.4)**. Doctor's permission is not required for discharging the patient under this section. Mentally ill person who requires treatment beyond 30 days should be reviewed by two psychiatrists.

Admission of a minor—Section 87
Nominated representative (NR) has to request the medical officer of the mental health establishment for the admission of minor. The minor shall be examined by two psychiatrists or one psychiatrist and one mental health personnel and if both conclude independently that admission is needed, minor shall be admitted. Admission is necessary if illness is severe enough to require admission, there is no other way to fulfill the clinical need, admission is in the best interest of the minor and all community alternatives have failed. All minor admissions are to be informed to the board within 72 hours. Minor can be discharged as and when nominated representative requests for it or when inpatient care is not necessary **(Figure 9.5)**.

Discharge of independent patients—Section 88
The medical officer or mental health professional in charge of a mental health establishment shall discharge from the mental health establishment any person admitted under Section 86.

2. Supported admission and discharge—
   Sections 89 and 90
When a person is unable to make treatment decisions independently, he or she will need a nominated representative (NR) in making decisions **(Box 9.4)**. Supported admission is limited to 30 days under Section 89. The medical officer or mental health professional in charge of mental health establishment shall admit every such person

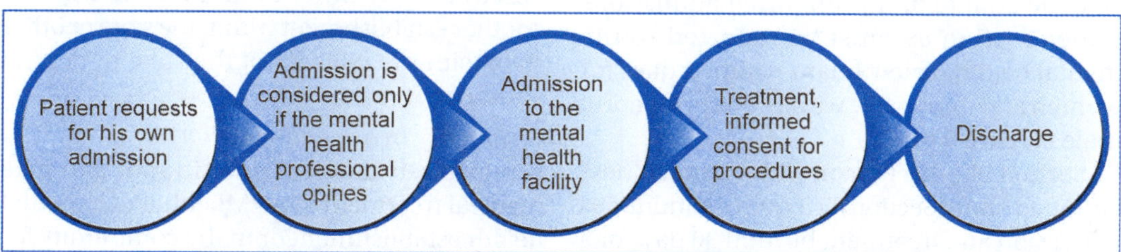

Figure 9.4: Independent admission and discharge (Section 86 and 88)

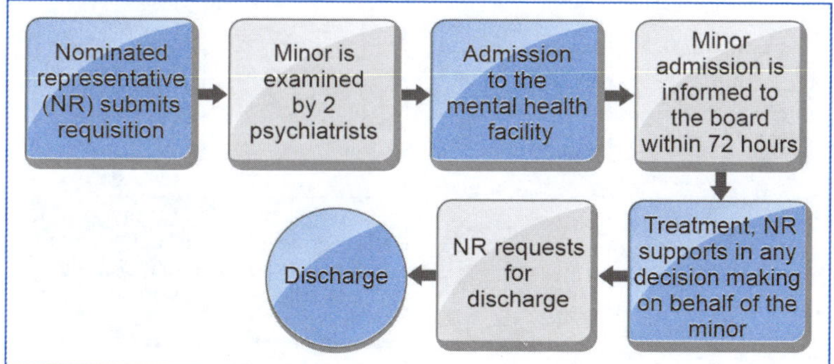

Figure 9.5: Admission of a minor and discharge (Section 87)

BOX 9.4: Example for supported admission

Mr Suresh is diagnosed with schizophrenia; he is unable to take care of himself. The nominated representative (NR) files an application for supported admission on his behalf.

to the establishment upon application by the nominated representative of the person under this section, if PMI

- has recently threatened or attempted or is threatening or attempting to cause bodily harm to himself
- has recently behaved or is behaving violently towards another person or has caused or is causing another person to fear bodily harm from him
- has recently shown or is showing an inability to care for himself to a degree that places the individual at risk of harm to himself

The person has been independently examined on the day of admission or in the preceding seven days by one psychiatrist and the other being a mental health professional or a medical practitioner, and both independently conclude that admission is needed, the person shall be admitted. All supported admissions under Section 89 must be reported to the mental health review board within 3 days for women and minor and within 7 days for adult male **(Figure 9.6)**.

Section 90—If a person with mental illness admitted under Section 89 requires continuous admission and treatment beyond 30 days or a person with mental illness discharged under sub-section (15) of that section requires readmission within 7 days of such discharge, he shall be admitted in accordance with the provisions of this section.

Leave of absence—Section 91
The medical officer or psychiatrist may grant leave of absence from mental health establishment to any PMI admitted under Sections 86, 87, 89 or 90 subject to consent from the NR.

Absence without leave or discharge— Section 92
Any person who absents himself without leave or without discharge from the mental health establishment shall be taken into protection by any police officer at the request of the medical officer or mental health professional and be sent back to the mental health establishment immediately.

Transfer of persons with mental illness from one mental health establishment to another mental health establishment—Section 93
A PMI admitted to a mental health establishment under Sections 87 or 89 or 90 or 103 may subject to any general or special order of the board be removed from such mental health establishment and admitted to any another establishment within the state or other state with the consent of the state or central authority.

Emergency treatment—Section 94
A registered medical practitioner can give medical treatment to a PMI either at a mental health establishment or in the community for a maximum period of 72 hours with informed

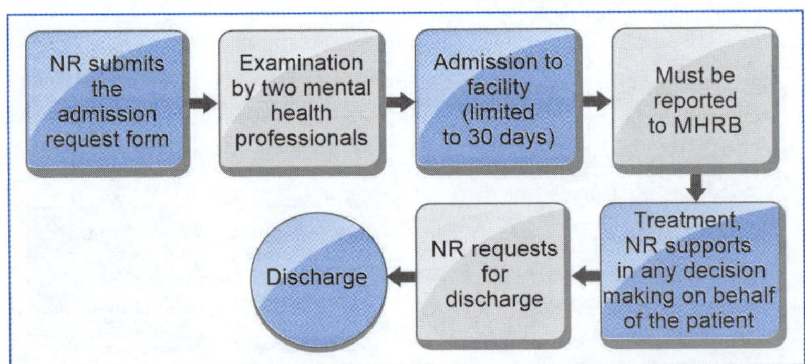

Figure 9.6: Supported admission and discharge (Section 89)

consent of NR in order to prevent death or irreversible harm to the person or causing serious damage to the property. ECT shall not be used as a form of emergency treatment.

Prohibitions and restrictions—Section 95
- ❖ ECT without anesthesia (direct ECT)
- ❖ ECT for minors
- ❖ Sterilization of men or women when such sterilization is intended as a treatment for mental illness
- ❖ Chained in any manner

Restriction on psychosurgery for persons with mental illness—Section 96
Psychosurgery shall not be performed as a treatment for mental illness unless approval from the concerned board and informed consent of the person has been obtained.

Restraints and seclusions—Section 97
A person with mental illness shall not be subjected to seclusion or solitary confinement. Physical restraint may only be used to prevent immediate harm to person concerned or to others.

Discharge planning—Section 98
Whenever a person undergoing treatment for mental illness in a mental health establishment is to be discharged into the community or to a different mental health establishment, the treating psychiatrist shall consult the person with mental illness, the nominated representative, the family member or care giver for discharge from the hospital.

Chapter XIII: Responsibilities of Other Agencies

It describes responsibilities of other agencies such as duties of police officers in respect of persons with mental illness, report to magistrate of person with mental illness in private residence who is ill-treated or neglected, admission of person with mental illness to mental health establishment by magistrate and prisoners with mental illness.

Chapter XIV: Restriction to Discharge Functions by Professionals not Covered by Profession

It deals with restriction to discharge functions by professional not covered by profession. No mental health professional or medical practitioner shall discharge any duty or perform any function not authorized by this act or specify or recommend any medicine or treatment not authorized by the field of his profession.

Chapter XV: Offences and Penalties

It deals with offences and penalties. While penalties relate to establishment or maintaining mental health establishment in contravention of provisions of this act, punishment is for contravention of provisions of the Act or rules or regulations made there under.

Chapter XVI: Miscellaneous

It describes miscellaneous issues such as power of central government to issue direction, special provisions for states in north east and hill states, presumption of severe stress in case of attempt to commit suicide (not a criminal offence if done due to mental illness).

RIGHTS OF MENTALLY ILL PATIENTS AND NURSE'S RESPONSIBILITIES

Chapter V of Mental Health Care Act 2017 describes rights of persons with mental illness **(Box 9.5)**: These are described as under:

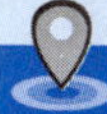

> **BOX 9.5:** Rights of mentally ill person according to MHCA 2017
>
> - Right to access mental healthcare services
> - Right to equality and non-discrimination
> - Right to personal contact and communication
> - Right to protection from cruel, inhuman and degrading treatment
> - Right to confidentiality
> - Right to information
> - Right to access medical records
> - Right to community living
> - Right to legal aid
> - Right to make complaints about deficiencies in provision of service

1. **Right to access mental healthcare services:** Every person has the right to access mental health care and treatment from government health services. The services should be affordable in cost,

of good quality and geographically accessible.

2. **Right to equality and non-discrimination:** All persons with mental illness must be treated equally and at par with persons with physical illnesses in the provision of medical care, and further cannot be discriminated against on any ground.

3. **Right to personal contacts and communication:** Right to receive or refuse visitors and communicate with others.

4. **Right to protection from cruel, inhuman and degrading treatment:** All mental health establishments have to comply with basic minimum standards to ensure people with mental illness are treated with dignity. This includes the right of a PMI to live in a safe and clean environment, right to have adequate and wholesome food, adequate sanitary conditions, right to have facilities for leisure, recreation, education and religious practices, right to have privacy and proper clothing, right to work with consent and appropriate payment, right to be protected from physical, verbal, emotional and sexual abuse and not be forced to shave their head.

5. **Right to confidentiality:** Every person has a right to confidentiality in respect of their mental health, treatment and physical health care subject to certain exceptions. Personal information shall not be provided to anyone else without the person's informed consent.

6. **Right to information:** Persons with mental illness and their nominated representative have a right to information regarding details of their admission, mental illness, treatment plan, etc.

7. **Right to access medical records:** A person with mental illness has the right to access their medical records unless disclosure would cause harm to the person or anyone else.

8. **Right to community living:** Persons with mental illness have a right to live in and be a part of society and cannot be segregated or excluded from their community.

9. **Right to legal aid:** All persons with mental illness have a right to receive free legal aid to exercise his or her rights under the MHCA.

10. **Right to make complaints about deficiencies in provision of services:** A person with mental illness has the right to complain about the deficiencies in the provision of care, treatment and services. Such a person can also seek a judicial remedy for violation of rights under any other law in force.

Civil Rights of the Mentally Ill

Due to global human right concerns, efforts have been made to safeguard the human rights of the mentally ill. A person who is supposed to look after the mentally ill person and does not take proper care and shows cruelty, may be summoned by the court on receipt of such an information either from the public or police. Stringent punishment has also been provided for those who subject the mentally ill to physical and mental indignity while in hospital. It has also been stated that the mentally ill person will not be used in research, except after obtaining proper consent from him and any communication or correspondence in any form shall not usually be censored or intercepted.

Nurse's Implications for Protecting Patient's Rights

Psychiatric patients are often the least capable of protecting their own rights. It is therefore one of the responsibilities of the nurse to guide the patients and relatives in matters related to their rights and protect the patient from any mistreatment.

❖ MHN should be aware of the rights of person with mental illness, ensure a safe and clean environment in the mental health establishment (MHE), keep environment in sanitary condition, provide adequate and wholesome food and facilities for leisure, recreation, education and religious practices. Ensure privacy, proper clothing, protect from physical, verbal, emotional and sexual abuse. Should not be forced to shave their head.

❖ MHN must ensure that a PMI shall have the right to receive free legal services and protection from all forms of abuse.

❖ She should ensure that ward procedures and policies should not violate patient's rights.

❖ Discussing these rights with the mental health team and including these rights in the nursing care plan is all part of her responsibility in protecting the patient's rights.

❖ Nurses should comply with principles of equality and non-discrimination while providing care.

❖ Nurses also can collect regular feedbacks from PMI regarding quality healthcare services.

LEGAL RESPONSIBILITIES OF A NURSE

Probably no other area of nursing specialty demands as great a need for knowledge of the law and ethics as does psychiatric mental health nursing. Psychiatric nurses are confronted on a daily basis with the interface of legal issues as they attempt to balance the rights of the patient with the rights of society. Nurses and other healthcare providers must never violate the rights of mentally ill patients. Nurses must be aware of:

❖ Both the laws in the state in which they practice

❖ Patient's rights

❖ Criminal and civil responsibilities of mentally ill patients

❖ Legal documentation

Thus, knowledge of the law regarding psychiatry in the area where the nurse is practicing helps her to protect herself from liability and the patient from unnecessary detention and mistreatment. The nurse should:

❖ Protect the patient's rights

❖ Keep legal records safely

❖ Maintain confidentiality of patient information

❖ Obtain informed/substitute consent from patient/relatives for any procedure

❖ Explain based on level of anxiety, span of attention and level of ability to decide

Nursing Malpractice

Malpractice involves the failure of professionals to provide proper and competent care that is given by the members of their profession resulting in harm to the patient.

For malpractice the following elements of nursing negligence must be proved:

❖ Nurse performed the duty negligently

❖ Damages were suffered by the plaintiff as a result

❖ Damages were substantial

Common Areas of Liability in Psychiatric Services

❖ Patient suicide

❖ Failure to diagnose

❖ Problems related to electroconvulsive therapy

❖ Misuse of psychoactive prescription drugs

❖ Breach of confidentiality

❖ Failure to obtain informed consent

❖ Inadequate supervision by trainers and employees

❖ Failure to report abuse

Steps to Avoid Liability in Psychiatric Services

❖ The nurse is responsible in reporting information to coworkers involved in patient care

❖ Maintain the records accurately and clearly

❖ Maintain confidentiality of patient information

❖ Practice within the scope of state laws and nurse practice act

❖ Collaborate with colleagues to determine the best course of action

❖ Use established practice standard to guide decisions and action

❖ Always put patient rights and welfare first

❖ Develop effective interpersonal relationship with patients and family

❖ Document all assessment data, treatment, interventions and evaluation of the patient's response to care accurately and thoroughly

Confidentiality

During the nurse patient relationship, a lot of information is gathered through direct and indirect sources which are both verbal and written. Keeping in view the ethics of nursing practice such information gathered is kept confidential and best used for providing enhanced care rather than for other purposes such as gossip or personal gain.

Confidentiality refers to the nondisclosure of private information related to one individual to another, such as from patient to nurse. Any breach of confidentiality could jeopardize the best interests of the patient, be it social or economic keeping in view the social stigma attached to mental illness.

Informed Consent

Informed consent is more than simply getting a patient to sign a written consent form. It is a process of communication between a patient and a nurse that results in patient's authorization or agreement to a specific medical intervention. Informed consent should include:

❖ Patient's diagnosis if known
❖ Nature and purpose of a proposed treatment or procedure
❖ Mode of administering the treatment
❖ Risk and benefit of a proposed treatment or procedure
❖ Alternate treatment procedures—risks and benefits
❖ Risks and benefits of not receiving treatment

However, in the case of psychiatric patients the ability to give informed consent as regards a procedure is highly debatable due to the nature of the problem. Though most of the patients perceive and act in their own best interests, some may not be capable of giving a valid consent. Due to such variations, patients have to be screened for following:

❖ Legal age and sound mind
❖ Intelligence and understanding ability
❖ Ability to express choices
❖ Capacity to comprehend the information given about the treatment

Substituted Consent

It refers to the situation where a patient is not capable of giving his own consent to the proposed treatment. In such cases authorization is given by another individual, being a guardian appointed by the court or the kith and kin on behalf of the patient.

Before getting the consent of the patient or his legal guardian, a full explanation is necessary in regard to the risks involved in the investigation, treatment and/or procedures administered to the patient.

Informed consent is to be obtained for following conditions:

❖ Admission of a person to a psychiatric hospital on a voluntary basis
❖ Procedures like ECT, psychosurgery and other invasive investigatory procedures like lumbar puncture, sphenoidal EEG, etc.
❖ Pentothal analysis (narcoanalysis)
❖ Drug treatments like disulfiram therapy and clozapine therapy
❖ Administration of any research drugs (drug trials)

Record Keeping

Nursing notes and progress records constitute legal documents and hence should be maintained carefully. They should be non-judgmental and the statements made should be objective in nature.

Specific Problems in Mental Hospitals

Specific problems that might arise in mental hospitals in everyday practice which may have legal implications are:

❖ Escape from mental hospital
❖ Death
❖ Pregnancy
❖ Unknown patient
❖ Mentally ill offender

Escape from mental hospital: In mental hospitals, escaping of mentally ill patient is a very common problem. As voluntary admissions increased incidences of escape of mentally ill patients decreased. Escape is more serious in case of involuntary admissions, admission on reception order, mentally ill offenders, mentally ill prisoners and women.

The reason for escape may include unsatisfactory living conditions in the mental hospital (inadequate food and absence of recreational facilities), severity of illness, attitude of the staff and, inadequate attention being given to the patient by doctors or the nursing staff.

In case of involuntary admission or admission under reception order, the escape of mentally ill offenders should immediately be intimated to the senior supervisor/medical superintendent by the ward staff. The medical superintendent should in turn inform either the local police station or the family (if necessary, details are available) or the concerned court (if admission through court orders) as the case may be.

Escape can be prevented by respecting the rights of the mentally ill person, rehabilitating the mentally ill patient in the community on recovery, providing safe and comfortable environment, arranging for the stay of family member with the patient in case of voluntary admission and collecting proper address and necessary details during admission.

Death: Patients admitted in a mental hospital may die due to a physical cause. Every attempt should be made to provide the best medical care possible to the patient. If needed, critically ill patient should be shifted to specialty hospitals. Once the death has already occurred, if the family members are staying along with the patient the body can be handed over to them. If the family members are not staying with the patient, the information of the death needs to be intimated immediately to them telephonically and the dead body kept in hospital mortuary till the family arrives. If no family member turns up for 3 days (72 hrs) or family details are not known, arrangements for last rites of the dead person should be confirmed according to his religion and handed over to municipal authorities. Postmortem is not mandatory in all cases. It is advisable only in suspected cases where death has occurred as a result of accident or an unnatural way. All the deaths occurring in a mental hospital should be discussed by conducting mortality review meetings involving the concerned people. It is done to not only ascertain the cause but also rule out negligence in medical care.

Pregnancy: Pregnancy in a female patient may occur under two different circumstances. One, wherein the patient is already pregnant at the time of admission, and the other wherein the patient becomes pregnant during her stay in the hospital. The second situation is more serious. Before admitting any female patient in the reproductive age group, the doctor should always ensure the presence or absence of pregnancy. In reception order cases, detailed gynecological examination should always be performed to rule out pregnancy.

When a pregnant unknown patient gets admitted in mental hospital, all efforts should be made to trace the family. If the pregnancy appears to be a result of rape and the patient is not in a position to take care of the child, it is advisable to terminate the pregnancy on humanitarian grounds. If the pregnancy is already in an advanced stage and the patient is not in a position to take care of the child in near future, also attempts at contacting the family fail then arrangements may be made to hand over the child to social welfare associations.

Unknown patient: Mentally ill patients wandering aimlessly may become unknown patients to mental hospitals. The nurse has to spend enough time with the patient to know the name and other details of the patient. Most of the time once his or her psychiatric or physical status improves the patient is usually able to recall and inform the details.

Mentally ill offender: In mental hospitals there should be a separate criminal or forensic ward with adequate security provided by the police. Mentally ill criminals may belong to any of the three groups: that incapable of standing trial, those acquitted by reason of being mentally ill, and prisoners who develop mental illness. Mentally ill criminals admitted to mental hospital based on court order should be treated just like any other patient. Security considerations and legal aspects need to be taken care of. For all reception order patients nurses recording should be done from time to time. Nurse's notes serve as a legal document in all such situations.

THE NARCOTIC DRUG AND PSYCHOTROPIC SUBSTANCES ACT OF 1985—ACT 61 (NDPSA)

It is an Act to consolidate and amend the law relating to narcotic drugs, to make stringent provisions for the control and regulation of operations relating to narcotic drugs and psychotropic substances. This Act 61 was enforced on 16th September 1985.

Contents

- ❖ The Act includes narcotic drugs (opium, poppy, straw, cannabis, cocaine, coca and all related synthesized drugs) and psychotropic substances (76 drugs and their derivatives, for example major tranquilizers, minor tranquilizers, pentazocine, barbiturates, etc.).
- ❖ In this act, if a person produces, possesses, transports, imports, sells, purchases or uses any narcotic drugs or psychotropic substances (except 'Ganja') he shall be punishable with:
  - ○ Rigorous imprisonment for not less than 10 years which may be extended up to 20 years and a fine of not less than 1 lakh rupees which may extend to two lakh rupees
  - ○ For repeat offence a rigorous imprisonment of not less than 15 years which may be extended up to 30 years and a fine of not less than 1.5 lakh rupees which may be extended up to 3 lakh rupees
  - ○ For handling 'Ganja' a rigorous imprisonment which may extend to 10 years and a fine up to 1 lakh rupees
  - ○ On carrying 'small quantities', for example, Heroin—250 mg, Opium—5 g, Cocaine—125 mg, Charas—5 g as were later specified in this act, the punishment may extend to 1 year or a fine or both. For Ganja (below 500 g) imprisonment is up to 6 months
  - ○ Under a specified court order there is a provision for detoxification of the patient
  - ○ Under a later enactment, the prevention of illicit traffic in Narcotic Drugs and Psychotropic Substances Act (NDPSA), 1988 (Act 46) was passed. Now there is a provision for preventive detention, seizure of property, death penalty if a person is bound to be trafficking more than or equal to 1 kg of pure heroin despite conviction and warning on the first attempt.

ADMISSION AND DISCHARGE PROCEDURES AS PER MHCA 2017

In MHCA, admission has been classified into two kinds: independent admission and supported admission.

1. **Independent admission:** When patient requests for his own admission (Section 86) or nominated representative (NR) requests for admission in case of minor (Section 87).
2. **Supported admission:** When NR requests for the admission (Sections 89 and 90)
   - ○ *Discharge of the independent patient (Section 88):* Discharge immediately when a patient admitted under Section 86 requests for. However, discharge can be prevented if the condition for supported admission (Section 89) gets fulfilled.
   - ○ *Emergency treatment (Section 94):* A registered medical practitioner can give medical treatment to a person with mental illness either at a mental health establishment or in the community for a maximum period of 72 hours with informed consent of NR in order to prevent death or irreversible harm to the health of person or person inflicting serious harm to himself or person causing serious damage to the property. All supported admissions under Section 90 must be reported to the mental health review board within 7 days.

Role of a Nurse in Admission Procedure

- ❖ Settling the patient in the ward
- ❖ Welcoming to the ward
- ❖ Introducing to the other staff members and patients

- Before assigning a bed, consider biological and emotional needs
- If any patient has suicidal ideation or is floridly psychotic, he should be located to a place where the patient can be closely observed
- The patient should be shown various facilities like availability of bathroom, recreation, refreshments, etc.
- Acquaint the patient with some of the ward rules, for example, meal time, ward activities, visiting hours, how to make appointments to see staff member, timings of any group meetings, etc.
- Provide appropriate information
- Head to foot observation for any injury
- Orientation towards structure, policies
- Find out whether patient had food before admission
- Enquire about any legal issue that the patient has prior to admission
- Perform history collection and MSE
- Write nurse notes; enter in admission register

Role of the Nurse in Leave of Absence (Parole)

Parole is the permission given to patients to perform certain rituals or attend certain family functions.

- Relatives are clearly instructed about the purpose for which the patient is being sent home and when he should be brought back

- Instruct the relatives on how to converse or behave with the mentally ill person duly complying to doctor's instructions
- If the patient is receiving any medications, insist on regularity and give necessary instructions to the family members about dosage, side effects, etc.
- Relatives should be asked to observe communication pattern, sleeping pattern, drug allergy, socialization, ability to perform role.

Role of the Nurse in Discharge Procedure

- Nurse must ensure that the patient leaves the unit with all his belongings and personal effects, has the appropriate medications with him, and appointment for followup has been made and understood.
- All necessary instructions especially regarding his medication regimen, side-effects, etc., must be clearly given to the patient and his family members.
- Any paper work including signing of documents should be completed. Hospital file along with all charts and notes should be sent to medical records section.
- The nurse should ascertain patient's travel plan and offer assistance if necessary.
- The nurse must bear in mind that the patient may have mixed feelings about leaving the hospital and going back to his home environment. She should help him cope with any distress about separating from his newfound friends and staff members.

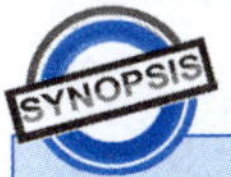

- The legal and ethical context of care is important for all psychiatric nurses because it focuses concern on the rights of patients and the quality care they receive.
- The Indian Lunacy Act 1912 is derived from English Lunacy Act, 1890 and contains 8 chapters and 100 sections.
- The Indian Mental Health Act (IMHA) 1987 came into effect in April 1993. The Act is divided into 10 chapters consisting of 98 sections.
- In India, the MHCA 2017 was passed on April 7, 2017 and enforced on May 29, 2018. It includes 16 chapters and 126 sections.
- Psychiatric patients are often the least capable of protecting their own rights. It is therefore one of the responsibilities of the nurse to guide the patients and relatives in matters related to their rights and protect the patient from any mistreatment.

❖ Forensic psychiatry is a subspecialty of psychiatry that practices at the intersection of mental health and the law.

❖ Probably no other area of nursing specialty demands as great a need for knowledge of the law and ethics as does psychiatric mental health nursing.

❖ Malpractice involves the failure of professionals to provide proper and competent care that is given by the members of their profession resulting in harm to the patient.

❖ Confidentiality refers to the nondisclosure of private information related to one individual to another, such as from patient to nurse.

❖ Informed consent is a process of communication between a patient and a nurse that results in patient's authorization or agreement to a specific medical intervention.

❖ Substitute consent refers to a situation where the patient is not capable of giving his own consent to the proposed treatment. Getting consent from the legal guardian is called substitute consent.

❖ Specific problems that might arise in mental hospitals are escape from mental hospital, death, pregnancy, unknown patient and mentally ill offender.

❖ The Narcotic Drug and Psychotropic Substances Act of 1985—Act 61 (NDPSA) is an Act to consolidate and amend the law relating to narcotic drugs, to make stringent provisions for the control and regulation of operations relating to narcotic drugs and psychotropic substances. This Act 61 was enforced on 16th September 1985.

❖ In MHCA, admission has been classified into two kinds: independent admission and supported admission.

REVIEW QUESTIONS

Long Essays

1. Explain in detail about Mental Health Care Act 2017 and describe the role of a nurse in admission procedures.

2. Describe types of admission in psychiatric hospitals—Role of a nurse.

3. Legal aspects of psychiatric nursing.

Short Essays

1. Rights of psychiatric patients.

2. Discharge procedure for a mentally ill patient according to MHCA 2017.

3. Role of a nurse in protection of rights of mentally ill patient.

Short Answers

1. What are prohibited/restricted procedures according to MHCA.

2. Nursing malpractice

3. Types of admissions according to MHCA 2017.

4. What is independent admission?

5. What is the meaning of supported admission?

Give the Meaning of the Following

1. Confidentiality

2. Informed consent

3. Leave of absence

4. Advance directive

5. Nominated representative

Fill in the Blanks

1. Temporary discharge of a patient from psychiatric hospital is termed as __________.

2. Indian Mental Health Act was passed in the year __________.
3. Indian Lunacy Act was passed in the year __________.
4. The Indian Mental Health Care Act was enacted in the year __________.

State the Following Statements are True or False

1. State mental health authority regulates and co-ordinates mental health services of the state government.
2. Every person has the right to access mental health services.
3. Non-disclosure of private information related to one individual to another is called informed consent.
4. When patient is not capable of giving own consent for proposed treatment, getting consent from the legal guardian is called substitute consent.
5. Nominated representative is appointed by hospital authorities.

Multiple Choice Questions

1. **The Indian Mental Health Act was passed during the year:**
   a. 1987
   b. 1947
   c. 1992
   d. 1942

2. **The Indian Lunacy Act was passed during the year:**
   a. 1910
   b. 1912
   c. 1920
   d. 1987

3. **The following are all key features of MHCA, *except*:**
   a. Decriminalization of suicide
   b. Protection of the human rights of mentally ill patients
   c. Provision for advanced directive
   d. Removal of misconceptions regarding mental illnesses in the public

4. **According to Mental Health Care Act 2017, 'Advance Directive' means:**
   a. It is a legal document that allows any adult to spell out their decisions in writing about their future mental health care
   b. It is the capacity to make mental health care and treatment decision
   c. A person is appointed by a PMI to discharge treatment related decisions
   d. It is a plan, design and program implementation for the promotion of mental health and preventive programs

5. **All minor admissions are to be informed to the mental health review board within _______ period.**
   a. 12 hours
   b. 24 hours
   c. 48 hours
   d. 72 hours

6. **Supported admission is required in all of the following conditions, *except*:**
   a. When a person is unable to make treatment decisions independently
   b. When a person is unable to take care of himself
   c. When a person's behavior is causing harm to self and others
   d. When a person has the capacity to make a decision on the treatment

7. **The Narcotic Drugs and Psychotropic Substances Act (NDPSA) was passed in the year:**
   a. 1985
   b. 1982
   c. 1995
   d. 2000

8. **Which of the following section decriminalized the attempt to die by suicide?**
   a. Section 309 of the IPC
   b. Section 114(b) of the IPC
   c. Section 115 of Mental Health Care Act
   d. Sections 328–339 of the IPC

9. **Nominated representative of Mr B submits request forms for admission. Mr B got admitted under which type of admission?**
   a. Independent admission
   b. Supported admission
   c. Admission of a minor
   d. Admission under special circumstances

10. **Which of the following procedures is restricted under Section 95 of MHCA?**
    a. Supportive psychotherapy
    b. ECT without anesthesia
    c. ECT with anesthesia
    d. Abreaction therapy

11. **The nurse on the evening shift of a psychiatric ward refuses to allow patients to wear their own clothes unless they participate in group meetings regularly. This practice violates which of the following?**
    a. The rights of mentally ill patients
    b. Ethical standards of nursing practice
    c. Nurse patient relationship
    d. State nurse practice acts

12. **All of the following represent appropriate maintenance of patient confidentiality by the psychiatric nurse, *except*:**
    a. Discussing patient's current problems and past history in treatment team meeting
    b. Explaining the patient's condition to family members
    c. Sending copy of patient's records to a referring agency without patient's written consent
    d. Telling a coworker that it is inappropriate to discuss patient's problems in the nurses' station

13. **Which of the following psychiatric treatments require that a psychiatric nurse obtain written informed consent from a patient?**
    a. Supportive psychotherapy
    b. Electroconvulsive therapy
    c. Behavioral therapy
    d. Group therapy

14. **Substitute consent is given in which of the following situations?**
    a. When the patient is not capable of giving his own consent
    b. When the family members are willing to arrange for treatment
    c. When the patient's behavior is not controllable
    d. When the patient is having legal problems

15. **All of the following are nursing malpractice, *except*:**
    a. Breach of confidentiality
    b. Failure to report abuse
    c. Failure to obtain informed consent
    d. Protection of patients' rights

16. **Nominated representative is:**
    a. Appointed by a PMI
    b. A minor
    c. Appointed by the police
    d. Appointed by the hospital authority

17. **Ms Lakshmi, a 30-year-old female diagnosed with depression having the capacity to take decision on her treatment wants to get admitted in the mental health establishment for further treatment. What type of admission does she require?**
    a. Supported admission
    b. Independent admission
    c. Minor admission
    d. Special admission

18. **Mr Lakshman, a 40-year-old male diagnosed with schizophrenia is experiencing worsening of symptoms for the past one month, is unable to take care of himself and lost the capacity to take any decision for his treatment. What type of admission does he require?**
    a. Supported admission
    b. Independent admission
    c. Minor admission
    d. Special admission

ANSWER KEY

Fill in the Blanks				
1. Leave of absence	2. 1987	3. 1912	4. 2017	

State the Following Statements are True or False				
1. True	2. True	3. False	4. True	5. False

Multiple Choice Questions				
1. a	2. b	3. d	4. a	5. d
6. d	7. a	8. c	9. b	10. b
11. a	12. c	13. b	14. a	15. d
16. a	17. b	18. a		

Appendices

HISTORY TAKING FORMAT IN PSYCHIATRIC NURSING

A. Identification Data

Name: Age: Sex:

Father/spouse:

Address: Mobile no.:   Aadhar no.:

Education: Occupation: Income:

Marital status: Religion:

Informant: Name of the informant, relationship and duration of acquaintance (Collate information if more than one informant)

Information: Reliable/not reliable, adequate/not adequate

B. Presenting Chief Complaint

(Salient complaints, with duration in chronological order, in patient's own words, avoid technical language, use informant's own words)

C. History of Present Illness

Duration (days/weeks/months/years):

Mode of onset: Abrupt (within 2 days)/acute (within 2 weeks)/subacute (2 weeks to one month)/insidious (months to years)

Course: Continuous/episodic/fluctuating/deteriorating/improving/unclear

Intensity: Same/increasing/decreasing

Precipitating factors: Yes/no, if yes explain

Description of present illness: Chronological description of abnormal behavior, start with the early symptoms and explain duration, context, frequency, increasing factors, decreasing factors, outcome of those symptoms, associated problems like suicide, homicide, disruptive behavior; thought content, speech, mood states, abnormal perception, biological functioning (sleep, appetite, libido, hygiene, bowel and bladder habits), social functioning (interaction with family members, friends, relatives and neighbors), occupational functioning (functioning, absenteeism, pending enquiry), changes in ADLs.

D. Negative History

Rule out organicity such as fever, head injury, vomiting, seizures, etc., any chronic illness and medication intake, substance abuse such as alcohol, cannabis, opioids, other psychotic symptoms, mood and anxiety symptoms.

E. Medical Illness
- Any past or present medical illness
- Any medication intake and details
- Any chronic medical conditions

    Surgical procedures/accidents/head injury/convulsions/unconsciousness/DM/HTN/CAD/venereal disease/HIV positivity/any other

F. Past Psychiatric History
- Number of previous episodes/hospitalization (psychiatric) with onset and course:
- Complete or incomplete remission:
- Duration of each episode:
- Treatment details and its side effects if any:
- Treatment outcome:
- Duration of treatment:
- Details of any precipitating factors if present:
- Substance use details:

G. Family History

Description (describe each family member briefly: age, education, occupation, health status, relationship with the patient, age at death, mode of death, history of medical or psychiatric disorder, living arrangement, family understanding of illness, family members attitude towards the patient, family stressors and discord).

Three generation genogram

H. Personal History

a. Perinatal History
- Antenatal period:
  - Maternal infections/exposure to radiation/any other
  - Check ups
  - Any complications
- Intranatal period
  - Type of delivery—normal/instrumental/cesarean
  - Any complications
- Birth: Full-term/premature/postmature
- Birth cry: Immediate/delayed
- Birth defects: Yes or no, if yes, specify
- Postnatal complications: Cyanosis/convulsions/jaundice/neonatal infections/any other
- Mile stones development: Normal or delayed

b. Childhood History
- Primary caregiver:
- Feeding: Breastfed/artificial mode of feeding
- Age at weaning:
  - Behavior and emotional problems: Thumb sucking/excessive temper tantrums/stuttering/head-banging/body rocking/nail biting/pica enuresis/morbid fears/night terrors/somnambulism.

- ◆ Illness during childhood: Specifically for CNS infections/epilepsy/neurotic disorders/malnutrition.

c. *Educational History*
   - ○ Age at beginning of formal education:
   - ○ Academic performance:
     (Specifically look for learning disability and attention deficit disorders)
   - ○ Extracurricular achievements, if any:
   - ○ Relationships with peers and teachers:
   - ○ School phobia: Yes/No
   - ○ Look for conduct disorders, for example, truancy/stealing: Yes/No
   - ○ Reason for termination of studies:

d. *Play History*
   - ○ Games played (at what stage and with whom):
   - ○ Relationships with playmates:

e. *Emotional Problems during Adolescence:* Running away from home/delinquency/smoking/drug-taking/any other (specify)

f. *Puberty*
   - ○ Age at appearance of secondary sexual characteristics:
   - ○ Anxiety related to puberty changes:
   - ○ Age at menarche:
   - ○ Reaction to menarche:
   - ○ Regularity of cycles, duration of flow:
   - ○ Abnormalities, if any (menorrhagia, dysmenorrhea, etc.):

g. *Obstetrical History*
   - ○ LMP:
   - ○ Number of children:
   - ○ Any abnormalities associated with pregnancy, delivery, puerperium:
   - ○ Termination of pregnancy, if any:
   - ○ Menopause (including any associated problems):

h. *Occupational History*
   - ○ Age at starting work:
   - ○ Jobs held in chronological order:
   - ○ Reasons for changes:
   - ○ Current job satisfaction: (including relationships with authorities, colleagues, subordinates)
   - ○ Whether job is appropriate to patient's background:

i. *Sexual and Martial History*
   - ○ Genogram (family of procreation—details of spouse and children):
   - ○ Type of marriage   :   Self-choice/arranged
   - ○ Duration of marriage   :
   - ○ Interpersonal and sexual relations   :   Satisfactory/unsatisfactory
   - ○ Extramarital relationship if any specify :

I. Premorbid Personality

(personality prior to the beginning of mental illness)
   - ○ Interpersonal relationships   :   Extrovert/introvert
   - ○ Family and social relationships   :
   - ○ Use of leisure time   :

- Predominant mood : Optimistic/pessimistic; stable/ fluctuating; cheerful/despondent
- Usual reaction to stressful events :
- Attitude to self and others: Self-appraisal of abilities, achievements and failures
- Attitude to work and responsibility:
- Religious beliefs and moral attitudes:
- Fantasy life: Daydreaming—frequency and content
- Habits
  - Eating pattern : Regular/irregular
  - Elimination : Regular/irregular
  - Sleep : Regular/irregular
  - Use of drugs, tobacco, alcohol, other substances:

MENTAL STATUS EXAMINATION FORMAT

A. General Appearance and Behavior

- *Appearance:* Looking one's age/looks older/younger than his/her age/underweight/overweight/physical deformity
- *Facial expression:* Anxious/blunted/pleasant/fearful
- *Level of grooming:* Normal/shabbily dressed/overdressed/idiosyncratically dressed
- *Level of cleanliness:* Adequate/inadequate/overtly clean
- *Level of consciousness:* Fully conscious and alert/drowsy/stuporous/comatosed
- *Mode of entry:* Came willingly/persuaded/brought using physical force
- *Behavior:* Normal/over friendly/preoccupied/aggressive
- *Co-operativeness:* Normal/more than so/less than so
- *Eye-to-eye contact:* Maintained/difficult/not maintained
- *Psychomotor activity:* Goal directed activity—increased/decreased; non-goal directed activity- restlessness
- *Rapport:* Spontaneous/difficult/not established
- *Gesturing:* Normal/exaggerated/odd
- *Posturing:* Normal posture/catatonic posture/stooped/stiff/guarded
- *Other movements:* Normal/stereotype/tremors/extrapyramidal symptoms/abnormal involuntary movements
- *Other catatonic phenomena:* Automatic obedience/negativism/excessive co-operation/waxy flexibility/echopraxia/echolalia
- *Conversion and dissociative signs:* Pseudoseizures/possession states/any other
- *Compulsive acts or rituals or habits (for example nail biting):*
- *Hallucinatory behavior:* Smiling or crying without reason/muttering or talking to self, odd gesturing.

B. Speech

- *Initiation:* Spontaneous/speaks when spoken to/minimal/mute
- *Reaction time (time taken to answer the question):* Normal/delayed/shortened/difficult to assess
- *Rate:* Normal/slow/rapid
- *Productivity:* Monosyllabic/elaborate replies/pressured
- *Volume:* Normal/increased (loud)/decreased (soft)
- *Tone:* Normal variation/high pitch/low pitch/monotonous
- *Relevance:* Fully relevant/sometimes off target/irrelevant
- *Stream:* Normal/circumstantial/tangential/blocking/verbigeration/stereotypies verbal/flight of ideas/clang associations (flow and rhythm of speech)
- *Coherence:* Fully coherent/loosening of associations (incoherent)
- *Others:* Echolalia/perseveration/neologism
- *Sample of speech (in response to open-ended questions, verbatim in 2 or 3 sentences, the questions may be tell me about favorite movie, family, agriculture, festivals, etc.):*

C. Mood and Affect

(Mood is longitudinal, affect is cross sectional)

- *Subjective report:*
- *Objective assessment:*

- *Predominant mood state*: Irritable/labile/blunted/anxious/fearful/panic/aggressive/cheerful/depressed
- *Congruent to the thought process:*
- *Appropriate* (relevance to the situation):
- *Range: Restricted/intact*
- *Reactivity: Absent/present*
- *Lability: Absent/present*

D. Thought

- *Stream (flow of thought, includes tempo and continuity):* Tempo—normal/racy thoughts (pressure of thought)/retarded thinking (poverty of thought)/circumstantiality; continuity-thought block/muddled or unclear thinking/perseveration.
- *Form (organization and expression of thought and formal thought disorder):* Normal/not understandable; Negative formal thought disorder—poverty of speech; positive formal thought disorder—derailment/omission/substitution
- *Possession* (ownership of thought):
  - Self-obsessions and compulsive phenomena: Thoughts/images/ruminations/doubts/impulsive rituals; phobias/imagery
  - External agency (thought alienation phenomena): Thought withdrawal/thought insertion/thought broadcasting

Content

- Delusions: Single/multiple; bizarre delusions/non-bizarre; fleeting or fixed; systematized or poorly systematized; mood congruent or not
- Describe any acting out behavior
- Specify type and give example—persecutory delusions/delusion of reference/delusion of influence or passivity/hypochondriacal delusions/delusion of grandeur/nihilistic delusions/delusion of infidelity/delusion of control
- Depressed cognition: Worthlessness/helplessness/hopelessness/guilt
- Suicidal ideations/death wishes: Intensity, frequency, plan, help sought
- Any preoccupations: Somatic/hypochondriacal/body image

E. Perception

- Hallucinations (specify type and give example): auditory/visual/olfactory/gustatory/tactile single/multiple hallucinations; continuous/intermittent; control/unable to control; commanding
- Illusions:
- Somatic passivity:
- Déjà vu/jamais vu:
- Depersonalization/derealization:

F. Cognitive Function (Neuropsychiatric Assessment)

- *Consciousness:* Alert/drowsy/stuporous
- *Orientation:*
  - Time: Appropriate time/day/night/date/day/month/year
  - Place: Place/area/city
  - Person: Self/close associates/hospital staff
  - Impression: Oriented/disoriented
- *Attention:*
  - Normally aroused/aroused with difficulty
  - Digit forward
  - Digit backward

- ○ *Concentration:*
  - ◆ Normally sustained/sustained with difficulty/distractible
  - ◆ Serial subtraction test: 20–1 (20 to 0 reversed in 15 seconds); 40–3 (37, 34, 31, etc., in 60 seconds) 100-7 (93, 86, 79, etc., in 120 seconds)
  - ◆ Mention number of mistakes and time taken
  - ◆ If illiterate ask: Names of months (backwards); Names of weekdays (backwards)
  - ◆ Impression: Aroused and sustained/difficult to arouse and sustain

Memory:
- ○ Immediate memory (same test as for attention):
- ○ Recent memory (recent happenings—last meal, visitors, etc.)
  - ◆ Verbal recall:
    - ▫ 3 unrelated objects (air, cap, cylinder)—ask after 5 minutes
    - ▫ Address test (imaginary address of 5 items)
    - ▫ Recall events in the last 24 hours
- ○ Remote memory:
  - ◆ Personal events (date of birth, marriage date, children's date of birth, etc.):
  - ◆ Impersonal events (year of COVID outbreak in India, year of independence, etc.):
  - ◆ Illness-related events (year of first episode/number of admissions, etc.):
- ○ Impression: Intact/impaired
  - ◆ Intelligence:
    - ▫ General information: Name of the present season/five nearby cities/local food grains/available vegetables, etc.
    - ▫ Arithmetic ability: Mental arithmetic/written sums
    - ▫ Comprehension test: Common questions such as what will you do when you are feeling very cold?
  - ◆ Abstraction
    - ▫ Normal/concrete
    - ▫ Interpretation of proverbs (give a proverb and ask the inner meaning, e.g., feathers of a bird flock together/rolling stones gather no mass):
    - ▫ Similarities between paired objects:
    - ▫ Dissimilarities between paired objects:
  - ◆ Impression of intelligence: Low/subnormal/average/above average
  - ◆ Judgment
    - ▫ Personal (future plans): Intact/impaired
    - ▫ Social (history of behavior over last one week): Intact/impaired
    - ▫ Test (present a situation and ask for response to the situation): Intact/impaired

G. Insight: (awareness of illness, attribution to the cause of illness, acceptance for treatment and change in behavior)
- ○ Insight is rated on a 6-point scale from 1 to 6:
  1. Complete denial of illness
  2. Slight awareness being sick but denial
  3. Awareness of being sick attributed to external or physical factor
  4. Awareness of being sick but due to something unknown in himself
  5. Intellectual insight: Aware about illness not ready to change behavior
  6. True emotional insight: Aware about illness and ready to change behavior
- ○ Impression: Absent/partial/present

Treatment

Drugs (name of the drug, dose, route, side-effects, if any):

ECT:

Psychotherapy:

Family therapy:

Rehabilitation:

Diagnostic Formulation

APPENDIX 3

MENTAL STATUS EXAMINATION OF UNCOOPERATIVE PATIENT

(Dr George H Kirby, 1921)

When the patient is uncooperative traditional mental status examination will not yield much information, the clinician should rely more on observations. Record the uncooperative patients till he or she becomes cooperative, without leaving any gap in clinical observation. A simple guide to evaluate the mental status examination for un-cooperative patient is given by Kirby (1921) is described below:

Aspects	Description
General reaction and posture	<ul><li>Spontaneous acts:<ul><li>– Any occasional show of activities or assaultiveness</li><li>– Is the patient tidy or untidy?</li><li>– Does the patient eat voluntarily or should be fed?</li><li>– Does the patient dress himself or require assistance?</li><li>– Does the patient have bowel and bladder control?</li><li>– Does the actions show initial slowness or consistent slowness throughout?</li></ul></li><li>Behavior towards the examiners: Resistive or evasive, irritable or apathetic or complaint</li><li>Voluntary postures:<ul><li>– Comfortable, natural or awkward or constrained</li><li>– What does the patient do when place in an awkward position?</li></ul></li><li>Is the behavior constant or changing with time?</li></ul>
Facial expression	<ul><li>Is the expression being alert, attentive, smiling, mask like, placid, sulky, anxious, perplexed, scowling, averse, distressed, tearful?</li><li>Is there any sign of tears, flushing, perspiration, smiles?</li><li>Is the facial expression constant or changing with time?</li><li>On what occasions?</li></ul>
Eyes and pupils	<ul><li>Are the eyes open or closed: Is there resistance to open the patient's eyes by examiner?</li><li>Does he give attention to examiner and move his eyes with that of object or light source?</li><li>Does he have fixed gaze or evasive gaze?</li><li>Is there blinking of eyes or flickering of eyelids?</li><li>Response to sudden movement of hand towards the patient eyes</li><li>Response of pupils to painful sensory stimulus and corneal reflex</li><li>Actively scanning the environment</li></ul>
Reaction to examiners questions and tests	<ul><li>What is the response to simple commands: asking to show tongue, lift right hand, grasp the hands?</li><li>Reaction to pin pricks</li><li>Presence of negativism—either active or passive uncooperativeness</li><li>Check for presence of automatic obedience, echolalia and echopraxia</li><li>Are the movements of limbs being slow or fast or interrupted?</li></ul>
Muscular reactions	<ul><li>Check for tone of muscles: look for rigidity, lead pipe or cogwheel type, waxy flexibility, negativism gegenhalten (resisting changes of position), mitgehen and mitmachen</li><li>Is there urinary or fecal incontinence?</li><li>Holding of saliva, drooling</li><li>Any abnormal movements</li></ul>

Aspects	Description
Emotional responsiveness	• Emotional response when family members speak or when personal facts are told or while describing sensitive issues of the history • Response to unexpected stimulus like clapping sound or by switching on lights • Do jokes elicit any response?
Speech	• Is there any spontaneous speech? • Is the patient mute, if so whether it is consistent present or not? • Is there any effort to speak or make sounds or whisper or lip movement, movement of head?
Writing	• Offer the patient a pencil and paper to write his wishes
Vitals	• Patient's pulse rate, blood pressure, temperature and respirator rate need to be measured at regular intervals • Input/output chart • Medications

NEUROLOGICAL EXAMINATION FORMAT

A. Level of Consciousness
- Alert/lethargic/stuporous/semi-comatose/comatose
- Score of Glasgow coma scale:

B. Mental Status Examination
- General appearance
- Speech
- Thought process
- Mood
- Cognitive functions:
  - Attention and concentration:
    - Digit span: Backward, forward
    - Serial 7
  - Orientation: Time, Place, Person
  - Memory:
    - Immediate
    - Recent
    - Remote
  - General knowledge
  - Abstract reasoning
  - Judgment
  - Insight

C. Special Cerebral Functions: Agnosia/apraxia/aphasia

D. Cranial Nerve Examination
- Olfactory nerve: Sense of smell—present/absent
- Optic nerve: Inspection of eye—inflammation/cataract/foreign bodies/any abnormalities
  - Visual acuity (Snellen's chart):
  - Visual field examination—Right eye

                        Left eye
  - Ophthalmoscope examination
  - Color vision: Present/absent
- Oculomotor, trochlear and abducent nerves
  - Pupillary reaction to light: Reacting/not reacting
  - Pupillary size: Equal/unequal
  - Eye movement in six directions: Normal/abnormal
  - Nystagmus: Present/absent
  - Diplopia: Present/absent
- Trigeminal nerve
  - Corneal reflex: Present/absent
  - Facial sensory response: Present/absent
  - Mandibular strength: Adequate/hypotonia
- Facial nerve
  - Facial expressions: Normal/hypotonia
  - Taste sensation: Present/absent

- ❍ Vestibule cochlear nerve:
    - ◆ Auditory acuity test
    - ◆ Air conduction
    - ◆ Bone conduction
- ❍ Glossopharyngeal and vagus nerve:
    - ◆ Gag reflex: Present/absent
    - ◆ Swallowing reflex: Present/absent
    - ◆ Position and movement of uvula and palate: Normal position/deviation
    - ◆ Sensation of taste: Present/absent
- ❍ Spinal accessory nerve:
    - ◆ Sternocleidomastoid muscle strength: Normal/hypotonia
    - ◆ Elevation of shoulders: Adequate strength/weakness
    - ◆ Turning of head: Adequate/inadequate
- ❍ Hypoglossal nerve: Tongue movement: Normal/abnormal

E. Motor Function Assessment
- ❍ Muscle size
- ❍ Muscle strength
- ❍ Muscle tone
- ❍ Muscle co-ordination
- ❍ Gait
- ❍ Movements of all the joints
- ❍ Deformities
- ❍ Abnormal movements

F. Sensory Function Assessment
- ❍ Pain sensation: Present/absent
- ❍ Temperature sensation: Present/absent
- ❍ Touch sensation: Present/absent
- ❍ Vibration sensation: Present/absent

G. Assessment of Cerebellar Function
- ❍ Finger to finger test: Normal/abnormal
- ❍ Finger to nose test: Normal/abnormal
- ❍ Romberg test: Normal/unable to perform
- ❍ Tandem walking test: Normal/unable to perform

H. Assessment of Reflexes
- ❍ Superficial reflexes: Present/absent
  Abdominal/plantar/corneal/pharyngeal/cremasteric/anal
- ❍ Deep tendon reflexes: Present/absent
  Biceps/triceps/brachioradial/patellar/Achilles
- ❍ Any abnormal reflexes: Present/absent

Summary

APPENDIX 5

PHYSICAL EXAMINATION FORMAT

A. Identification Data

Name: Age: Sex:

House no: Marital status:

Occupation:

Address:

Chief complaints

B. Present Medical History:

C. Past Medical and Surgical History:

D. General Examination:

Temp:

Pulse:

Resp:

BP:

CVS, peripheral pulsations:

Respiratory system:

Abdomen:

Musculoskeletal system:

Lymph nodes:

Breasts:

Pelvic examination:

Any other signs:

APPENDIX 6

GLASGOW COMA SCALE

Best eye-opening response (Record 'C' if eyes are closed by swelling)	Spontaneously	4
	To speech	3
	To pain	2
	No response	1
Best motor response To painful stimulus (Record best upper limb response)	Obeys verbal command	6
	Localizes pain	5
	Flexion—withdrawal	4
	Flexion—abnormal	3
	Extension—abnormal	2
	No response	1
Best verbal response (Record 'E' if endotracheal tube in place. 'T' if tracheostomy tube in place)	Oriented to time, place, person	5
	Conversation confused	4
	Speech inappropriate	3
	Sounds incomprehensive	2
	No response	1
	Total score 15	

Scores range between 3–15 (score of 3 indicates patient is unresponsive, score of 15 indicates patient is alert and obeys commands).

PROCESS RECORDING FORMAT

A. Identification Data:

Name: Age: Sex:

Religion: Marital status: Educational status:

Occupation: Income per month: Languages known:

IP no.:   Ward: Diagnosis:

Address:

Date of admission: Date and time of process recording:

Brief summary of the patient problem:

B. Place of Interaction:

C. Description of the Environment:

D. Reason for Selecting the Patient:

E. Objectives:

1.

2.

3.

Nurses' response		Patients' response			
Verbal	Non-verbal	Verbal	Non-verbal	Technique	Inference

Conclusion: Fixing the time and place for the next interview
Summary: List of inferences
                Care plans made according to inference
                Any special difficulties faced during the inference
                Techniques used to overcome difficulties

Signature

APPENDIX 8

MINI-MENTAL STATUS EXAMINATION (MMSE) FORMAT

Component description	Patient score	Points
A. Orientation		
Which year is it right now?		1
Season?		1
Date?		1
Day?		1
Month?		1
Which is your state?		1
Country?		1
Town or city?		1
Hospital?		1
Floor?		1
B. Attention and Calculation		
Spell "world" backwards; Give 1 point for each letter that is in the right place (for example, DLROW = 5, DLORW = 3). Alternatively, do serial 7s (ask the person to count backwards from 100 in blocks of 7, i.e., 93, 86, 79, 72, 65). Stop after five subtractions. Give one point for each correct answer.		5
C. Registration		
Name three objects (for example, apple, table, pen) taking one second to utter each one. Ask the individual to repeat the names of all three objects. Give one point for each correct answer. Repeat the names of all three objects till they are learned.		3
D. Recall		
○ Ask for the three objects repeated above (for example, apple, table, pen) ○ Give one point for each correct object		3
E. Language		
○ Point to a pencil and ask the person to name the object (1 point) ○ Do the same thing with a wrist watch (1 point)		2
○ Ask the person to repeat the following. No 'ifs' and/or 'buts' (1 point) ○ Allow only one trial		1

Give the person a piece of blank white paper and ask them to follow a three stage command. Take a paper in your right hand, fold in half and put it on the floor (1 point for each part that is correctly followed).	3
Write 'CLOSE YOUR EYES' in large letters and show it to the patient. Ask him or her to read the message and do what it says (give 1 point if they actually close their eyes).	1
Ask the individual to write a sentence of their choice on a blank piece of paper. The sentence must contain a subject and a verb, and must make sense. Spelling punctuation and grammar are not important (1 point).	1
Show the person a drawing of two pentagons which intersect to form a quadrangle. Each side should be about 1.5 cm. Ask them to copy the design exactly as it is (1 point). All 10 angles need to be present and the two shapes must intersect to score 1 point. Tremor and rotation are ignored.	1
Total score	**30**

Interpretation: Maximum score for MMSE is 30. A score of 25 or higher is classified as normal. If the score is below 24, the result is usually considered to be abnormal, indicating possible cognitive impairment (Adapted from Folstein, et al. 1975).

APPENDIX 9

ALCOHOLISM HISTORY COLLECTION FORMAT

A. Demographic Data

Name: Age: Sex:

Occupation: Income: Education:

Marital status: Married/Single/Widow

IP no.:   Address: Mobile no.:

Informant:

Information: Reliability/adequacy

B. Chief Complaints (in chronological order with duration):

C. History of Present Illness
- First drink causes:
- First experience with alcohol:
- The type and volume of first drink—Hard drink/Regular drink:
- Current drinking pattern: Every day?/Weekends?
- Time of day: Morning/evening/all day
- Quantity of alcohol use in an average day:
- Type and place of drinking:
- Situations that make you drink more or less in a day:
- Money spent on alcohol:
- Withdrawal symptoms (If you stop drinking, do you get tremors/sweating/feel sick/notice any physical change?):
- Craving (Do you feel a compulsion or need to drink?):
- Tolerance (Do you have to drink more than you used to, to get the same effects?):
- Reasons for excessive consumption of alcohol:
- Diet: Adequate intake/type of food/eating pattern
- History of any other substance abuse:
- Last use (in hours or days):
- Motivation level:

D. Past Medical History
- Medical problems associated with alcoholism: Liver disease/peptic ulcers/pancreatitis/heart disease
- Psychiatric problems associated with alcoholism:
- Any history of admission and treatment for alcoholism:
- Previous history of abstinence with duration:
- Reasons for relapse:

E. Family History
- Family history of similar problems:
- Interpersonal relationship in the family:
- Family coping:
- Any domestic violence:
- Family history of psychiatric disorders:
  - Psychosis

- ◆ Mood disorders
- ◆ Neurotic disorders
- ◆ Substance abuse
- ◆ Epilepsy
- ○ Genogram (family of origin, three generations)

F. Personal History
- ○ Birth and early development
- ○ Behavioral disorders during childhood (ADHD, conduct disorder, any other issues)
- ○ Educational history (specific learning disorders, truancy, educational performance, etc.)
- ○ Occupational history
- ○ Menstrual history

G. Marital History
- ○ Role reversal
- ○ Emotional disorders in children
- ○ History of exposure to extramarital relationship
- ○ Sexual dysfunction

H. Premorbid Personality
- ○ Personality prior to the beginning of alcohol use: Dependence/anankastic/passive aggressive/antisocial/any other
- ○ Social relations
- ○ Taking up responsibilities
- ○ Coping with stress
- ○ Intellectual activities
- ○ Hobbies
- ○ Habits
- ○ Internet use/gambling

I. Complications (focus on finding relationship with substance abuse)
- ○ Medical complications: Accidents/head injury/seizures/myopathy/liver diseases/peptic ulcers/pancreatitis/heart disease, etc.
- ○ Psychiatry complications: Psychosis/depression/bipolar affective disorders/anxiety disorders/personality disorder/suicide attempt
- ○ Legal complications: Violence/stealing/FIR
- ○ Social/economical complications: Loan/property issues/job loss/fights with family members/fights with friends and relatives
- ○ Civil complications: Divorce/disciplinary actions

CHILD AND ADOLESCENT PSYCHIATRY ASSESSMENT FORMAT

A. Demographic Data

Name: Age: Sex:

Address:

Income: Residence: Urban/Semi-Urban/Rural

Hospital no.:

Informant: Mother/Father/Others

B. Chief Complaints (with duration in brief)

C. History of Present Illness

Describe each symptom in chronological order, describe symptoms at home, school and other social situations, describe each symptom with duration, context, frequency, increasing and decreasing factors, progression of symptoms, outcome of each symptom.

Description of associated symptoms such as biological functioning (sleep, appetite, hygiene, bowel and bladder habits), school or college functioning (regularity, absenteeism, academic performance), social functioning (interaction with friends, relatives and neighbors).

D. Family History

- Nuclear/non-nuclear
- Consanguineous marriage/non-consanguineous marriage
- History of mental illness/epilepsy/mentally retarded/any other
- Genogram (three generations):
- Significant other parent figures: Grandparents/aunt/other caregivers
- Parenting style: Authoritative/permissive/uninvolved

E. Personal History

- Antenatal history: Nutritional deficiencies, teratogenic exposure, infections, hypertension, diabetes, immunizations
- Perinatal history: Normal labor/cesarean section/premature birth/any fetal distress
- Birth cry: Immediate/delayed
- Birth weight:
- Postnatal history: Infections/seizures/jaundice
- Milestones development: Motor development, cognitive development, social development, language development, current level of development

F. Past History

- Psychiatric illness: Number of past episodes, treatment sought, medication history, side effects if any, response to treatment, duration of treatment, psychosocial interventions
- Others

G. Current Level of Functioning

- Intelligence: Above average/average/below average
- School performance: Above average/average/below average
- Self-help: Age appropriate
  - Toilet: Yes/No
  - Dressing: Yes/No
  - Eating: Yes/No
  - Bathing/Washing: Yes/No

H. Schooling History
- Age at starting schooling
- School refusal
- Academic performance

I. Menstrual and Sexual History
- Body image concern:
- Menstrual history: Age at menarche, last menstrual history, reaction to menarche

J. Temperamental History
- Activity level
- Adaptability to environment
- Impulsivity
- Regularity in biological functioning
- Intensity of reaction
- Quality of mood
- Shy, fearful and anxious of certain places: Yes/No
- Excessive tantrums: Yes/No
- Excessive clinging behavior: Yes/No

K. Physical Examination
- Vision
- Hearing
- CNS
- Respiratory system
- Cardiovascular system
- Gastrointestinal system
- Genitourinary system

L. Treatment History Till Date

M. Mental Status Examination
- Attention and concentration
- Activity level
- Motor behavior
- Speech and language ability
- General intelligence
- Mood and affect
- Thought processes
- Perception

Summary

APPENDIX 11

GERIATRIC HISTORY COLLECTION FORMAT

A. Demographic Data

Name:	Age:	Sex:
Occupation:	Income:	Education:
Marital status: Married/Single/Widow		IP no.:

Address

Informant

B. Chief Complaints

C. Precipitating Factors: Head injury/infection/sensory handicaps/retirement/bereavement/ any other

D. History of Present Illness
- Stress:
- Qualitative or quantitative changes in routine activities:
- Cognitive function:
- Habits and others:

E. Past Medical History

F. Past Psychiatric History

G. Family History
- Joint or nuclear family
- Monthly family income
- Socioeconomic status
- Family history of mental or physical health
- Genogram

H. Personal History
- Developmental history
- Educational history
- Occupational history pre-retirement
- Source of income: Employment/pension/assistance from family/other financial problems if any
- Residence:
  - Living at home/alone/with spouse/with children
  - Own/rented house
  - Any problems with living situation

I. Marital History
- Sexual/menstrual history
- Genogram

J. Premorbid Personality
- Specific traits
- Social functioning
- Occupational functioning

- o Biological functioning
- o Interest/hobbies, alcohol and other drug abuse

K. Community Involvement: Members of organization/club/political activities/voluntary work

L. Social Support

M. Attitude towards Aging and Death

N. Mental Status Examination

O. Summary

P. Investigations

Q. Treatment

APPENDIX 12

NURSING CARE PLAN FORMAT IN PSYCHIATRIC NURSING

A. Identification Data

Name of the patient: Age: Sex:

Religion: IP no.:   Ward:

Marital status: Education: Occupation:

Income per month:

Address:

Informant:

B. Presenting Chief Complaints

C. History of Present Illness

D. Past Psychiatric and Medical History

E. Family History

F. Personal History

G. Premorbid Personality

H. Mental Status Examination
- General appearance and behavior
- Speech
- Mood
- Thought
- Perception
- Cognitive function
- Insight
- Judgment
- Diagnostic formulation

I. Physical Examination

J. Treatment

K. Nursing Management
- Nursing assessment (objective data, subjective data)
- List of nursing diagnosis

Nursing Care Plan

Assessment	Nursing diagnosis	Goal/objective	Intervention	Implementation	Rationale	Evaluation

L. Health Education

M. Conclusion

APPENDIX 13

CASE STUDY/CASE PRESENTATION FORMAT IN PSYCHIATRIC NURSING

A. Identification Data

Name of the patient:　　　　Age:　　　　Sex:

Religion:　　　　IP no.:　　　　Marital status:

Education:　　　　Occupation:

Address:

Informant:

B. Presenting Chief Complaints

C. History of Present Illness

D. Past Psychiatric and Medical History

E. Family History

F. Personal History

G. Premorbid personality

H. Mental Status Examination
- General appearance and behavior
- Speech
- Mood
- Thought
- Perception
- Cognitive function
- Insight
- Judgment
- Diagnostic formulation

I. Physical Examination

J. Treatment

Book Picture of Disease Condition
- Introduction
- Definition
- Incidence
- Etiology

Book picture	Patient picture

❖ Psychopathology
❖ Clinical manifestations

Book picture	Patient picture

❖ Investigations and diagnoses

Book picture	Patient picture

❖ Treatment

Book picture	Patient picture

❖ Nursing management:
  ○ Nursing assessment
  ○ List of nursing diagnoses
  ○ Nursing interventions (according to book)
  ○ Nursing evaluation

Nursing Care Plan

Assessment	Nursing diagnosis	Goal/objective	Intervention	Implementation	Rationale	Evaluation

Health education:

Conclusion:

References:

ECT HISTORY COLLECTION FORMAT

A. Identification Data

Name of the patient: Age: Sex:

Religion: IP no.:   Marital status:

Education: Occupation:

Address:

Informant:

B. Presenting Chief Complaints

C. History of Present Illness

D. Past Psychiatric and Medical History

E. Family History

F. Personal History

G. Mental Status Examination
- General appearance and behavior
- Speech
- Mood
- Thought
- Perception
- Cognitive function
- Insight
- Judgment
- Diagnostic formulation

H. Physical Examination

I. Treatment

J. Assessment of patient's and family's knowledge of indications, side effects, therapeutic effects and risks associated with ECT

K. Pre-ECT Care Checklist
- Informed consent
- Assess vital signs
- Nil by mouth (6–8 hours)
- Withhold night dose of drugs
- Withhold oral medications in the morning
- Head shampooing
- Remove jewelry, prosthesis, dentures, contact lens, etc.
- Remove tight clothing
- Empty bladder and bowel just before ECT
- Pre ECT medications

L. Intraprocedure Care Checklist
- Place the patient comfortably on ECT table
- Stay with the patient
- Insert mouth gag

- ○ Apply gel and electrodes
- ○ Monitor voltage intensity and duration of electrical activity
- ○ Monitor seizure activity
- ○ Monitor vital signs

M. Postprocedure Care Checklist
- ○ Place the patient in sideline position
- ○ Monitor vital signs
- ○ Oxygen administration
- ○ Assess for post-ictal confusion
- ○ Use of side rails to prevent falls
- ○ Reorient the patient after recovery
- ○ Recording the case

PSYCHOTHERAPY FORMAT

A. Demographic Data

Name of the patient: Age: Sex:

Religion: IP no.:   Marital status:

Education: Occupation:

Address:

Informant:

B. Brief Description of Present Illness

C. Brief Description of Mental Status Examination

D. Treatment History

E. Indications for Psychotherapy

F. Problems Identified for Work-up

G. Brief description of psychotherapy given to the patient
- Session no.
- Place
- Time
- Psychotherapy approach
- Techniques used by the therapist
- Plan for next session
- Home works, if any (given to the patient)
- Outcome of the session

Summary

APPENDIX 16

OCCUPATIONAL THERAPY FORMAT

A. Demographic Data

Name of the patient: Age: Sex:

Religion: IP no.:   Marital status:

Education: Occupation:

Address:

Informant:

B. Brief Description of Present Illness

C. Brief Description of Mental Status Examination

D. Treatment

E. Objective for Occupational Therapy

F. Evaluation of the Patient
- Current level of functioning
- Social functioning
- Behavioral problems

G. Description of Occupational therapy (Activities) Planned or Provided for Patient

Description of activities	Therapeutic value

- Difficulties faced by the patient during occupational therapy
- Outcome of the session
- Plan for the next session

APPENDIX 17

BEHAVIOR THERAPY FORMAT

A. Demographic Data

Name of the patient:	Age:	Sex:
Religion:	IP no.:	Marital status:
Education:	Occupation:	
Address:		
Informant:		

B. Brief Description of Present Illness

C. Brief Description of Mental Status Examination

D. Treatment

E. Indications for Behavioral Therapy

F. Techniques Used by the Therapist

Summary

APPENDIX 18

RECREATION/PLAY THERAPY FORMAT

A. Demographic Data

Name of the patient:	Age:	Sex:
Religion:	IP no.:	Marital status:
Education:	Occupation:	
Address:		
Informant:		

B. Brief Description of Present Illness

C. Brief Description of Mental Status Examination

D. Treatment

E. Indications for Therapy

F. Advantages of Therapy for the Patient

G. Outcome of the Session

H. Plan for Next Session

GROUP THERAPY FORMAT

Purposes of group therapy:

Size of group:

Selection of patients:

Indications for group therapy:

Topics addressed in the group therapy:

Techniques used in the group therapy:

Problems encountered in the group therapy:

Plan for the next session:

Summary of therapy:

APPENDIX 20

HEALTH EDUCATION FORMAT

Name of the topic:

Group and number:

Place:

Date:

Time:

Duration of health education:

Name of the student:

Name of the supervisor:

Method of the teaching:

AV aids:

General objective:

Specific objective:

Specific objective	Content	AV aids	Evaluation

References

APPENDIX 21

DRUG BOOK FORMAT

Pharmaco-logical name and trade name	Dose and route	Mechanism of action	Indications	Contraindications	Adverse effects	Nurses' responsibility

References

APPENDIX 22

PSYCHIATRIC OPD LOGBOOK

Sl. No.	Name of the patient, age, sex, address	Occupation- and education	Chief complaints and diagnosis	Past history	Treatment	Health education

APPENDIX 23

ADMISSION PROCEDURE FORMAT

Date:	Address:
Name:	Education:
Age:	Occupation and income:
Sex:	Marital status:
Date of admission:	Hospital no.:
Diagnosis:	

Nursing interventions given to patient
Type of admission
Mention whether consent was given by patient/family member/any other
Brief description of patient condition
Brief description on preparation of patient unit
Describe the preparation of patient record with all the information like unit, bed number, weight, vital signs, MSE and general condition, etc., and write the admission note with details such as time of patient arrival to ward, mode of arrival, patient's complaints, and any other significant information
Describe the orientation given to the patient regarding physical set up of the ward, hospital policies regarding meal time, ward activities, visiting hours, gate pass, attendant staying with the patient and restrictions in the ward
List the investigations advised such as urine, blood or any other
List the medications ordered by the psychiatrist with details (dose, route and frequency)

Name and Signature of Student   Name and Signature of Supervisor

APPENDIX 24

DISCHARGE PROCEDURE FORMAT

Date: Address:

Name: Education:

Age: Occupation and income:

Sex: Marital status:

Date of admission: Hospital no.:

Diagnosis:

Nursing interventions given to patient
Type of discharge
Check for physician's discharge order
Assess and describe the patient's healthcare needs at the time of discharge
Write a note on discharge summary
List the medications prescribed to the patient as ordered by the psychiatrist
Write a note on follow-up visits
Brief description of health education provided to the patient
Summary of nurse's notes

Name and Signature of Student   Name and Signature of Supervisor

APPENDIX 25

DRUG GUIDE

Haloperidol

Trade Names
Serenace, Triperidol, Senorm-LA, Haldol

Classification
Dopamine receptor antagonists–butyrophenone

Dose
Oral: 0.5–5 mg, Parental: 5–100 mg/mL

Mechanism of Action
An antipsychotic, antiemetic and antidyskinetic agent that competitively blocks postsynaptic dopamine receptors, interrupts nerve impulse movement and increases turnover of dopamine in the brain. Peripheral effects include anticholinergic properties and alpha adrenergic blockage.

Indications
Acute psychotic episodes in schizophrenia and schizoaffective disorders, mania, depression with psychotic symptoms, delusional disorders, borderline personality disorder, and substance induced psychotic disorder, delirium and dementia, mental disorders due to a medical condition, pervasive developmental disorder, Tourette's syndrome, Huntington's disease.

Contraindication
Angle-closure glaucoma, CNS depression, myelosuppression, Parkinson's disease, severe cardiac or hepatic disease.

Side Effects
* **Frequent:** Blurred vision, constipation, orthostatic hypotension, dry mouth, peripheral edema.
* **Occasional:** Difficulty urinating, decreased thirst, dizziness, decreased sexual function, drowsiness, nausea, vomiting, photosensitivity, lethargy.
* **Serious reactions:** Extrapyramidal symptoms (EPS)—akathisia, acute dystonia, tardive dyskinesia, and drug-induced Parkinsonism.

Nurse's Responsibility
* Assess patient behavior and emotional status.
* Children are more susceptible to dystonias. Haloperidol use is not recommended for children younger than three years.
* A decreased dosage is recommended for the elderly who are more susceptible to extrapyramidal and anticholinergic effects, orthostatic hypotension and sedation.
* Use haloperidol cautiously in patients with cardiovascular disease, hepatic or renal dysfunction or a history of seizures. Haloperidol may be given undiluted by IV push.
* Give IV push at a rate of 5 mg/minute.
* Prepare haloperidol decanoate IM injection using a 21-guage needle. Slowly inject the drug deep into the upper outer quadrant of the gluteus maximus.
* Keep the patient in recumbent position (head low and legs raised) for 30–60 minutes after administration to minimize hypotensive effects.
* Monitor the patient for fine tongue movements, mask-like facial expression, rigidity and tremor.

- ❖ The therapeutic serum level for haloperidol is 0.2–1 μ/mL and the toxic serum level is >1 μ/mL.
- ❖ Caution the patient against abruptly discontinuing haloperidol after long-term use.
- ❖ Inform the patient that drowsiness generally subsides with continued therapy.
- ❖ Warn the patient to avoid tasks that require mental alertness or motor skills until his response to the drug has been established.
- ❖ Urge the patient to avoid alcohol during haloperidol therapy.
- ❖ Urge the patient to avoid exposure to sunlight and any condition that may cause dehydration or overheating because they may increase the risk of heat stroke.
- ❖ Suggest taking sips of water or chewing sugarless gum to help relieve dry mouth.
- ❖ Instruct the patient to rise slowly from a lying or sitting position.
- ❖ Monitor blood pressure lying and standing frequently. Document and report significant changes.

Chlorpromazine

Trade Name
Largactil, thorazine

Classification
Dopamine receptor antagonists—phenothiazine

Dose
Oral: 300–1500 mg per day in divided doses, Parental: 25–100 mg per day IM only.

Mechanism of Action
Chlorpromazine blocks dopamine neurotransmission at postsynaptic dopamine receptor sites. Possesses strong anticholinergic, sedative and antiemetic effects, moderate extrapyramidal effects and slight antihistamine action.

Indications
Acute psychotic episodes in schizophrenia and schizoaffective disorders, mania, depression with psychotic symptoms, delusional disorders, borderline personality disorder, and substance-induced psychotic disorder, delirium and dementia, mental disorders due to a medical condition, pervasive developmental disorder, Tourette's syndrome, Huntington's disease.

Contraindication
Comatose states, myelosuppression, severe cardiovascular disease, severe CNS depression, subcortical brain damage.

Side Effects
- ❖ **Autonomic side effects**: Dry mouth, constipation, urinary retention, orthostatic hypotension, impotence
- ❖ **EPS**: Akathisia, acute dystonia, rabbit syndrome, drug-induced Parkinsonism
- ❖ **CNS side effects**: Seizures, sedation
- ❖ **Metabolic and endocrine side effects**: Weight gain
- ❖ **Allergic side effects**: Cholestatic jaundice, agranulocytosis, mild leukopenia
- ❖ **Cardiac side effects**: Tachycardia
- ❖ **Dermatological side effects**: Contact dermatitis, photosensitivity reaction

Nurse's Responsibility
- ❖ Assess patient behavior and emotional status

- Use chlorpromazine cautiously in patients with alcoholism, glaucoma, history of seizures, hypocalcemia (increases susceptibility to dystonias), impaired cardiac, hepatic, renal or respiratory function, benign prostate hyperplasia or urine retention.
- Avoid skin contact with the oral concentrate and syrup to prevent contact dermatitis.
- Do not give chlorpromazine by the subcutaneous route because severe tissue necrosis may occur.
- To prevent irritation at the injection site, dilute the injection solution with sodium chloride.
- Monitor the patient's blood pressure for hypotension, advice the patient to get up from the bed or chair slowly. Monitor blood pressure lying and standing frequently. Document and report significant changes.
- Advise the patient to take sips of water frequently.
- Apply glycerin to the lips.
- Advise high fiber diet and more water intake.
- Monitor patient for EPS.
- Regularly check patient's CBC as ordered for evidence of blood dyscrasias.
- Monitor patient's serum drug level. Therapeutic serum level for chlorpromazine is 50–300 µ/mL and toxic serum level >750 µg/mL.
- Advise the patient that urine may darken.
- Inform the patient that drowsiness generally subsides with continued therapy.
- Warn the patient to avoid tasks that require mental alertness or motor skills until his response to the drug has been established.
- Urge the patient to avoid alcohol and excessive exposure to sunlight while taking chlorpromazine.
- Ensure that patient wears protective sun screens, clothing and sunglasses while spending in outdoors.
- Evaluate the patient's fine tongue movement for signs of tardive dyskinesia. These symptoms are potentially irreversible. The drug should be withdrawn at the first sign which is usually vermiform movements of the tongue.

Fluphenazine Hydrochloride

Trade Name
Permitil, Prolixin, Prolixin Decanoate

Classification
Dopamine receptor antagonists—phenothiazine

Dose
Oral: 1–30 mg/day, Parental: 25 mg/mL once in 2–4 weeks

Mechanism of Action
A phenothiazine that antagonizes dopamine neurotransmission at synapses by blocking postsynaptic dopaminergic receptors in the brain.

Indications
Schizophrenia, mania with psychotic symptoms, organic brain syndrome, chronic schizophrenia.

Contraindications
Angle-closure glaucoma, myelosuppression, severe cardiac or hepatic disease, severe hypertension or hypotension.

Side Effects

❖ **Frequent:** Hypotension, dizziness and syncope (occur frequently after first injection, occasionally after subsequent injections and rarely with oral doses).

❖ **Occasional:** Somnolence, dry mouth, blurred vision, lethargy, constipation or diarrhea, nasal congestion, peripheral edema, urine retention.

❖ **Serious reactions:** EPS-akathisia, acute dystonia, parkinsonian symptoms, tardive dyskinesia, abrupt discontinuation after long-term therapy may precipitate nausea, vomiting, gastritis, dizziness and tremors. Fluphenazine may lower the seizure threshold. Blood dyscrasias particularly agranulocytosis and mild leukopenia may occur.

Nurse's Responsibility

❖ Assess patient behavior and emotional status.

❖ Avoid skin contact with the oral concentrate and syrup to prevent contact dermatitis.

❖ Monitor the patient's blood pressure for hypotension and complete blood count for blood dyscrasias.

❖ Administer deep injection in large muscle mass.

❖ Evaluate the patient's fine tongue movement for signs of tardive dyskinesia. These symptoms are potentially irreversible. The drug should be withdrawn at the first sign which is usually vermiform movements of the tongue.

❖ Inform the patient that drowsiness generally subsides with continued therapy.

❖ Warn the patient to avoid tasks that require mental alertness or motor skills until his response to the drug has been established.

Trifluoperazine Hydrochloride

Trade Name

Stelazine, Terfluzine, Solazine, Flurazine

Classification

Dopamine receptor antagonists—phenothiazine

Dose

Oral: 2–5 mg/day up to 40 mg/day, parental: IM 1–2 mg up to 10 mg/day

Mechanism of Action

A phenothiazine derivative that blocks dopamine at postsynaptic receptor sites. Possess strong extrapyramidal and antiemetic effects and weak anticholinergic and sedative effects.

Indications

Acute psychotic episodes in schizophrenia and schizoaffective disorders, mania, depression with psychotic symptoms, delusional disorders, borderline personality disorder, and substance-induced psychotic disorder, delirium and dementia, mental disorders due to a medical condition, pervasive developmental disorder, Tourette's syndrome, Huntington's disease.

Contraindications

Angle-closure glaucoma, myelosuppression, severe cardiac or hepatic disease, severe hypertension or hypotension.

Side Effects

❖ **Frequent:** Hypotension, dizziness and syncope (occur frequently after first injection, occasionally after subsequent injections and rarely with oral doses).

❖ **Occasional**: Drowsiness during early therapy, dry mouth, blurred vision, lethargy, constipation or diarrhea, nasal congestion, peripheral edema, urine retention.
❖ **Serious reactions**: EPS—akathesia, acute dystonia, parkinsonian symptoms, tardive dyskinesia, abrupt discontinuation after long-term therapy may precipitate nausea, vomiting, gastritis, dizziness and tremors. Trifluoperazine may lower the seizure threshold. Blood dyscrasias, particularly agranulocytosis and mild leukopenia may occur.

Nurse's Responsibility

❖ Assess patient behavior and emotional status
❖ Use trifluoperazine cautiously in patients with Parkinson's disease or seizure disorders.
❖ Give oral drugs along with food to decrease GI effects.
❖ Administer deep injection in large muscle mass.
❖ Monitor the patient's BP for hypotension.
❖ Observe the patient for extrapyramidal symptoms such as gait changes, tremors, and abnormal movement in the trunk, neck or extremities.
❖ Monitor the patient's WBC count for blood dyscrasias such as anemia, neutropenia, pancytopenia and thrombocytopenia.
❖ Monitor the patient for fine tongue movement, an early sign of tardive dyskinesia. These symptoms are potentially irreversible. The drug should be withdrawn at the first sign which is usually vermiform movements of the tongue.
❖ Assess the patient for signs of a therapeutic response.
❖ Inform the patient that drowsiness generally subsides with continued therapy.
❖ Warn the patient to avoid tasks that require mental alertness or motor skills until his response to the drug has been established.
❖ Instruct the patient not to take antacids within one hour of trifluoperazine.
❖ Urge the patient to avoid alcohol and excessive exposure to artificial light and sunlight during trifluoperazine therapy.
❖ Instruct the patient to rise slowly from a lying or sitting position to prevent hypotension. Monitor blood pressure lying and standing frequently. Document and report significant changes.

Risperidone

Trade Name
Sizodon

Classification
Atypical antipsychotic—serotonin dopamine antagonists

Dose
Oral: 0.5–6 mg/day

Mechanism of Action
Antiserotonergic, antiadrenergic and antihistaminergic actions. It has less action as antidopaminergic especially D2 receptors.

Indications
Positive and negative symptoms of schizophrenia, other psychosis, schizoaffective symptoms.

Contraindications
Hypersensitivity, heart diseases, epilepsy, hyperprolactinemia, parkinsonism, renal and hepatic impairment.

Side Effects

- ❖ **CNS**: Somnolence, seizures, headache.
- ❖ **CVS**: Orthostatic hypotension, dizziness, tachycardia and syncope.
- ❖ **Other adverse reactions**: Weight gain, constipation, erectile dysfunction, vomiting, rash, abdominal pain. Rare reactions include tardive dyskinesia (characterized by tongue protrusion, puffing of the cheeks, and chewing or puckering of the mouth) and neuroleptic malignant syndrome (marked by hyperpyrexia, muscle rigidity, change in mental status, irregular pulse or blood pressure, tachycardia, diaphoresis, cardiac arrhythmias and acute renal failure).

Nurse's Responsibility

- ❖ Before beginning risperidone therapy assess for blood urea nitrogen levels and serum alkaline phosphatase, bilirubin, creatinine, renal and hepatic functions.
- ❖ Assess for behavioral and emotional status.
- ❖ The elderly are more susceptible to orthostatic hypotension. They may require a dosage adjustment because of age-related renal or hepatic impairment.
- ❖ Monitor patient's BP, heart rate, liver function test results, and weight gain.
- ❖ Observe the patient for fine tongue movement which may be the first sign of irreversible tardive dyskinesia.
- ❖ Monitor the patient for neuroleptic malignant syndrome.
- ❖ Take measures to reduce constipation.
- ❖ Urge the patient to notify the physician if he or she experiences altered gait, difficulty in breathing, palpitations, pain or swelling in breasts, severe dizziness or fainting, trembling fingers, unusual movements, rash or visual changes.
- ❖ Inform the patient that risperidone may cause dizziness or drowsiness. Warn the patient to avoid tasks that require mental alertness or motor skills until his response to the drug has been established.
- ❖ Instruct the patient to change positions slowly to minimize the drug's hypotensive effects
- ❖ Urge the patient to avoid alcohol during risperidone therapy.

Olanzapine

Trade Name

Zyprexa

Classification

Atypical antipsychotic—serotonin dopamine antagonists

Dose

Oral: 5–10 mg/day

Mechanism of Action

Antagonizes alpha-adrenergic, dopamine histamine muscarinic and serotonin receptors. Produces anticholinergic, histaminic and CNS depressant effects.

Indications

Positive and negative manifestations of schizophrenia, schizoaffective disorders, bipolar mania.

Contraindications

Narrow angle glaucoma, paralytic ileus, urinary outflow obstruction.

Side Effects

- ❖ **CNS**: Somnolence, agitation, insomnia, headache, nervousness, hostility.
- ❖ **CVS**: Orthostatic hypotension, tachycardia, syncope, dizziness.
- ❖ **Other adverse reaction**: Weight gain, constipation.
- ❖ Rare reactions include seizures, neuroleptic malignant syndrome, EPS.

Nurse's Responsibility

- ❖ Obtain liver function test results as ordered before beginning olanzapine treatment.
- ❖ Assess patient's behavior and emotional status.
- ❖ Use olanzapine cautiously in patients with a hypersensitivity to clozapine, hepatic impairment, cerebrovascular disease, cardiovascular disease, history of seizures and conditions predisposing patients to hypotension such as dehydration, hypovolemia, use of antihypertensives.
- ❖ Monitor the patient for blood pressure.
- ❖ Instruct the patient to take olanzapine as ordered. Caution the patient against abruptly discontinuing the drug or increasing the dosage.
- ❖ Inform the patient that drowsiness generally subsides with continued therapy.
- ❖ Caution the patient to notify the physician if she becomes pregnant or intends to become pregnant during olanzapine therapy.
- ❖ Warn the patient to avoid tasks requiring mental alertness or motor skills until his response to the drug has been established.
- ❖ Advise the patient to avoid dehydration particularly during exercise; exposure to extreme heat; and concurrent use of medications that cause dry mouth or other drying effects.
- ❖ Suggest taking sips of tepid water and chewing sugarless gum to help relieve dry mouth.
- ❖ Instruct the patient to maintain a healthy diet and exercise program to prevent weight gain.
- ❖ Administer or instruct patient to take drug early in the day to reduce insomnia, instruct to avoid caffeinated drinks or food.

Olanzapine Injection

Trade Names
Zyprexa, Zyprexa Relprevv, Olanzapine Pamoate Depot Injection

Classification
Atypical antipsychotic

Dose
- ❖ Available intramuscular powder for injection 10 mg.
- ❖ Olanzapine depot injection is given every 2 or every 4 weeks as an injection into the buttock muscle only.

Mechanism of Action
Olanzapine pamoate is an antipsychotic depot formulation for injection. It is designed to release olanzapine slowly from the intramuscular site. Helps restore the chemical imbalances in the brain. It improves thoughts, behavior and enhances the quality of life.

Indications
Schizophrenia, mania, bipolar affective disorder

Contraindications

Liver disease, heart disease, low blood pressure, high cholesterol, stroke, narrow-angle glaucoma, diabetes and an enlarged prostate. Not recommended for children aged below 18 years, pregnancy and lactating mother.

Side Effects

Weight gain, sleepiness, increased blood sugar levels, hypercholesterolemia. Post injection syndrome includes sedation, drowsiness, dizziness, confusion, disorientation, slurred speech, aggression, ataxia, hypertension, seizures and weakness. Initial signs and symptoms of post injection syndrome appear within one hour following injection. In most cases, full recovery is expected to occur within 24–72 hours after injection.

Nurse's Responsibility

- ❖ Instruct the patient not to drive or operate heavy machines rest of the day after the injection.
- ❖ Reconstitute with diluent provided to form a suspension. Administer by deep IM gluteal injection only, every 2 weeks or every 4 weeks.
- ❖ Do not rub or massage the injection site after injection. Do not inject into a vein or under the skin.
- ❖ Patient should be watched carefully for first 3 hours after the injection for post injection syndrome. These symptoms include:
  - ○ Severe dizziness, light-headed feeling, drowsiness or weakness
  - ○ Trouble walking or talking, nervousness
  - ○ Seizures
- ❖ Discuss potential risk with patients each time they receive injection.
- ❖ It may increase the weight of the patient, blood sugar and cholesterol. Hence instruct the patient to eat healthy, exercise regularly and monitor blood sugar levels regularly.
- ❖ To reduce the chance of feeling dizzy, instruct the patient to rise slowly.
- ❖ Instruct the patient not to stop injection abruptly.

Clozapine

Trade Name

Sizopine

Classification

Atypical antipsychotic—serotonin dopamine antagonists

Dose

Oral: Initially 25 mg, 1–2 times per day. This can be gradually increased to 300 mg per day in 2–3 divided doses.

Mechanism of Action

Antagonizes alpha-adrenergic, dopamine histamine muscarinic and serotonin receptors. Produces anticholinergic, histaminic and CNS depressant effects.

Indications

Positive and negative manifestations of schizophrenia, schizoaffective disorders, schizophrenia not responding to traditional antipsychotic drugs, patient who cannot tolerate the side effects of traditional antipsychotics, management of severely ill schizophrenic patients.

Contraindications

Bone marrow suppression, lactation, hypersensitivity, CNS depression, coma, below 16 years age.

Side Effects
- ❖ **Clozapine-induced agranulocytosis**: Decreased WBC count specifically polymorphonuclear leukocytes, seizures, tachycardia, hypotension.
- ❖ **Other side effects** are sedation, fatigue, sialorrhea, weight gain, constipation, anticholinergic effects.

Nurse's Responsibility
- ❖ Great risk period is first 6 months, explain treatment risks. Agranulocytosis is a life-threatening side effect which should be informed to the family members.
- ❖ Before starting therapy test blood for TC, DC, LFT and RFT
- ❖ For the first 6 months of continuous therapy obtain patient's WBC count on a weekly basis, then biweekly for patients with acceptable WBC count. If the WBC is below $1500/mm^3$ clozapine should be stopped.
- ❖ Instruct the patient to notify symptoms such as sore throat, fever, lethargy, weakness like symptoms to the physician promptly.
- ❖ Take precautions for seizure
- ❖ Use clozapine cautiously in patients undergoing alcohol withdrawal and in those with cardiovascular disease, glaucoma, history of seizures, benign prostate hyperplasia, myocarditis, urine retention or impaired hepatic, renal or respiratory function.
- ❖ Caution the patient against abruptly discontinuing clozapine.
- ❖ Inform the patient that drowsiness generally subsides with continued therapy.
- ❖ Warn the patient to avoid tasks that require mental alertness or motor skills until his response to the drug has been established.
- ❖ Urge the patient to avoid alcohol during clozapine therapy.

Aripiprazole

Trade Name
Abilify, Aripiprex

Classification
Psychotropic drug—atypical antipsychotic, dopamine, serotonin agonist and antagonist

Dose
Available forms
Tablets: 10, 15, 20, 30 mg
Adults: 10–15 mg/day PO
Pediatric patients: Safety and efficacy not established

Mechanism of Action
Acts as an agonist at dopamine and serotonin sites and antagonist at other serotonin receptor sites; this combination of actions is thought to be responsible for the drug's effectiveness in treating schizophrenia though the mechanism of action is not understood.

Pharmacokinetics
Usual administration is oral route. Metabolized in the liver, may cross placenta; may pass into breast milk, excretes through urine and feces.

Indications
Used in the treatment of schizophrenia, bipolar disorder, major depressive disorder (as an add on to other treatment), tic disorders, and irritability associated with autism.

Contraindications

Contraindicated in the presence of allergy to aripiprazole during lactation period. Use cautiously in the presence of suicidal ideation, pregnancy, cerebral vascular disease, known cardiovascular disease, seizure disorders, patients with Alzheimer's disease, dysphagia (risk for aspiration pneumonia).

Side Effects

Weight gain, headache, agitation, insomnia, anxiety, nausea and vomiting, akathisia (a sense of unease and restlessness that presents itself with anxiety), light-headedness, constipation.

Nurse's Responsibility

- ❖ Monitor blood pressure
- ❖ Protect the patient from extreme of heat (avoid heavy exercise, dehydration)
- ❖ Provide plenty of oral fluids
- ❖ Explain about side effects
- ❖ Report severe dizziness, trembling, light-headedness, suicidal thoughts, and blurred vision

Paliperidone

Trade Name

Invega, Invega sustenna

Classification

Atypical antipsychotic

Dose

Paliperidone comes as an extended-release (long-acting) tablet to be taken by mouth once a day in the morning with or without food. Usual dose is 3–6 mg per day orally, 6 mg for subjects weighing <51 kg and 12 mg for subjects weighing >51 kg.

Mechanism of Action

Paliperidone is the primary active metabolite of the older antipsychotic risperidone. Specific mechanism of action is unknown; it is believed that paliperidone and risperidone act via similar if not the same pathways. The drug's therapeutic activity in schizophrenia is mediated through a combination of central dopamine type 2 (D2) and serotonin type 2 (5HT2A) receptor antagonism. Paliperidone was approved by the FDA for treatment of schizophrenia on December 20, 2006.

Pharmacokinetics

The absolute oral bioavailability of paliperidone following administration is 100%. Peak plasma levels of drug occur 1 hour after administration. Paliperidone is 90% plasma protein bound. Excreted in urine.

Indications

Treatment for schizophrenia, schizoaffective disorders, bipolar affective disorder and depression.

Contraindications

- ❖ Allergic to any ingredient in paliperidone or to risperidone
- ❖ Moderate to severe kidney problems, liver problems
- ❖ History of irregular heartbeat
- ❖ Taking certain antiarrhythmics (e.g., amiodarone, procainamide, quinidine, sotalol)
- ❖ Taking certain antipsychotic medicines (e.g., chlorpromazine, thioridazine)
- ❖ Pregnancy and breastfeeding
- ❖ History of seizures, heart problems, heart failure, abnormal ECG

- High blood cholesterol or triglycerides
- High or low blood pressure
- History of neuroleptic malignant syndrome, tardive dyskinesia, suicidal thoughts, alcohol abuse or dependency
- Reye syndrome, diabetes, Alzheimer disease, dementia, Parkinson's disease, high blood prolactin levels
- History of certain cancers (e.g., breast, pancreas, pituitary)

Side Effects

Constipation; diarrhea; dizziness; drowsiness; dry mouth; headache; light-headedness; mild pain, swelling, or redness at the injection site; mild stomach pain or discomfort; nausea; restlessness; trouble sleeping; vomiting; weakness; weight gain.

Nurse's Responsibility

Instruct the patient or family on following aspects:

- Drinking extra fluids while taking this drug are recommended.
- Tell your doctor or dentist that you are taking paliperidone before taking any medical or dental care or emergency care or surgery.
- Do not drive or perform unsafe tasks while taking drug because paliperidone may cause drowsiness, dizziness or light-headedness.
- Do not drink alcohol.
- Do not change dose or stop medication without doctor's advise.
- Do not become overheated in hot weather.
- Diabetic patients should check blood sugar levels closely.
- Inform doctor of any signs of infection like fever, sore throat, rash or chills.
- Monitor weight regularly.
- Take medicine at around the same time everyday. Swallow the tablet whole with plenty of water or other liquid.
- Take the missed dose as soon as you remember it. However, if it is almost time for the next dose, skip the missed dose and continue your regular dosing schedule. Do not take a double dose to make up for a missed one.

Amisulpride

Trade Names

Amgrace, Cyam, Bipo Life, Zonapride, Zulpride, Solian

Classification

Second generation atypical antipsychotic

Dose

It comes as a tablet to be taken by mouth on an empty stomach. IM injection should be given into large muscle. For adult <15 years, the recommended dose is 400–800 mg/day in divided doses PO. Maximum dose is 1.2 g/day. For intramuscular (IM) injection, the recommended dose is 400 mg/day.

Mechanism of Action

Amisulpride, a substituted benzamide derivative is a second-generation (atypical) antipsychotic. Amisulpride binds selectively to D2 dopaminergic receptors and D3 receptors but does not have any affinity for D1, adrenergic, cholinergic, serotonergic or H1 histaminergic receptors. It shows greater affinity for limbic dopaminergic receptors than for striatal structures suggesting better neurological tolerability compared with classical neuroleptics which block all dopamine receptors equally. High doses (400–800 mg) inhibit hyper-dopaminergic symptomatology and control psychotic symptoms, low doses (50–300 mg) have an effect on negative symptoms.

Pharmacokinetics

Amisulpride is absorbed rapidly, within 3–4 hours of oral administration. Drug is excreted through urine mainly as unchanged drug, the elimination half-life is approximately 12 hours, plasma protein binding is low.

Indications

For treatment of schizophrenia, schizoaffective disorders, bipolar affective disorders and other psychotic disorders.

Contraindications

Caution should be exercised in patients with history of diabetes, epilepsy, brain damage, Parkinson's disease, heart disease, stroke, dementia, high blood pressure, alcoholism, elderly, pregnancy and lactation period.

It should not be used in following patients: Those allergic to amisulpride, having breast cancer or tumor on their adrenal gland (prolactine dependent tumors), taking levodopa medicines, during pregnancy and lactation period, children before the onset of puberty.

Side Effects

Extrapyramidal symptoms, hyperprolactinemia, insomnia, anxiety agitation, weight gain, dizziness, restlessness, stiffness in arms or legs, increased salivation, changes in blood sugar level and cholesterol level, rash, changes in menstrual cycle.

Nurse's Responsibility

- ❖ Caution should be exercised in patients with history of sugar, epilepsy, brain damage, Parkinson's disease, heart disease, abnormal heart rhythm, disturbances in blood electrolytes level, stroke, dementia, high blood pressure, smoking habit, alcoholism, elderly, and during pregnancy.
- ❖ Drug may cause drowsiness, advice the patient not to drive a car or operate machinery while taking medication.
- ❖ Inform patient and family members to consult doctor if patient develops abnormal movements, particularly of the face, lips, jaw and tongue while taking medication.
- ❖ Monitor blood sugar level, ECG, weight, waist circumference regularly while taking medication.
- ❖ Inform patient and family members about neuroleptic malignant syndrome and tardive dyskinesia symptoms like high fever, sweating, muscle stiffness, faster breathing and drowsiness or sleepiness. Consult doctor immediately if these symptoms appear.
- ❖ Explain to the patient that if he forgets to take the drug, he may take it as soon as he remembers it. However, if it is nearly time for the next dose, skip the missed dose. Do not take a double dose to make up for a forgotten dose.
- ❖ Advice the patient not to stop the drug abruptly as stopping the treatment suddenly may cause withdrawal effects such as feeling sick, sweating, difficulty in sleeping, muscle stiffness or unusual body movements.

Quetiapine

Trade Name
Serequel

Dose

Children and adolescents 100–350 mg/day, adults—300–400 mg in 2–3 divided doses in a day.

Classification

Atypical antipsychotic agent, dibenzothiazepine

Mechanism of Action

Exact mechanism of action is unknown. It has been proposed that this drug's antipsychotic activity is mediated through a combination of dopamine type 2 (D2) and serotonin type 2 (5-HT2) antagonism.

Pharmacokinetics

Pharmacokinetics absorbed orally, protein binding plasma 83%, primarily metabolized in liver, excreted through urine and feces.

Indications

Treatment of schizophrenia, schizoaffective disorders, mania, bipolar disorders, autism, psychosis.

Contraindications

Use with caution in patients with Parkinson's disease, hemodynamic instability, prior myocardial infarction, hypercholesterolemia, thyroid disease, seizures, hepatic impairment, renal or respiratory diseases. Should not be used for patients with hypersensitivity to quetiapine, bone marrow suppression, blood dyscrasias, severe hepatic disease or coma.

Side Effects

Headache, somnolence, weight gain, tachycardia, palpitations, postural hypotension, dizziness, rash, abdominal pain, constipation, anorexia, weakness, in rare conditions diabetes mellitus, hyperlipidemia, hypothyroidism, vertigo.

Nurse's Responsibility

- ❖ Monitor for side effects
- ❖ Instruct the patient to take medication along with food at the same time regularly
- ❖ Do not stop the medicine suddenly
- ❖ Drug may cause drowsiness, avoid driving, doing other activities until you see how this medicine affects you.
- ❖ Avoid alcohol, take plenty of oral fluids.

Ziprasidone

Trade Name

Zeldex, Ziprasidone Hydrochloride, Ziprasidone Mesylate

Dose

Adults—20–100 mg twice daily orally, intramuscular injection 10 mg in every 2 hours or 20 mg in every 4 hours.

Classification

Atypical antipsychotic D(3) dopamine receptor antagonist

Mechanism of Action

Ziprasidone's antipsychotic activity is likely due to a combination of its antagonistic function at D2 receptors in the mesolimbic pathways and at 5HT2A receptors in the frontal cortex.

Alleviation of positive symptoms is due to antagonism at D2 receptors while relief of negative symptoms is due to 5HT2A antagonism.

Pharmacokinetics
Well absorbed orally, metabolized in the liver, excreted through feces and urine, protein binding 99%.

Indications
Schizophrenia, acute mania, bipolar affective disorder, also used for depression, anxiety, aggression, dementia, attention-deficit hyperactivity disorder, obsessive-compulsive disorder, autism, post-traumatic stress disorder.

Contraindications
Hypersensitivity to ziprasidone, recent myocardial infarction, history of arrhythmias, heart failure, use of antiarrhythmics. Use with caution in patients with seizures.

Side Effects
Somnolence, headache, nausea, hypertension, postural hypotension, extrapyramidal symptoms, rash, dysmenorrheal, constipation, abdominal pain.

Nurse's Responsibility
❖ Monitor serum potassium and magnesium levels
❖ Potential for extrapyramidal symptoms, fever, confusion, stiffness should be promptly evaluated for neuroleptic malignant syndrome.
❖ Drug should not be administered to a patient who recently had heart attack or congestive heart failure.

Imipramine

Trade Name
Antidep, Tofranil

Classification
Tertiary tricyclic antidepressant drugs

Dose
75–300 mg per day orally

Mechanism of Action
The tricyclic antidepressants are also called as monoamine reuptake inhibitors (MARIs). Their main modes of action are:
❖ Blocking the reuptake of norepinephrine (NE) and serotonin (5-HT) at the nerve terminals thus increasing NE and 5-HT level at receptor site.
❖ Regulation of the β adrenergic receptors.

Indications
Depressive episodes, depression with psychotic symptoms, dysthymia, reactive depression, secondary depression due to hypothyroidism, Cushing's syndrome, abnormal grief reaction.

Childhood psychiatric disorders, enuresis, phobia, separation anxiety, somnambulism, night terrors. Other psychiatric disorders like panic attacks, agoraphobia, social phobia, obsessive-compulsive disorder, aggression in elderly, post-traumatic stress disorder, depersonalization. *Medical disorders*: Chronic pain, migraine, peptic ulcer.

Contraindications

Cardiac disorders, acute recovery period after MI, use within 14 days of MAOIs.

Side Effects

- ❖ **Autonomic**: Dry mouth, constipation, urinary retention, mydriasis, orthostatic hypotension, impotence, delirium, blurred vision, urinary hesitancy
- ❖ **CNS**: Sedation, tremors, withdrawal syndrome, seizures
- ❖ **CVS**: Tachycardia, arrhythmias, direct myocardial depression
- ❖ **Allergic**: Agranulocytosis, cholestatic jaundice
- ❖ **Other reactions**: Weight gain, tiredness, drowsiness, insomnia, acute organic syndrome

Nurse's Responsibility

- ❖ Perform CBC, blood serum chemistry tests to specifically assess the blood glucose level, and liver and renal function tests prior to and periodically during long-term therapy.
- ❖ Plan to perform a baseline ECG if the patient is at risk for arrhythmias.
- ❖ Use of drug is not recommended for children younger than 6 years.
- ❖ Expect to administer a lower dosage to elderly patients because they are at risk for drug toxicity.
- ❖ Use cautiously in patients with cardiac disease, diabetes mellitus, glaucoma, hiatal hernia, history of seizures, history of urinary obstruction, hyperthyroidism, benign prostatic hyperplasia, renal or hepatic disease.
- ❖ Make sure at least 14 days elapse between the use of MAOIs and imipramine.
- ❖ Give with food or milk if GI distress occurs.
- ❖ Do not crush or break film-coated tablets.
- ❖ Closely monitor suicidal patients during early therapy. As depression lessens, the patient's energy level generally improves, increasing the likelihood of suicide attempts.
- ❖ Assess the patient's pattern of daily bowel activity and stool consistency.
- ❖ Assess the patient's appearance, behavior, level of interest, mood and sleep pattern before and during therapy.
- ❖ Monitor the patient's BP and pulse rate to detect hypotension and arrhythmias.
- ❖ Palpate the patient's bladder for evidence of urine retention.
- ❖ Caution the patient against abruptly discontinuing medication.
- ❖ Inform the patient that improvement may occur 2–5 days after starting therapy but that the full therapeutic effect will likely occur within 2–3 weeks.
- ❖ Instruct the patient to change positions slowly to help prevent dizziness.
- ❖ Warn the patient to avoid tasks that require mental alertness or motor skills until his response to the drug has been established.
- ❖ Inform the patient that taking sips of tepid water and chewing sugarless gum may relieve dry mouth.
- ❖ Advise the patient to take high fiber diet.

Clomipramine

Trade Name

Anafranil

Classification

Tertiary tricyclic antidepressant drugs

Dose

150–250 mg/day orally

Mechanism of Action

A tricyclic antidepressant that blocks the reuptake of neurotransmitters such as norepinephrine and serotonin at CNS presynaptic membranes, increasing their availability at postsynaptic receptor sites.

Indications

Obsessive compulsive disorder, depression, panic disorder, phobias, pain disorders

Contraindications

- Cardiac disorders, acute recovery period after MI, use within 14 days of MAOIs.
- Should be avoided during pregnancy, the drug should be given cautiously in patients with hepatic and renal disease.

Side Effects

Somnolence, fatigue, dry mouth, blurred vision, constipation, sexual dysfunction, ejaculatory failure, impotence, weight gain, delayed micturition, orthostatic hypotension, diaphoresis, impaired concentration, increased appetite, urine retention, GI disturbances, seizures, orthostatic hypotension, dizziness, tachycardia, palpitation and arrhythmias and hyperpyrexia.

Nurse's Responsibility

Same as that for imipramine

Amitriptyline Hydrochloride

Trade Name

Elavil, Endep, Levate

Classification

Tertiary tricyclic antidepressant drugs

Dose

30–100 mg/day orally, may increase up to 150–300 mg/day.

Mechanism of Action

A tricyclic antidepressant that blocks the reuptake of neurotransmitters such as norepinephrine and serotonin at CNS presynaptic membranes, increasing their availability at postsynaptic receptor sites.

Indications

Depression, relief of neuropathic pain such as experienced by patients with diabetic neuropathy or post therapeutic neuralgia, treatment of bulimia nervosa.

Contraindications

Cardiac disorders, acute recovery period after MI, use within 14 days of MAOIs.

Side Effects

Dizziness, somnolence, dry mouth, orthostatic hypotension, headache, increased appetite, weight gain, nausea, unusual fatigue, unpleasant taste, blurred vision, confusion, constipation, arrhythmias, fine muscle tremors, anxiety, diarrhea, diaphoresis, heartburn, insomnia.

Nurse's Responsibility

- Perform CBC, blood serum chemistry tests specifically to assess the blood glucose level, and liver and renal function tests before and periodically during long-term therapy.

❖ Plan to perform a baseline ECG if the patient is at risk for arrhythmias.

❖ Amitriptyline use is not recommended for children younger than 10 years. Children are more sensitive to an acute overdose and are at an increased risk for amitriptyline toxicity.

❖ Elderly patients are more sensitive to the drug's anticholinergic effects and are at an increased risk for amitriptyline toxicity.

❖ Use amitriptyline cautiously in patients with cardiac disease, diabetes mellitus, glaucoma, hiatal hernia, history of seizures, history of urinary obstruction, hyperthyroidism, and benign prostatic hyperplasia, renal or hepatic disease.

❖ Make sure at least 14 days elapse between the use of MAOIs and clomipramine.

❖ Give amitriptyline with food or milk if GI distress occurs.

❖ Closely monitor suicidal patients during early therapy. As depression lessens, the patient's energy level generally improves increasing the likelihood of suicide attempts.

❖ Assess the patient's pattern of daily bowel activity and stool consistency.

❖ Assess the patient's appearance, behavior, level of interest, mood and sleep pattern before and during therapy.

❖ Monitor the patient's BP and pulse rate to detect hypotension and arrhythmias.

❖ Palpate the patient's bladder for evidence of urine retention.

❖ Instruct the patient to change positions slowly to help prevent dizziness.

❖ Warn the patient to avoid tasks that require mental alertness or motor skills until his response to the drug has been established.

❖ Inform the patient that taking sips of tepid water and chewing sugarless gum may relieve dry mouth.

❖ Advise the patient to take high fiber diet.

❖ Inform the patient that the drug's full therapeutic effect may be noted in 2–4 weeks.

❖ Inform the patient that he may develop sensitivity to sunlight.

❖ Urge the patient to report any visual disturbances.

Fluoxetine Hydrochloride

Trade Name

Auscap, Fluohexal, Lovan, Novo-Fluoxetine, Prozac

Classification

Antidepressant: Serotonin—specific reuptake inhibitors

Dose

Initially, 20 mg each morning. If therapeutic improvement does not occur after 2 weeks, gradually increase to a maximum of 80 mg/day in two equally divided doses in morning and at noon.

Mechanism of Action

Selectively inhibits serotonin uptake in the CNS enhancing serotonergic function.

Indications

Depression, obsessive-compulsive disorder, panic disorder and other anxiety disorders, bulimia nervosa, premenstrual dysphoric disorder, treatment of hot flashes.

Contraindications

Hypersensitivity, severe hepatic or renal impairment, pregnancy, lactation and history of seizures.

Side Effects

Headache, nervousness, insomnia, drowsiness, anxiety, seizures, rarely EPS, apathy, anorexia, nausea, diarrhea, dyspepsia, and sexual dysfunction.

Nurse's Responsibility
- ❖ Perform CBC, liver and renal function tests before and periodically during long-term therapy.
- ❖ Use cautiously in patients with cardiac dysfunction, diabetes, or seizure disorder and in patients at high risk of suicide.
- ❖ Give with food or milk, if GI distress occurs.
- ❖ Avoid administration at night, instruct the patients to take the last dose of the drug before 4 PM to avoid insomnia.
- ❖ Assess the patient's pattern of daily bowel activity and stool consistency.
- ❖ Closely monitor suicidal patients during early therapy. As depression lessens, the patient's energy level generally improves, increasing the likelihood of suicide attempts.
- ❖ Assess the patient's appearance, behavior, level of interest, mood and sleep pattern before and during therapy.
- ❖ Inform the patient that the drug's full therapeutic effect may be noted in 2–4 weeks.
- ❖ Warn the patient to avoid tasks that require mental alertness or motor skills until his response to the drug has been established.
- ❖ Urge the patient to avoid alcohol.
- ❖ Caution the female patient to notify the physician if she becomes pregnant.
- ❖ Instruct the patient to report fatigue, headache, sexual dysfunction or tremor.
- ❖ Suggest the patient to take sips of tepid water or chew sugarless gum to relieve dry mouth.

Sertraline Hydrochloride

Trade Name
Zoloft

Classification
Antidepressant: Serotonin—specific reuptake inhibitors.

Dose
50–200 mg

Mechanism of Action
Selectively inhibits serotonin uptake in the CNS enhancing serotonergic function. It blocks the reuptake of the neurotransmitter serotonin at CNS neuronal presynaptic membranes increasing its availability at postsynaptic receptor sites.

Indications
Depression, obsessive-compulsive disorder, panic disorder and other anxiety disorders, bulimia nervosa, premenstrual dysphoric disorder, treatment of hot flashes.

Contraindications
Hypersensitivity, severe hepatic or renal impairment, pregnancy, lactation and history of seizures.

Side Effects
Headache, nervousness, insomnia, drowsiness, anxiety, seizures, rarely EPS, apathy, anorexia, nausea, diarrhea, dyspepsia, and sexual dysfunction.

Nurse's Responsibility
Same as that for fluoxetine hydrochloride

Escitalopram

Trade Name

Lexapro

Classification

Antidepressants: Selective serotonin reuptake inhibitors (SSRI)

Dose

It is available in solution and tablet form. Oral solution at a concentration of 1 mg/mL and tablets in 5 mg, 10 mg, or 20 mg strengths.

The initial dose of medication is 10 mg with an option to increase after 1 week for symptom management.

Mechanism of Action

Selectively inhibits the reuptake of serotonin in the CNS.

Indications

Major depressive disorder, generalized anxiety disorder, panic disorder, obsessive-compulsive disorder, post-traumatic stress disorder, social anxiety disorder, premenstrual dysphoric disorder.

Contraindications

Hypersensitivity to citalopram, concurrent use of MAOIs or use within 14 days of discontinuing MAOIS; pregnancy, lactation, children below 18 years. Cautious use in dehydration, renal or hepatic insufficiency, older adults, cardiovascular disease, history of seizures and suicidal tendencies.

Side Effects

- ❖ **CNS**: Dizziness and drowsiness
- ❖ **GI**: Diarrhea, nausea, abdominal pain, dry mouth, constipation
- ❖ **Endocrine**: Syndrome of inappropriate secretion of antidiuretic hormone (SIADH) causes increased water retention leading to low sodium concentration (hyponatremia), dysmenorrhea
- ❖ **Dermatology**: Increased sweating
- ❖ **Genitourinary**: Erectile dysfunction
- ❖ **Serotonin syndrome**: It is a potential life-threatening adverse effect, results from excess serotonin in both peripheral and central nervous system. This syndrome is more likely to be seen in patients who take a high dose of SSRIs or multiple serotonergic drugs or combining SSRI with a monoamine oxidase inhibitor. The symptoms of serotonin syndrome include tachycardia, hypertension, dizziness, diaphoresis, flushing, mydriasis, increased temperature, nausea, vomiting, diarrhea and mental status changes. Neuromuscular signs such as incoordination, rigidity, hyperreflexia, tremors and hypertonicity.

Nurse's Responsibility

- ❖ Assess dizziness and drowsiness that might affect gait, balance and other functional activities. Caution the patient and family to guard against falls and trauma.
- ❖ Monitor signs of fluid and electrolyte imbalance due to SIADH and hyponatremia. The symptoms of hyponatremia include confusion, lethargy, weakness, myoclonus and depressed reflexes.
- ❖ Monitor periodically hepatic function, CBC, serum sodium
- ❖ Monitor heart rate and blood pressure

❖ Instruct patient not to engage in hazardous activities, avoid using alcohol while taking escitalopram, avoid other CNS depressants, do not breast feed while taking this drug.

❖ Advise the patient that antidepressant effects may not occur immediately, it may take 2–3 weeks before an improvement in mood is observed.

❖ Advise patient to report severe nausea, diarrhea, constipation, abdominal pain.

❖ Instruct patient to report other troublesome side effects. Caution the patient not to discontinue drug abruptly.

❖ Before attempting another antidepressant therapy, a 4 week weaning off period is recommended to prevent the risk of serotonin syndrome.

Venlafaxine

Trade Names
Effexor

Classification
Antidepressant: Serotonin and norepinephrine reuptake inhibitor (SNRI)

Dose
Venlafaxine comes in an oral tablet and capsule. Dose between 75–150 mg per day in divided doses.

Mechanism of Action
Selectively inhibits the reuptake of both serotonin and norepinephrine at the presynaptic terminal. This results in increased levels of neurotransmitters available at the synapse that can stimulate postsynaptic receptors.

Indications
Major depressive disorder, generalized anxiety disorder, social anxiety disorder, panic disorder in adults, migraine, vasomotor symptoms associated with menopause.

Contraindications
Contraindicated in concurrent use of monoamine oxidase inhibitors, seizure disorder patient uncontrolled angle-closure glaucoma, pregnancy, breastfeeding. Caution is advisable in heart failure patients, hyperthyroidism and those with recent myocardial infarction.

Side Effects
Headache, nausea, insomnia, dizziness, hypotension, anorexia, constipation, diarrhea, abdominal pain, weight loss, impotence, hypercholesterolemia, hyponatremia, serotonin syndrome, seizures.

Nurse's Responsibility
❖ Monitor vital signs and blood pressure, report to physician if sustained increase in BP.

❖ Monitor depressive symptoms, anxiety, agitation, confusion and emotional lability. Inform physician if these symptoms are troublesome.

❖ Monitor and immediately report signs of serotonin syndrome.

❖ SNRIs are contraindicated with MAOIs or within 14 days of use of an MAOI.

❖ Elderly patients are at greater risk for developing hyponatremia use with caution.

❖ Patients are instructed to take medications as prescribed. The dose should be tapered prior to discontinuation.

❖ Instruct the patient to avoid use of alcohol or other CNS depressant drugs.

❖ Instruct family members to monitor patient carefully for suicidality.

Tranylcypromine Sulfate

Trade Name
Parnate

Classification
Antidepressants—monoamine oxidase inhibitors (MAOI)

Dose
Oral: 10–60 mg per day

Mechanism of Action
An MAOI that inhibits the activity of the enzyme monoamine oxidase at CNS storage sites leading to increased levels of neurotransmitters epinephrine, norepinephrine, serotonin and dopamine at neuronal receptor sites.

Indications
Depression refractory to or intolerant of other therapy.

Contraindications
Cardiac disorders, children younger than 16 years, pheochromocytoma, severe hepatic or renal impairment, uncontrolled hypertension.

Side Effects
- ❖ **Frequently**: Orthostatic hypotension, restlessness, GI upset, insomnia, dizziness, lethargy, weakness, dry mouth, peripheral edema.
- ❖ **Occasional**: Flushing, diaphoresis, rash, urinary frequency, increased appetite, transient impotence.
- ❖ **Serious reactions**: Hypertensive crisis occurs rarely and is marked by severe hypertension, occipital headache radiating frontally, neck stiffness or soreness, nausea, vomiting, diaphoresis, fever or chills, clammy skin, dilated pupils, palpitations, tachycardia or bradycardia and constricting chest pain.

Nurse's Responsibility
- ❖ Monitor blood pressure both lying and standing every 2–6 hours when initiating therapy.
- ❖ Monitor liver function test and complete blood count.
- ❖ Determine patient's medical history. Ask the patient if he takes CNS depressants, meperidine and other antidepressants. Tranylcypromine should not be used within 14 days of taking selective serotonin reuptake inhibitors (SSRI).
- ❖ Use tranylcypromine cautiously within several hours of ingestion of a contraindicated substance such as tyramine-containing food.
- ❖ Assess patient's behavior and emotional status.
- ❖ Monitor patient's blood pressure, temperature and weight.
- ❖ Evaluate the patient for an occipital headache radiating frontally and neck stiffness or soreness which may be the first symptoms of an impending hypertensive crisis. If hypertensive crisis occurs, administer phentolamine 5–10 mg IV as prescribed.
- ❖ Discontinue tranylcypromine immediately, if the patient experiences frequent headaches or palpitations.
- ❖ Tell the patient that depression may start to lift during the first week of therapy and that the drug's full therapeutic benefit will occur within 3 weeks.
- ❖ Instruct the patient to change position slowly and to dangle the legs momentarily before standing to avoid dizziness.

❖ Urge the patient to avoid foods that require bacteria or molds for their preparation or preservation (such as yogurt and aged cheese); foods containing tyramine (such as bananas, broad beans, meat, liver, smoked or pickled meats and fish, papayas, figs, raisins, sour cream, soy sauce, beer, wine, and yeast extracts); and excessive amounts of caffeine-containing foods or beverages (including chocolate, coffee and tea).

Lamotrigine

Trade Name
Lamictal

Classification
Central nervous system agent; anticonvulsant

Dose
Available forms: 25 mg, 100 mg, 150 mg, 200 mg tablets; 2 mg, 5 mg, 25 mg chewable tablets.
Adults: 25–200 mg/day PO in two divided doses.
Pediatric patients: Safety and efficacy not established.

Mechanism of Action
The exact mechanism of action is unknown; thought to act by inhibiting the release of glutamate, an excitatory neurotransmitter at voltage-sensitive sodium channels. Stabilizing the neuronal membrane and modulating calcium-dependent presynaptic release of excitatory amino acids.

Pharmacokinetics
Usual administration is oral route. Metabolized in the liver, may cross placenta; may pass into breast milk, excretes through urine.

Indications
❖ Adjuvant therapy in the treatment of partial seizures in adults with epilepsy
❖ Monotherapy in adults with partial seizures
❖ Generalized tonic—clonic, absence, or myoclonic seizures in adults, treatment of bipolar disorder

Contraindications
❖ Contraindicated with allergy to drug, lactation and pregnancy.
❖ Use cautiously with impaired hepatic, renal, or cardiac function; patients aged <16 years.

Side Effects
Skin rash, Stevens-Johnson syndrome, toxic epidermal necrolysis with multiorgan failure, dizziness, insomnia, headache, somnolence, ataxia, diplopia, blurred vision, nausea, vomiting.

Nurse's Responsibility
❖ Monitor renal and hepatic function before and during therapy.
❖ Monitor patient for any sign of skin rash; discontinue lamotrigine immediately if rash appears.
❖ Do not discontinue drug abruptly or change the dosage without medical advice.
❖ Taper drug slowly over a 2-week period when discontinuing.
❖ Advise the patient not to breastfeed while taking drug.
❖ Advise the patient for periodic ophthalmologic examination with long-term use.
❖ Advise the patient to report yellowing of skin, abdominal pain, changes in color of urine or stools, fever, sore throat, mouth sores, unusual bleeding or bruising, rash

Alprazolam

Trade Name
Alprax, Apo-Alpraz, Novo-Alprazol

Classification
Antianxiety agents, sedatives/hypnotics—benzodiazepines

Dose
Oral: Adults—0.25–0.5 mg, 2–3 times daily

Mechanism of Action
Antianxiety agents may increase the inhibiting effects of gamma aminobutyric acid (GABA), an inhibitory neurotransmitter. Benzodiazepines reduce anxiety by stimulating the action of the inhibitory neurotransmitter GABA in the limbic system. The limbic system plays an important role in the regulation of human behavior. Dysfunction of GABA neurotransmission in the limbic system may be linked to the development of certain anxiety disorders.

Indications
Anxiety disorders, panic disorder, premenstrual syndrome, insomnia, irritable bowel syndrome

Contraindications
Acute alcohol intoxication with depressed vital signs, acute angle closure glaucoma, myasthenia gravis, severe COPD, hypersensitivity, pregnancy and lactation.

Side Effects
❖ **Frequent**: Ataxia, light-headedness, transient mild somnolence, slurred speech
❖ **Occasional**: Confusion, depression, blurred vision, constipation, diarrhea, dry mouth headache, nausea
❖ **Serious reactions**: Abrupt or too-rapid withdrawal may result in pronounced restlessness, irritability, insomnia, hand tremors, abdominal and muscle cramps, diaphoresis, vomiting and seizures. Overdose results in somnolence, confusion, diminished reflexes and coma.

Nurse's Responsibility
❖ Assess the patient for motor responses such as agitation, tension and trembling, and autonomic responses such as cold, clammy hands and diaphoresis.
❖ Chronic use of alprazolam during pregnancy may produce withdrawal symptoms in the patient and CNS depression in the neonate.
❖ Use alprazolam cautiously in patients with impaired renal or hepatic function.
❖ Caution the patient not to stop taking alprazolam abruptly after long-term therapy.
❖ Inform the patient that drowsiness usually disappears with continued therapy.
❖ Instruct the patient to change positions slowly from recumbent to sitting before standing to prevent dizziness.
❖ Caution the patient to avoid tasks that require mental alertness or motor skills until his response to the drug has been established.
❖ Urge the patient to avoid alcohol during therapy.
❖ Encourage the patient to stop smoking because smoking reduces alprazolam's effectiveness.
❖ Urge the female patient on long-term therapy to use effective contraception during therapy and notify the physician immediately if she becomes or even suspects to be pregnant.
❖ Inform the patient that sour hard candy, gum, or sips of tepid water may relieve dry mouth.

Chlordiazepoxide

Trade Name
Librium, Novopoxide

Classification
Antianxiety agents, sedatives/hypnotics—benzodiazepines

Dose
Oral: 15–100 mg per day in 3–4 divided doses. Parental: 25–50 mg IV or IM

Mechanism of Action
Antianxiety agents may increase the inhibiting effects of gamma aminobutyric acid (GABA), an inhibitory neurotransmitter. Benzodiazepines reduce anxiety by stimulating the action of the inhibitory neurotransmitter GABA in the limbic system. The limbic system plays an important role in the regulation of human behavior. Dysfunction of GABA neurotransmission in the limbic system may be linked to the development of certain anxiety disorders.

Indications
Alcohol withdrawal symptoms, anxiety, panic disorder, tension headache, tremors.

Contraindications
Comatose patients, pre-existing CNS depression, uncontrolled severe pain, narrow angle glaucoma, acute alcohol intoxication.

Side Effects
- **Frequent**: Pain at IM injection site, somnolence, ataxia, dizziness, confusion
- **Occasional**: Rash, peripheral edema, GI disturbances
- **Serious reactions**: IV administration may produce painful swelling, thrombophlebitis and carpal tunnel syndrome. Abrupt or too-rapid withdrawal may result in pronounced restlessness, irritability, insomnia, hand tremors, abdominal or muscle cramps, diaphoresis, vomiting and seizures. Overdose results in somnolence, confusion, diminished reflexes and coma.

Nurse's Responsibility
- Assess patient's BP, pulse rate and respiratory rate, rhythm and depth immediately before giving chlordiazepoxide.
- Assess the patient for motor responses such as agitation, tension and trembling, and autonomic responses such as cold, clammy hands and diaphoresis.
- Keep the patient recumbent for up to 3 hours after parenteral administration to reduce the drug's hypotensive effect.
- Assist the patient with ambulation if he experiences ataxia or drowsiness.
- Know the therapeutic serum level for chlordiazepoxide is 1–3 µg/mL and toxic serum level is > 5 µg/mL.
- Inform the patient that IM injection may produce discomfort.
- Inform the patient that drowsiness usually disappears with continued therapy.
- Instruct the patient to change positions slowly from recumbent to sitting before standing to prevent dizziness.
- Caution the patient to avoid tasks that require mental alertness or motor skills until his response to the drug has been established.
- Warn the patient to avoid alcohol during therapy.
- Encourage the patient to stop smoking during therapy as it reduces drug's effectiveness.

Diazepam

Trade Name
Valium, Valpam

Classification
Antianxiety agents, sedatives/hypnotics—benzodiazepines

Dose
Oral: 2–10 mg, 2–4 times a day. Parental: 2–10 mg, may repeat in 3–4 hours if needed

Mechanism of Action
May potentiate the effects of gamma-aminobutyric acid (GABA) and other inhibitory neurotransmitters by binding to specific benzodiazepine receptors in the limbic and cortical areas of the CNS. GABA inhibits excitatory stimulation which helps control emotional behavior. Diazepam suppresses the spread of seizure activity caused by seizure-producing foci in the cortex, thalamus and limbic structures.

Indications
Anxiety, skeletal muscle relaxation, preanesthesia, alcohol withdrawal, status epilepticus, control of increased seizure activity in patients with refractory epilepsy who are on stable regimens of anticonvulsants, treatment of panic disorder, tension, headache, tremors.

Contraindications
Angle closure glaucoma, coma, pre-existing CNS depression, respiratory depression, severe uncontrolled pain.

Side Effects
Dizziness, drowsiness, lethargy, hangover, paradoxical excitation, mental depression, headache, hypotension, rashes, blurred vision, nausea, vomiting, diarrhea, constipation, venous thrombosis, phlebitis, respiratory depression, psychological dependency.

Nurse's Responsibility
- Assess the patient's BP, pulse rate and respiratory rate, rhythm and depth immediately before giving diazepam.
- Assess the patient for motor responses such as agitation, tension and trembling, and autonomic responses such as cold, clammy hands and diaphoresis.
- Keep the patient recumbent for up to 3 hours after parenteral administration to reduce the drug's hypotensive effect.
- Inform the patient that drowsiness usually disappears with continued therapy.
- Instruct the patient to change positions slowly from recumbent to sitting before standing to prevent dizziness.
- Administer with food to minimize gastric irritation.
- Advise the patient to take medication exactly as directed. Abrupt withdrawal may cause insomnia, irritability and sometimes even seizures.
- Explain about adverse effects and advise him to avoid activities that require alertness.
- Caution the patient to avoid alcohol or any other CNS depressants along with benzodiazepines; also instruct him not to take any over-the-counter (OTC) medications.
- If IM administration is preferred give deep IM.
- For IV administration do not mix with any other drug. Give slow IV as respiratory or cardiac arrest can occur; monitor vital signs during IV administration. Prevent extravasations since it can cause phlebitis and venous thrombosis.

Phenergan

Generic Name

Promethazine HCl

Brand Name

Phenergan

Classification

Sedative/hypnotics

Dose

25–50 mg (sedation); 10–25 mg every 4 hours as needed (antiemetic) (1amp).

Mechanism of Action

Antiemetics, antihistamines, sedative/hypnotics. Selectively blocks H1 receptors, diminishing the effects of histamine on cells of the upper respiratory tract and eyes, and decreasing the sneezing, mucus production, itching and tearing that accompany allergic reactions. Blocks cholinergic receptors in the vomiting center that are believed to mediate the nausea and vomiting caused by gastric irritation.

Indications

Preoperative sedation, treatment and prevention of nausea and vomiting, adjunct to anesthesia and analgesia.

Contraindications

Hypersensitivity, comatose patient, prostatic hypertrophy, bladder neck obstruction, narrow angle glaucoma.

Side Effects

- Confusion, disorientation, sedation, dizziness, extrapyramidal reaction, fatigue, insomnia, nervousness
- Bradycardia or tachycardia; hypotension or hypertension
- Constipation, drug-induced hepatitis, dry mouth
- Blood dyscrasias
- Blurred vision, diplopia, tinnitus, photosensitivity, rashes

Nurse's Responsibility

- Assess level of sedation after administration.
- Monitor pulse, respirations and blood pressure frequently.
- Assess for nausea or vomiting before and after administration.
- Give IM injections deep into muscles, administration into subcutaneous muscle causes tissue necrosis.
- Arteriospasms and gangrene of artery may occur when administered intra-arterially.

Donepezil

Brand Name

Aricept

Classification

Acetylcholinesterase inhibitor

Dose

5–10 mg per day

Mechanism of Action

The precise mechanism of action of donepezil in patients with Alzheimer's disease is not fully understood. In Alzheimer's disease, there is a substantial loss of the elements of the cholinergic system and it is generally accepted that the symptoms of Alzheimer's disease are related to this cholinergic deficit, particularly in cerebral cortex and other areas of the brain. In normal function, acetylcholine is an essential neurotransmitter and plays an important role in cognitive function including memory storage and retrieval. Loss of cholinergic neurons of the central nervous system has been found to correlate with the severity of cognitive impairment. Donepezil inhibits acetylcholinesterase, an enzyme responsible for the destruction of one neurotransmitter, acetylcholine. This leads to increased concentrations of acetylcholine in the brain which in turn is believed to be responsible for the improvement seen during treatment with donepezil. Cholinesterase inhibitors do not alter Alzheimer's disease but may stabilize the elder at the current level of dementia or lessen the symptoms.

Pharmacokinetics

It has an oral bioavailability of 100% and easily crosses the blood-brain barrier. Biological half-life is about 70 hours. Excretes through urine.

Indications

Treatment of mild to moderate dementia of the Alzheimer's type.

Contraindications

Donepezil should not be used for people who are allergic to ingredients in donepezil or to another piperidine derivates, use with caution in people with cardiac disease, chronic obstructive pulmonary disease, asthma, severe cardiac arrhythmias, patients with gastrointestinal disorders and seizures.

Side Effects

Headache, generalized pain, fatigue, dizziness, bradycardia, nausea, vomiting, diarrhea, anorexia, abdominal pain, vivid dreams, weight loss, muscle cramping, joint pain, increased frequency of urination.

Nurse's Responsibility

- Assess cognitive ability of the patient.
- Monitor heart rate as bradycardia may occur
- Emphasize the importance of taking medication every day.
- Monitor side effects like gastrointestinal disturbances and sleep disturbances.
- Explain family members that donepezil may cause dizziness and the patient may need to take medication before going to bed.
- Emphasize to take medicine along with food and drinking plenty of liquids.
- Explain patient not to take alcohol, other medicines like sedatives, tranquilizers, mood stabilizer.
- Advise small frequent meals, frequent mouth care, sucking hard candy or chewing gum which may help to reduce nausea.
- Advise the patient to intimate physician about suicidal thoughts, nervousness, loss of appetite, severe dizziness, vomiting, dark urine, yellow eyes or skin rash.

Acamprosate

Trade Name

Acamprol

Classification

Anticraving medication

Dose

Acamprosate is available as 333 mg tablets. The recommended daily dose for adults is four to six tablets (1332–1998 mg) in three divided doses. Usual practice is to start at half of these doses and increase by one tablet a week.

Mechanism of Action

Acamprosate enhances the GABA neurotransmitter system which is reduced in persons with chronic exposure to alcohol and interferes with glutamate action in different pathways. Acamprosate also acts on the calcium channels and reduces central nervous system hyper-excitability caused by cessation of alcohol intake. Acamprosate is thought to work by decreasing craving related to conditioned withdrawal.

Indications

Treating alcoholism

Pharmacokinetics

Only 10% of acamprosate is absorbed of which 90% is excreted unchanged into urine. It can be used in patients of alcohol dependence with mild to moderate liver dysfunction since it is not metabolized in the liver.

Contraindications

Acamprosate is contraindicated in patients with known hypersensitivity to the drug, renal insufficiency or cirrhosis with severe hepatic dysfunction, but patients with mild to moderate liver dysfunction may take it safely. Safety during pregnancy and lactation has not been established.

Side Effects

Transient diarrhea, occasional headaches, dizziness, paresthesia, decreased libido, confusion, rash and pruritus.

Nurse's Responsibility

Explain the following to family members and patients:

- Do not miss any doses.
- Drug may cause dizziness, do not drive, operate machinery or perform any other dangerous activities until the patient knows how he reacts to acamprosate.
- Do not drink alcohol while taking drug.
- Alcohol dependent patients should be monitored for the development of depression or suicidal thinking.
- Monitor mood changes.
- Contact or report to healthcare provider if any of the following effects occur or worsen: anxiety, restlessness or irritability, panic attacks, suicidal ideations, unusual changes in the behavior or mood.

Alcohol Deterrent Therapy

Deterrent agents are those which are given to desensitize the individual to the effects of alcohol and maintain abstinence. The most commonly used drug is disulfiram (tetraethyl thiuram disulfide) or antabuse.

Disulfiram

Disulfiram is used to ensure abstinence in the treatment of alcohol dependence. Its main effect is to produce a rapid and violently unpleasant reaction in a person who ingests even a small amount of alcohol while taking disulfiram.

Dosage

Disulfiram is supplied in tablets of 250 and 500 mg. The usual initial dose is 500 mg/day orally for the first 2 weeks, followed by a maintenance dosage of 250 mg/day. The dosage should not exceed 500 mg/day.

Mechanism of Action

Disulfiram is an aldehyde dehydrogenase inhibitor that interferes with the metabolism of alcohol and produces a marked increase in blood acetaldehyde levels. The accumulation of acetaldehyde (to a level of 10 times more than that which occurs in the normal metabolism of alcohol) produces a wide array of unpleasant reactions called the disulfiram ethanol reaction (DER) characterized by nausea, throbbing headache, vomiting, hypotension, flushing, sweating, thirst, dyspnea, tachycardia, chest pain, vertigo, blurred vision and a sense of impending doom associated with severe anxiety. The reaction occurs almost immediately after the ingestion of even one alcoholic drink and may last up to 30 minutes.

Therapeutic Indications

The primary indication for disulfiram use is as an aversive conditioning treatment for alcohol dependence.

Side Effects

The adverse effects of disulfiram in the absence of alcohol consumption include fatigue, dermatitis, impotence, optic neuritis, mental changes, acute polyneuropathy and hepatic damage.

With alcohol consumption the intensity of the disulfiram-alcohol reactions varies with each patient. In extreme cases, it is marked by convulsions, respiratory depression, cardiovascular collapse, myocardial infarction and death.

Contraindications

* Pulmonary and cardiovascular disease
* Should be used with caution in patients with nephritis, brain damage, hypothyroidism, diabetes, hepatic disease, seizures, poly-drug dependence or an abnormal electroencephalogram.
* Patients at high risk of alcohol ingestion.

Nurse's Responsibility

* An informed consent should be taken before starting treatment.
* Ensure that at least 12 hours have lapsed since the last ingestion of alcohol before administering the drug.
* Patient must be instructed that ingestion of even the smallest amount of alcohol brings on a disulfiram-ethanol reaction with all its unpleasant effects; he should therefore be strictly warned not to intake any alcoholic drink.
* The patient should also be warned against ingestion of any alcohol-containing preparations such as cough syrups, drops of any kind, and alcohol-containing foods and sauces. Advice against use of alcohol based aftershave lotions and inhalation of paints, varnishes, etc., containing alcohol. Any topical applications containing alcohol should also be avoided.
* Caution patient against taking CNS depressants or any OTC (over-the-counter) medications during disulfiram therapy.

- ❖ Instruct patient to avoid driving or other activities requiring alertness until response to drug is known.
- ❖ Patients should be warned that the disulfiram-alcohol reaction may continue for as long as 1–2 weeks after the last dose of disulfiram.
- ❖ Patients should carry identification cards describing disulfiram-alcohol reaction and listing the name and telephone number of the physician to be called.
- ❖ Emphasize the importance of follow-up visits to the physician to monitor progress in long-term therapy.

Memantine

Trade Names
Axura, Ebixa, Marixino, Namenda, Namenda 49 Titration Pack, Namzaric

Classification
N-methyl-D-aspartate (NMDA) receptor antagonist

Dose
Oral: Starting dose—5 mg once daily, target dosage—20 mg once daily

Mechanism of Action
Binds to CNS-methyl-D-aspartate (NMDA) receptors sites, preventing binding of glutamate an excitatory neurotransmitter.

Indications
Treatment of moderate to severe Alzheimer dementia, mild to moderate vascular dementia, chronic pain, mild cognitive impairment.

Contraindications
Patients with hypersensitivity to memantine, renal impairment, hepatic impairment, pregnancy, lactation and children.

Side Effects
Dizziness, headache, confusion, diarrhea, constipation, vomiting, abdominal pain, weight gain, hallucinations, hypertension, fatigue, urinary frequency, anemia.

Nurses' Responsibility
- ❖ Frequently assess blood pressure, report to physician any increase in BP.
- ❖ Monitor signs of anemia such as pallor, fatigue, shortness of breath, etc.
- ❖ Assess for dizziness that might affect balancing gait, caution the patient and family to guard against falls and trauma.
- ❖ Check weight regularly, report weight gain to the physician.
- ❖ Instruct patient and caregivers to report severe or prolonged headache, skin rash or urinary frequency.

Atomoxetine

Trade Name
Strattera

Classification
Selective norepinephrine reuptake inhibitor.

Dose

❖ Initial dosing for adults is 40 mg per day and can be increased after a minimum of 3 days to achieve therapeutic effects. A maximum daily dose is 100 mg per day.

❖ Initial dosing for children older than six years and < 70 kg is 0.5 mg/kg per day. The maximum daily dose of 1.4 mg/kg per day or 100 mg, whichever is less.

❖ Atomoxetine is available in 10 mg, 18 mg, 25 mg, 40 mg, 60 mg, 80 mg, and 100 mg capsules as a hydrochloride salt.

Mechanism of Action

Atomoxetine is a potent and selective inhibitor of the norepinephrine transporter (NET) which prevents cellular reuptake of norepinephrine throughout the brain which is thought to improve the symptoms of attention deficit hyperactivity disorder (ADHD).

Indications

It is a selective norepinephrine reuptake inhibitor (SNRI) used in the treatment of ADHD.

Contraindications

❖ Hypersensitivity to atomoxetine

❖ Use of MAOIs within the past 14 days

❖ Narrow-angle glaucoma

❖ Hypertension, tachycardia

❖ Cerebrovascular disease

❖ Pregnancy and lactation

Side Effects

Headache, nausea, vomiting, constipation, sleepiness, decreased appetite, abdominal pain, increased heart rate, high blood pressure, dizziness, impotence, dry mouth, mood changes.

Nurse's Responsibility

❖ Do not use atomoxetine if the patient has used monoamine oxidase inhibitor in the past 14 days as it causes dangerous drug interaction.

❖ Monitor blood pressure and vital signs.

❖ Monitor growth of children on long-term atomoxetine therapy.

❖ Administer drug before 6 PM to prevent night time sleep disturbances.

❖ If a woman of child-bearing age is using this drug suggest use of contraceptives.

❖ Educate the patient to take drug exactly as prescribed.

❖ Avoid the use of alcohol and over the counter drugs including nose drops, cold remedies and herbal therapies while taking this drug.

❖ Educate the patient to report palpitations, dizziness, weight loss, severe dry mouth and difficulty swallowing and pregnancy.

APPENDIX 26

ABBREVIATIONS

5-HT	Serotonin
AA	Alcoholic Anonymous
ACTH	Adrenocorticotropic Hormone
ADHD	Attention Deficit Hyperactivity Disorder
AHNA	American Holistic Nurse's Association
AIDS	Acquired Immunodeficiency Syndrome
ALI	American Law Institute
AMEND	Association for Mentally Disabled
AMTA	American Massage Therapy Association
ANA	American Nurses Association
APA	American Psychiatric Association
ARDSI	Alzheimer's and Related Disorders Society of India
BAERs	Brain Stem Auditory Evoked Responses
BPAD	Bipolar Affective Disorder
CA	Chronological Age
CAM	Complementary Alternative Medicine
CBCL	Child Behavior Checklist
CCRAS	Central Council for Research in Ayurveda and Sidda
CDT	Carbohydrate Deficient Transferrin
CID	Critical Incident Debriefing
CMHN	Community Mental Health Nurse
CNS	Central Nervous System
CRH	Corticotropin-releasing Hormone
CROMP	Centre for Rehabilitation of Mental Patients
CT	Computed Tomography
DIMHANS	Dharwad Institute of Mental Health and Neurosciences
DMHT	District Mental Health Team
DMHP	District Mental Health Program
DOES	Disorder of Excessive Somnolence
DPN	Diploma in Psychiatric Nursing
DSM	Diagnostic and Statistical Manual
ECT	Electroconvulsive Therapy
EEG	Electroencephalogram
EMG	Electromyogram
EPS	Extrapyramidal Syndrome
GABA	Gamma Amino Butyric Acid
GAD	Generalized Anxiety Disorder

GAF	Global Assessment of Functioning
GAS	General Adaptation Syndrome
GGT	Gamma Glutamyl Transpeptidase
GI	Gastrointestinal
GHRH	Growth Hormone-releasing Hormone
GTS	Gilles de Tourette's Syndrome
HGH	Human Growth Hormone
HIV	Human Immunodeficiency Virus
HPA	Hypothalamic Pituitary Axis
HT	Healing Touch
ICD	International Statistical Classification of Disease
IEC	Information Education Communication
ILA	Indian Lunacy Act
IMHA	Indian Mental Health Act
INC	Indian Nursing Council
IQ	Intelligent Quotient
ISM&H	Indian System of Medicine and Homeopathy
ISMO	International Society for Mental Health Online
ISPN	Indian Society for Psychiatric Nurses
ITAQ	Insight and Treatment Attitude Questionnaire
LSD	Lysergic Acid Diethylamide
MA	Mental Age
MAO	Monoamine Oxidase
MAOIs	Mono Amino Oxidase Inhibitors
MARIs	Monoamine Reuptake Inhibitors
MDP	Manic Depressive Psychosis
MHA	Mental Health Act
MHCA	Mental Health Care Act
MMSE	Mini Mental Status Examination
MPA	Medico Pastoral Association
MR	Mental Retardation
MRI	Magnetic Resonance Imaging
MSE	Mental Status Examination
NACO	National Aids Control Organization
NAMI	National Alliances for the Mentally Ill
NANDA	North American Nursing Diagnoses Association
NCCAM	National Centre for Complementary and Alternative Medicine
NE	Norepinephrine
NIMHANS	National Institute of Mental Health and Neurosciences
NMHP	National Mental Health Program

NMS	Neuroleptic Malignant Syndrome
NNMC	National Nursing Midwifery Council
NOS	Nothing Otherwise Specific
NOSIE	Nurses Observation Scale for Impatient Evaluation
NREM	Non-rapid Eye Movement Sleep
OCD	Obsessive-compulsive Disorders
OTC	Over-the-counter
PANSS	Positive and Negative Symptoms Scale
PCLN	Psychiatric Consultation Liaison Nurse
PDD	Pervasive Development Disorders
PET	Positron Emission Tomography
PPP	Postpartum Psychosis
PTSD	Post-traumatic Stress Disorders
RAS	Reticular Activating Symptom
REM	Rapid Eye Movement
SDD	Specific Development Disorders
SFRS	Schneider's First Rank Symptoms of Schizophrenia
SSRIS	Selective Serotonin Reuptake Inhibitors
TCAs	Tricyclic Antidepressants
TCL	Training in Community Living
THP	Trihexyphenidyl
TLE	Temporal Lobe Epilepsy
TMD	Transitory Mood Disorder
TMS	Transcranial Magnetic Stimulation
TRADA	Total Response to Alcohol and Drug Abuse
TRH	Thyrotropin Releasing Hormone
TT	Therapeutic Touch
UNESCO	United Nations Educational, Scientific and Cultural Organization
VNS	Vagus Nerve Stimulation
WAIS	Wechsler Adult Intelligence Scale
WFMH	World Federation for Mental Health
WHO	World Health Organization
WISC	Wechsler Intelligence Scale for Children

Index